ANNALS *of* THE NEW YORK ACADEMY OF SCIENCES

T0344760

DIRECTOR AND EXECUTIVE EDITOR
Douglas Braaten

PROJECT MANAGER
Steven E. Bohall

The New York Academy of Sciences
7 World Trade Center
250 Greenwich Street, 40th Floor
New York, NY 10007-2157

annals@nyas.org
www.nyas.org/annals

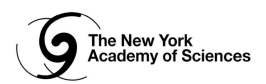

**The New York
Academy of Sciences**

Published by Blackwell Publishing
On behalf of The New York Academy of Sciences

Boston, Massachusetts
2010

ANNALS *of* THE NEW YORK ACADEMY OF SCIENCES

VOLUME 1208

ISSUE

Psychiatric and Neurologic Aspects of War

Published in cooperation with the Association for Research in Nervous and Mental Disease

ISSUE EDITORS
Jack D. Barchas and JoAnn Difede

This volume presents manuscripts stemming from the 89th Annual Conference of the Association for Research in Nervous and Mental Disease, entitled "Psychiatric and Neurologic Aspects of War," held December 16, 2009 at The Rockefeller University, New York, New York.

TABLE OF CONTENTS

Become a Member Today of the New York Academy of Sciences

The New York Academy of Sciences is dedicated to identifying the next frontiers in science and catalyzing key breakthroughs. As has been the case for 200 years, many of the leading scientific minds of our time rely on the Academy for key meetings and publications that serve as the crucial forum for a global community dedicated to scientific innovation.

 Select one FREE *Annals* volume and up to five volumes for only $40 each.

 Network and exchange ideas with the leaders of academia and industry.

 Broaden your knowledge across many disciplines.

 Gain access to exclusive online content.

Join Online at **www.nyas.org**

Or by phone at **800.344.6902** (516.576.2270 if outside the U.S.).

ANNALS OF THE NEW YORK ACADEMY OF SCIENCES

Issue: *Psychiatric and Neurologic Aspects of War*

Background and acknowledgments

The Association for Research in Nervous and Mental Disease was founded in 1920 by a group of members of the New York Neurological Society who sought to promote research in nervous and mental disease. They formed an organizing committee consisting of Drs. Walter Timme, Charles L. Dana, Frederick Tilney, J. Ramsay Hunt, Smith Ely Jelliffe, Forster Kennedy, Bernard Sachs, and Israel Strauss. The first meeting of the organization was held February 10, 1920, at Dr. Timme's home. Their desire was to advance research on various neurological and psychiatric disorders and to see that the results were presented in a coordinated manner. Today, under the guidance of its board of trustees, the association continues the work it began almost a century ago. The unique format of the conferences provides an up-to-date and in-depth analysis of current topics not provided by other research-oriented professional societies. In short, the ARNMD, as it usually is called, has become an important tradition and a significant force in contemporary neurology and psychiatry.

More than a century ago, there was little distinction between neurology and psychiatry. Great physician-scientists, such as Jackson, Charcot, Kraepelin, and Freud, made crucial observations linking abnormalities of perception, cognition, emotion, and behavior to brain dysfunction. Freud had great insights into the workings of the human mind. However, he knew that he lacked the neuroscientific tools to understand its neurobiological substrate. Perhaps as a result, psychiatry and neurology drifted apart. Today, after an explosion of neuroscientific investigation involving advances in both biological research and behavioral research through the past few decades, those tools now exist. With them, there is no longer the need for dichotomous conceptions of diseases as purely "neurologic" or "psychiatric," and patients are better served by both professions depending upon their specific problems and disorders.

Over the past several decades ARNMD has organized some of the most important brain-behavior symposia. Through a collaborative effort with the New York Academy of Sciences and The Rockefeller University, we present to you the proceedings of the 89th Annual Conference, *Psychiatric and Neurologic Aspects of War*. The conference coordinators were JoAnn Difede, associate professor of psychology in psychiatry, and director of the Program for Anxiety and Traumatic Stress, Weill Cornell Medical College; and Jack D. Barchas, Barklie McKee Henry Professor, and chair of the Department of Psychiatry, Weill Cornell Medical College, and psychiatrist-in-chief, New York Presbyterian Hospital, Weill Cornell Medical Center.

All conferences of ARNMD result from discussions of the Board of Trustees. In this instance, we owe special thanks to Professor Albert J. Stunkard, former chair of psychiatry at the University of Pennsylvania and a long-standing and extremely helpful member of the board. He presented a strong case for the timeliness of this topic. We also are appreciative of Dr. David Hamburg of Weill Cornell for his conception of the broad nature of the topic and agreeing to be the keynote speaker.

The program was made possible through a grant received from the Bob Woodruff Foundation. We would especially like to thank Gilbert Sanborn, civilian aide to the Secretary of the Army for the State of Connecticut, who has been very supportive not only of our program, but also of a range of efforts around the country to support National Guard and veterans of Operation Iraqi Freedom/Operation Enduring Freedom (OIF/OEF).

The ARNMD conferences are also supported by the institutions whose departments are represented on the Board of Trustees. Those institutions

doi: 10.1111/j.1749-6632.2010.05794.x

are therefore able to send their trainees to the meeting, permitting it to serve a broad educational function. Additional support was received from the Department of Psychiatry at Weill Cornell and the DeWitt Wallace Fund of New York-Presbyterian Hospital and Weill Cornell Medical College.

We are deeply appreciative to Professor Bruce McEwen of The Rockefeller University whose work on stress was relevant to many of the presenters. He directly facilitated work with our partners in this conference at The Rockefeller University and the New York Academy of Sciences.

The New York Academy of Sciences has been very helpful. We particularly wish to thank the staff of the *Annals of the New York Academy of Sciences* for their patience and thoughtfulness as the volume was put together. Their high level of expertise has proven very important.

We are very appreciative of Pamela Trester, Brittany Mello, and Kathy Rosenberg of the Weill Cornell Department of Psychiatry for their editing assistance in the final stages of this effort. Their attention to detail and grace under pressure facilitated the elegant execution of this volume.

In this and other activities of the ARNMD, Francis Lee, a member of the board and secretary-treasurer, has proven invaluable. He has a rare capacity to deal with complex situations and materials and possesses superb judgment.

A word of special thanks from our entire board to Annlouise Goodermuth, the executive director of the ARNMD, who has dealt with many problems with grace, creativity, and commitment through the years in order to make sure that these meetings run in a smooth and efficient manner.

Jack D. Barchas, MD
for the Association for Research in Nervous and Mental Disease

Conflicts of interest

Jack Barchas owns stock in Lilly, Elan, and Neuocrine.

Ann. N.Y. Acad. Sci. ISSN 0077-8923

Psychiatric and neurologic aspects of war: an overview and perspective

JoAnn Difede and Jack D. Barchas

Department of Psychiatry, Weill Cornell Medical College, New York, New York

Address for correspondence: JoAnn Difede, Ph.D., Department of Psychiatry, Weill Cornell Medical College, 525 East 68th Street, Box 200, New York, New York 10065. jdifede@med.cornell.edu

The growing number of soldiers returning home with psychiatric and neurologic disorders, notably posttraumatic stress disorder (PTSD) and traumatic brain injury (TBI), underscores the need for an interdisciplinary framework for understanding the emergent consequences of combat. Among the challenges facing the scientific community is the development of effective treatment strategies for TBI from blast and other injuries, given the confounding effects of comorbid psychological symptoms on accurate diagnoses. At the individual level, emerging technologies—including virtual reality, the use of genetic biomarkers to inform treatment response, and new brain imaging methodology—are playing an important role in the development of differential therapeutics to best address a soldier's particular clinical needs. At the macro level, new approaches toward understanding the political, cultural, and ideological contexts of mass conflict, the decision to join in violence, and ways of preventing genocide are discussed.

Keywords: posttraumatic stress disorder; traumatic brain injury; veterans; technology; methodology; virtual reality; valor; terrorist behavior; genocide prevention; mass violence

Introduction to the scope of the conference and proceedings

Though war is a universal and timeless event, documented in the historical record from the earliest days of humanity, each conflict is unique, defined by the specific sociopolitical context of the time.[1] A range of questions from the scientific to the logistical beset those who grapple with the problems of warfare, requiring a multiplicity of perspectives. The Association for Research in Nervous and Mental Disease (ARNMD) conference, "Psychiatric and Neurologic Aspects of War," brought together distinguished scientists, clinicians, and scholars to discuss some of the issues and potential solutions that have emerged from the U.S. engagement in Iraq and Afghanistan.

One generation's solutions often create the next generation's problems. The structure of any given conflict, from the combatants to how the war is waged to the nature of its consequences, is partially defined by the knowledge base of that time. Just as the science and art of warfare have undergone

vast changes since as recently as World War II, so have the costs of war for the individual soldier and his or her family. Advances in the sciences and art of war, such as the body armor used by American soldiers, and the medical advances allowing for the treatment of shock from injuries while on the battlefield, has meant the survival of many more soldiers who suffered traumatic blast injuries today than would have been possible even as recently as the Desert Storm conflict, and most certainly since Vietnam. Thus, unlike prior conflicts, the two most common medical problems emerging from Operation Iraqi Freedom (OIF) and Operation Enduring Freedom (OEF) requiring medical intervention are neuropsychiatric in nature: posttraumatic stress disorder (PTSD) and traumatic brain injury (TBI).

The Association for Nervous and Mental Disorders is a venerable organization with a long-standing interest in bringing together persons in psychiatry and psychology with those in neurology and related disciplines, including neuroscience. Through the years, the organization has taken a broad look

doi: 10.1111/j.1749-6632.2010.05795.x
Ann. N.Y. Acad. Sci. 1208 (2010) 1–9 © 2010 Association for Research in Nervous and Mental Disease.

at multiple fields and presented conferences that aim to connect current problems to potential future developments. In this case, the topic of psychiatric and neurologic aspects of war gave rise to a remarkable range of issues. For this meeting, the ARNMD has partnered with The Rockefeller University and the New York Academy of Sciences. To adequately capture the complexity of the issues, the conference was organized to have a keynote session as well as multiple roundtable discussions. The roundtable discussions were thoughtfully and creatively moderated by Timothy Pedley, chair of neurology at Columbia[2] and Charles Marmar, chair of psychiatry at New York University.[3] Our contributors come from a range of backgrounds including psychiatrists, psychologists, neurologists, neurosurgeons, and neuroscientists, as well as scholars from public health, international relations, and political science—many from the armed forces.

Because the detailed aspects of pharmacological and psychological treatment of various neuropsychiatric disorders have been addressed in other information sources in psychiatry, psychology, and neurology, we have chosen to highlight aspects and areas that are extraordinarily important but considered less frequently, including broad issues of war and conflict, before turning to the use of research from clinical neuroscience areas to elucidate issues of specific disorders and the interaction of psychiatric and neurologic problems. Included are new approaches to diagnosis and treatment and the roles of emerging technologies from biological to psychosocial—all of which have promise to aid veterans and their families and that thereby also have implications for the entire population. We have tried to provide a broader framework than has traditionally been included within concerns on psychiatric and neurologic aspects of war. We hope that the papers provide both current and promising approaches to issues that need scientific knowledge and its implementation. The following materials are organized in the themes of the conference with information on invited presenters, to provide a sense of the broad backgrounds of the participants.

Many contributors have worked extensively with veterans and offer a lively discussion across dimensions from the biological to the psychosocial. We hope our readers will agree the presentations are in the tradition of the ARNMD as a path-leading source of knowledge.

Broad perspectives: new approaches to prevention of mass conflict, the minds of warriors, jihadists, and political extremists

The core issue is how humanity can prevent mass violence and genocide. Much has been written describing humankind's horrible history of demonizing others. There has been little consideration to ways to prevent these aspects of savagery. The keynote speaker, David Hamburg, was president of the Institute of Medicine, then subsequently president of the Carnegie Corporation and co-chair of its Commission on Preventing Deadly Conflict. He has chaired separate special commissions of the United Nations and the European Union on genocide and has received the Presidential Medal of Freedom. His approach takes lessons from public health and behavioral sciences, further developed during the past decade as a DeWitt Wallace Distinguished Scholar at Weill Cornell. He has authored several volumes including *Preventing Genocide*[4] and, with Dr. Beatrix Hamburg, *Learning to Live Together*,[5] which deals with teaching children not to hate. He emphasizes the new dangers of the 21st century, including the easy availability of weapons of mass destruction and proposes a series of pillars of prevention including ways of providing help to troubled nations, fostering democracy, aiding equitable socioeconomic development, education starting at the earliest stages, mechanisms to reduce human rights violations, and training in preventive diplomacy. He focuses on proactive steps rather than waiting till conflict has become unmanageable, and on how each step can become a new reality.

While the dominant effort in psychiatry has been to tend to the wounds of the warrior, the nascent field of political psychiatry has endeavored to understand the mind of the warrior, on both sides of the conflict. What motivates a fellow human being to aspire to terrorism and to sacrifice his life as a martyr to advance the cause of his people? Jerrold Post, a psychiatrist and political scientist, now a professor of clinical psychiatry at George Washington University, is a founder of modern political psychology and has authored several significant and well-received volumes. Much as Hannah Arendt startled readers with her thesis regarding the banality of evil in World War II,[6] Dr. Post unsettles by suggesting the apparent normalcy of a terrorist when placed in the appropriate social and historical context.[7] His insights suggest a series of strategies to diffuse terrorism that may prove critical for consideration by policy makers.

Political extremism within a nation can lead to violence including the threat of terror and provides a model that may have applicability to the study of divisions within and between cultures. Using an Israeli population, a view of this problem is provided by Nathanial Laor, professor of psychiatry and philosophy at Tel Aviv, clinical professor at the Yale Child Study Center, and director of the Cohen-Harris Center for Trauma and Disaster Intervention in Israel, who has written extensively on trauma and resilience. He and his colleagues look at the mind of extremists, building upon a stress and trauma model using research to compare persons from the far left and far right political wings. They demonstrate the powerful play of ideological and morbid transcendence with the finding that both political extremes report threat, though their type and content differ.

Of great importance is the question, Who are the young men and women who choose to defend our nation? At a time when military service is voluntary, insight into this unique group is imperative and may lead to further insights that will allow us to develop more effective training and support of our warriors. In Jonathan Shay's approach, our warriors are likened to the familiar heroes from the Homeric epics, *The Iliad* and *The Odyssey*, providing the foundation for a hermeneutics of healing.[8] A psychiatrist, Dr. Shay has worked with veterans in a Veterans Health Administration hospital and has been the recipient of a MacArthur Foundation Award.

For the conference, Matthew Bogdanos, Colonel, U.S. Marine Corps; homicide prosecutor, New York City; recipient of the National Humanities Medal; and winner of the Bronze Star, provided an account of aspects of the mind of current American warriors and their multiple roles, including efforts to rebuild society. In this case, the exhilarating and dangerous effort to find and bring together artifacts removed from the museum in Iraq is described in a compelling volume that he authored.[9]

Neurologic aspects and TBI

TBI and concussions represent major areas requiring intensive scientific and clinical efforts to address the gaps in our knowledge base. Owing to advancements in battlefield critical care, a greater proportion of service members deployed to OIF/OEF have survived their blast injuries to return home with TBI, ranging from the mild (concussion) to the severe, than in prior conflicts.

The RAND report[10] found that 19.5% of OIF/OEF veterans reported experiencing a probable mild TBI (mTBI) during deployment. Of those experiencing TBI, over a third also had overlapping PTSD or depression—320,000 veterans may have experienced at least a mild mTBI. As Ref. 11 (p. xiii) notes,

> The symptoms of comorbid mental health conditions such as PTSD or depression (associated with intrusive thoughts, concentration difficulty, and poor sleep) interfere with normal cognitive functioning. On the other hand, the cognitive impairment and emotional control problems associated with TBI are likely detrimental to the resilience essential to overcome PTSD.

Thus, the warrior with TBI and comorbid PTSD or depression presents a complex clinical picture challenging us to develop strategies for accurate differential diagnosis and therapeutics. The presentations illuminate problems in diagnosing and treating TBI and challenges in living facing warriors who have suffered TBI.

The change in emphasis from direct penetrating traumatic injury to closed traumatic injury in warriors is presented by Louis French, M.D., chief of the Traumatic Brain Injury Center at Walter Reed. He notes the high percentages of individuals with these problems, including as many as 20% with concussions and considers the still uncertain issues with the designation of "blast" injuries, the wide range of comorbid problems, as well as emotional and cognitive difficulties, including PTSD.[12]

The cross-cutting paper of Thomas McAllister, Millennium Professor of Psychiatry and director of neuropsychiatry at Dartmouth considers problems in adequately characterizing the range of psychological and TBIs as a prelude to developing effective treatment strategies. The paper raises the question of what neuropsychiatric after effects are associated with which type of trauma and demonstrate that chronic effects are associated with a significant overlap of symptoms.

Jamshid Ghajar, professor of clinical neurosurgery, Weill Cornell, and director of the Brain Trauma Foundation, and his colleagues further illuminate the diversity of symptoms drawing from extensive preclinical and clinical research with civilians who have experienced TBI with a particular emphasis on mTBI. They unify the range of symptoms through brain imaging and behavioral studies including visual tracking and note the widespread specific microstructural changes including damage to frontal white matter tracts caused by shearing injuries. They propose specific rapid tests that may lead to better diagnosis and therapeutic interventions.

Psychiatric aspects of war

Recent Institute of Medicine (IOM) reports,[13,14] commissioned by the Department of Defense (DoD) and the Veterans Administration (VA), concluded that the evidence base for the treatment of PTSD is severely lacking. They noted that only one psychological intervention, prolonged exposure therapy, had sufficient data to warrant consideration as a first-line treatment for PTSD. "Exposure therapy" refers to behavioral and cognitive behavioral treatments that involve confronting feared but safe thoughts, images, objects, situations, or activities to reduce pathological (unrealistic) fear, anxiety, and anxiety disorder symptoms. No pharmacological treatments have been deemed efficacious to date, though clinicians have believed that some seem to be helpful in certain patients. A review suggests that less than 50% of patients improve with selective serotonin reuptake inhibitors,[15] the only class of medication with Food and Drug Administration approval for the treatment of PTSD. Taken another way, the data suggest the possibility of subtypes of illness with different neuronal and psychological mechanisms that could ultimately lead to more specific treatments. Information dealing with the current status and new developments of pharmacological and psychological treatments of PTSD was given throughout the sessions on psychiatric aspects by Professor Charles Marmar, former president of the International Society for Traumatic Stress Studies and currently chair of psychiatry at New York University; he is noted for his comprehensive scholarly work on the mental health impact of combat[16-20] and moderated those sessions with a magical touch. Judith Cukor, assistant professor of psychology in psychiatry at Weill Cornell provides a cogent summary of both the current evidence-based treatment approaches for PTSD as well as promising psychotherapeutic and psychopharmacological

treatments that are in the nascent stages of developing a persuasive evidence base.

If we look to the recent history of the disciplines, dealing with PTSD, the state of these fields is not surprising. Nancy Andreasen, professor of psychiatry at the University of Iowa, a recipient of the Presidential Medal of Science, was one of those key to development of the formal concept of PTSD and its incorporation into the Diagnostic and Statistical Manual of the American Psychiatric Association. She presents an engrossing history of a long-standing concept based on many types of stressors but that has only been in the formal diagnostic nomenclature for a short time. As recently as the Vietnam War, the diagnosis of PTSD was the subject of vitriolic debate. The psychotherapeutic community's emphasis on intrapsychic events was not yet tempered by empirical advances in the clinical and preclinical sciences in psychiatry. The zeitgeist in clinical psychiatry and psychology has shifted toward greater acceptance of the legitimacy of the diagnosis of PTSD and from an emphasis on the theoretical to an emphasis on the empirically substantiated, opening the door to the potential to teach the next generation of clinicians from a vastly improved evidence base.

A keynote overview of PTSD and traumatic stress has been provided by Robert Ursano and his colleagues. Professor Ursano, chair of psychiatry, Uniformed Services University, heads the Center for the Study of Traumatic Stress. They present extensive data demonstrating the substantial rates of behavioral alterations, including PTSD, due to war exposure. The paper provides information on the impacts of disorders including depression, suicide, and aggression/violence—major problems that influence not only the veteran but their families and loved ones. Some potential biological factors and biomarkers that might lead to new treatments and diagnostic methods are presented as well as psychological treatments, including psychotherapy.

The topic of evidence-based treatments for PTSD and new directions in such treatments has been covered by Judith Cukor and her colleagues. She has worked with patients from a wide range of severe trauma situations and has worked with the Army and Air Force providing training in specialized treatments for PTSD. The paper includes multiple approaches within both biological and psychological modalities and combinations of those methods as well as emerging possibilities. The authors include a useful discussion of the barriers to the implementation of evidence-based treatments.

Although PTSD is one of the most common psychiatric problems consequent to war, others are also important. The RAND survey[10] found that 18.5% of returning service members met criteria for either PTSD or depression.

Unlike PTSD, where a paucity of treatment options is the norm, there are numerous effective psychological and pharmacological interventions, as well as the combination of approaches for the treatment of various forms of depression.[21–25] Both cognitive behavioral therapy and interpersonal psychotherapy have substantial empirical support as having a role in the treatment of some forms of depression across the adult lifespan, and many other forms of psychotherapy are under study in controlled experiments. There is a wealth of pharmacological alternatives including drugs that may act on various neurotransmitter systems or other fundamental neuroregulator processes. Multiple studies have documented successful strategies with first-line antidepressants.[26] Other biological treatments including electroconvulsive shock and emerging techniques involving various forms of brain stimulation are under investigation and use. Examples of other methods include light therapy, sleep deprivation, as well as new classes of medications based on cellular communication processes, various hormonally based medications, and novel rapid-acting drugs that act on specific neuronal systems, such as ketamine. Again, more needs to be known as to the varying subtypes of illness to define new diagnostic criteria and new treatment approaches and to determine biomarkers that will help to predict which treatment or combination of treatments will prove most effective with a given patient.

Despite available treatments that are effective in many patients, less than half of those in need of care seek it,[27] underscoring the added need to develop strategies to overcome barriers to care, such as stigma. Issues of psychiatric disorders in veterans and their families including depression, anxiety, suicide, psychosis, and substance abuse with particular attention to peer-to-peer treatment programs are considered by John Greden and his colleagues. Professor Greden is professor and former chair of the Department of Psychiatry at the University of Michigan, founder and director of the National Centers for Depression, and is a scientific founder and site director of the Welcome Back Veterans Initiative. Psychosocial solutions discussed include the Buddy-to-Buddy program that offers a strategy targeted toward reducing the stigma of mental illness and suicide prevention. In this peer-to-peer model, as developed with the Michigan National Guard, every soldier returning from OIF/OEF is contacted by peers identified by the Guard leadership and trained by clinical staff from the University of Michigan. It is hypothesized that such models may ameliorate the stigma of mental illness and motivate soldiers for treatment thereby bridging the chasm between returning soldiers and the available systems of care, such as VA and DoD facilities. They have developed methods for reaching large numbers of individuals in a model private–public partnership.

Issues of suicide in those who have served in the recent operations in Iraq and Afghanistan are considered by Martha Bruce, professor of sociology in psychiatry at Weill Cornell and a member of the VA Blue Ribbon Panel on Suicide Prevention. She offers her perspective as a leading expert in health services delivery on strategies for the prevention of suicide. Suicide has a significant association with PTSD, depression, and TBI and is a significant concern, highlighting the need to develop suicide prevention strategies. Since 2003, rates of suicide in active military personnel have been increasing and surpass age- and gender-matched nonveterans. The VA is undertaking special programs toward suicide prevention and those are described, including the barriers and problems with their implementation.

The options for treatment of PTSD and for comorbid conditions, such as depression, make the issue of stigma and impediments to care more apparent as highlighted by Steven Lindley and Alan Schatzberg and their colleagues from Stanford. Lindley is director of outpatient mental health of the Palo Alto Hospital, a faculty member at Stanford, and a member of the Stanford node of the Welcome Back Veterans Initiative while Schatzberg is Norris Professor and has been chair of psychiatry at Stanford, has served as president of the American Psychiatric Association, and is a scientific founder and site director of the Welcome Back Veterans Initiative. Their paper highlights the characteristics and predictors for seeking or not seeking help including factors ranging from nature of the provider to diagnosis, with depression being particularly problematic. The work emphasizes the importance of close continual monitoring to reveal ways to improve care.

New technologies: from media to telecommunications to developments in psychology and biology

Technological advances provide examples of ways to change the paradigms of understanding and of dealing with severe neuropsychiatric disorders. Promising research follows the theoretical line of inquiry that views PTSD as a disorder of learning and plasticity. Early results from one area of investigation center around enhancing exposure therapy with virtual reality simulations of combat-related trauma to facilitate emotional engagement and extinction learning. Two papers present this approach. Albert Rizzo, associate director of the Center for Creative Technologies and research professor of psychiatry at the University of Southern California, provides background on virtual reality methods to treat PTSD and describes the use of customizable virtual scenarios, such as a convoy or a city situation, in a successful open clinical trial. Barbara Rothbaum, professor of psychiatry and director of the Trauma Recovery Center at Emory University in Atlanta and colleagues provide information on methods leading to virtual reality methodology and its potential uses including versions suitable for specific trauma situations. Advantages and disadvantages are presented including the ability to control the exact "dose" of therapy and high acceptance among the "digital generation." In a radical departure from the conventional use of psychopharmacological agents, early data using D-cycloserine (an antibiotic approved decades ago to treat tuberculosis that we now know acts on specific neuronal systems) to enhance the effects of exposure therapy is also presented.

Another advance in electronic technology is demonstrated by the use of telemedicine as presented by JoAnn Difede and her colleagues. She is associate professor of psychology in psychiatry and director of the program for Anxiety and Traumatic Stress at Weill Cornell and a scientific founder and co-site director of the Welcome Back Veterans Initiative. Rizzo, Reger, Rothbaum, and Difede recently received the American Psychological Association Trauma Division "Award for Outstanding Contributions to the Practice of Trauma Psychology" for their work developing, testing, and disseminating the virtual reality-based treatment for combat-related PTSD. Rural Americans enlist in the military and serve at much higher rates than urban Americans, disproportionately representing today's veteran population.[28,29] Veterans in rural areas who need mental health services are much less likely to have access to care. They describe links to provide care in remote regions with potential solutions to a range of problems.

National shortages of trained mental health clinicians, coupled with this increasing number of U.S. service members requiring mental health treatment, are driving the need for the development of innovative technologies, such as telemedicine, as well as research to demonstrate its efficacy as a treatment modality. The increasing number of military members in need of mental health care demands the development and use of novel vehicles to deliver quality psychological therapies, regardless of clinician and patient location. Telemedicine technologies offer a unique potential to expand services to those in great need. While now broadly accepted in concept, telemedicine is a recent new technology with potential to impact large numbers of persons with serious problems.

While technology has changed warfare, both how it is waged and the consequences suffered by those who wage it, the history of innovation is marked by resistance to change. Though the human capacity for imagination allows us to envision uses of technology to solve extant problems, such as access to care, education of medical providers, and development of new treatments, our resistance to change remains among the most significant impediments to their implementation. Yet, several studies have noted the resistance to the use of telemedicine and evidence-based treatments on the basis of myths and fears, not on any hard evidence pointing to their detrimental nature.[30–33]

Biological advances include transformative technologies for mental illness. The power of brain imaging technologies, which depend upon electronic, mechanical, mathematical, statistical, and behavioral advances to study brain activity, is being applied to problems, such as PTSD. Michael Roy, Colonel, Medical Corps, U.S. Army; director, division of military internal medicine, and professor of medicine at the Uniformed Services University and his colleagues provide encouraging data using functional magnetic resonance imaging with suggestive early evidence of improvement of cerebral function following completion of evidence-based treatments for PTSD. Combined with other studies using brain imaging in these proceedings, the results underscore the potential of the emerging forms of imaging technology.

Technologies involving genetics and molecular neurobiology are bursting forth with expectations of applications to neuropsychiatric disorders. Francis Lee is a recipient of a White House Award for Excellence, a psychiatrist and neurobiologist, and vice-chair for research at Weill Cornell. He and his colleagues provide a theoretical model of an approach centered on the fact that it is currently impossible to predict who will respond to therapeutics. The model is based on genetic variants of the gene encoding brain derived neurotrophic factor. The investigators have shown links to anxiety and learned fear memory in studies in mice and humans, behaviors core to PTSD. They propose a nascent foundation for a differential therapeutics of PTSD that may lead to the ability to match a patient to the appropriate treatment on the basis of their genetic profile before the treatment is undertaken. In broad perspective, such work is likely to lead to a paradigm shift in neuropsychiatric diagnoses and treatments.

In a far reaching presentation, Rachel Yehuda, professor of psychiatry and neurobiology and director of the Traumatic Stress Studies Division of Mount Sinai School of Medicine, provides an elegant methodology for the discovery of biomarkers for PTSD, which will hopefully lead to a more precise diagnostic picture and targeted treatments. She and her colleagues ask core questions dealing with the potential of using biological markers to inform clinically meaningful treatment response. They ask about the comparison between PTSD in civilian populations and veteran populations where the criteria and outcomes seem quite different, areas that call out for further study. They note the poorer responses to treatment in the veteran population. They consider the range of possible biological markers including hormonal and stress measures and the issues involved in correlating multiple biological and behavioral markers in a variety of populations and illness presentations at different time points. The framework that is presented has the potential to lead to new diagnostic systems and improved and specified treatments.

Final conclusions and perspectives

A range of strategies was discussed in the conference and this symposium volume that offer hope. In his summary, David Silbersweig, a psychiatrist, neurologist, clinical neuroscientist, specialist in functional brain imaging, and now chair of psychiatry and director of the Neuroscience Initiative at Brigham and Women's Hospital of Harvard, provides an integration of the broad data sets we will need to advance these important problems. In his presentation, the various anatomic areas involved in patterns of symptoms are considered and the possibilities for new diagnostic schemes that also include genetics and behavior become clearer. In this powerful look at the future, he also considers ways in which later behavior is impacted.

Our "marching orders" are clear. We need to work on broad, overlapping issues of war at the same time that we support work on specific neuropsychiatric problems. The conference could touch on only a few of the broader issues that represent the tip of the iceberg. Many important topics require further inquiry, such as impacts of war on large human populations and the experiences of refugees, families, and survivors whether or not they have been in battle. We as professionals in clinical neurosciences with knowledge of aspects of behavior—and we as members of a civilization—will need to consider issues in the domain of the social sciences including group psychology, sociology, economics, political science, and international relations as well as their interaction with issues of public health and public policy. Those efforts have often been neglected by persons in our domains but are now critical to a new concept of public health that has become central to all areas of medicine. Research, scholarship, and implementation in those areas must deal with the multiple societies and their components that make up our current world and that can influence the likelihood of conflict. Such study will require intense effort and courage but is already being undertaken in an encouraging and surprising development by persons associated with the medical field—as seen in the proceedings, we have much to offer and can influence policy. The problems of societies, cultures, and individuals (including the impacts of severe personality disorders in leaders or followers), must be dealt with if we, as humans, are to survive—thus the rationale for the broad perspective of this conference on psychiatric and neurologic aspects of war.

As described in the concluding chapter and from the proceedings as a whole, taking the issues of specific neuropsychiatric problems, one of the striking themes is the likelihood of subtypes of the illnesses including PTSD, depression, and TBI. The finding that only a few are helped by treatments could be an important clue, indicating one or more subtypes that are specifically helped. The goal must be to identify markers that permit determination of the biological and psychological subtypes for each illness including the neuronal mechanisms, such as multiple learned fear pathways, and to find the biological and psychological treatments or combinations of therapies that aid specific subtypes. Developing technologies of all types will have dramatic impacts as is already being seen for PTSD and depression. For TBI much of the current work involves refining diagnosis and mechanisms but new technologies including cell growth, migration, remodeling, stem cells, and brain stimulation, as well as new behavioral mechanisms and re-learning may dramatically change the outcome. The overall paucity of interventions requires a major effort in each of the disorders to rectify this shortcoming as noted by our contributors.

The degree of overlap, comorbidity, in the same individual between one or more induced neuropsychiatric or behavioral conditions—concussion, mild or severe TBI, cognitive problems, PTSD, anxiety, depression, demoralization, family problems, aggression, and suicide—calls out for further integrated study. The specific neuropsychiatric issues must be studied separately and together at basic, translational, and clinical levels, in order to best help veterans and their families.

Much as the U.S. military partnered with private universities, such as New York City's own Rockefeller University, to solve the crisis created by the pandemic flu outbreak during World War I,[34] a partnership between academic medical centers and government agencies should be developed to address current problems. This new knowledge will have enormous impacts also on neuropsychiatric diagnosis and treatment for entire populations. Thus, in collaboration with government institutions, such as the VA and the DoD, we must endeavor to bring the unparalleled research and clinical resources of university medical centers to bear on the neuropsychiatric problems confronting warriors and their families.

Conflicts of interest

Jack Barchas owns stock in Lilly, Elan, and Neuocrine.

References

1. Gombrich, E.H. 2008. *A Little History of the World*. Yale University Press. New Haven, CT.
2. Rowland, L.P. & T.A. Pedley, Eds. 2009. *Merritt's Neurology*. 12th edn. Lippincott Williams & Wilkins. Philadelphia, PA.
3. Bremner, J. & C. Marmar, Eds. 1998. *Trauma, Memory and Dissociation*. APA Press. Washington, DC.
4. Hamburg, D. 2008. *Preventing Genocide: Practical Steps Toward Early Detection and Effective Action*. 1st edn. Paradigm Publishers. Boulder, CO.
5. Hamburg, D. & B. Hamburg. 2004. *Learning to Live Together: Preventing Hatred and Violence in Child and Adolescent Development*. Oxford University Press. New York; Macquarie University edition.
6. Arendt, H. 1994. *Eichmann in Jerusalem: A Report on the Banality of Evil*. Penguin Classics. New York.
7. Post, J.M. 2008. *The Mind of the Terrorist: The Psychology of Terrorism from the IRA to Al-Qaeda*. Palgrave Macmillan. New York.
8. Shay, J. 2002. *Odysseus in America: Combat Trauma and the Trials of Homecoming*. Scribner. New York.
9. Bogdanos, M. & W. Patrick. 2006. *Thieves of Baghdad*. Bloomsbury Publishing PLC. New York and London.
10. Tanielian, T. & L.H. Jaycox, Eds. 2008. *Invisible Wounds of War: Psychological and Cognitive Injuries, Their Consequences, and Services to Assist Recovery*. RAND. Santa Monica, CA.
11. Lew, H.L., R.D. Vanderploeg, D.F. Moore, *et al.* 2008. Overlap of mild TBI and mental health conditions in returning OIF/OEF service members and veterans. [Guest Editorial]. *J. Rehabil. Res. Dev.* **45:** xi–xvi.
12. French, L.M. & G.W. Parkinson. 2008. Assessing and treating veterans with traumatic brain injury. *J. Clin. Psychol.* **64:** 1004–1013.
13. Institute of Medicine (IOM). 2006. Posttraumatic stress disorder: diagnosis and assessment. http://www.nap.edu/catalog/11674.html
14. Institute of Medicine (IOM). 2008. *Treatment of Posttraumatic Stress Disorder: An Assessment of the Evidence*. The National Academies Press. Washington, DC.
15. Foa, E.B., M.E. Franklin & J. Moser. 2002. Context in the clinic: how well do cognitive-behavioral therapies and medications work in combination? [Comparative Study Review]. *Biol. Psychiatry* **52:** 987–997.
16. Cohen, B., K. Gima, D. Bertenthal, *et al.* 2009. Mental health diagnoses and utilization of VA non-mental health medical services among returning Iraq and Afghanistan veterans. *J. Gen. Intern. Med.* **25:** 18–24.
17. Marmar, C. 2009. Mental health impact of Afghanistan and Iraq deployment: meeting the challenge of a new generation of veterans. *Depress. Anxiety* **26:** 493–497.

18. Seal, K., D. Bertenthal, C. Miner, *et al*. 2007. Mental health disorders among 103 788 US veterans returning from Iraq and Afghanistan seen at Department of Veterans Affairs Facilities. *Arch. Intern. Med.* **167:** 476–482.

19. Seal, K., S. Maguen, B. Cohen, *et al*. 2010. VA mental health services utilization in Iraq and Afghanistan veterans in the first year of receiving new mental health diagnoses. *J. Trauma. Stress* **23:** 5–16.

20. Seal, K., T. Metzler, K. Gima, *et al*. 2009. Trends and risk factors for mental health diagnoses among Iraq and Afghanistan veterans using department of veterans affairs health care, 2002–2008. *Am. J. Public Health* **99:** 1651–1658.

21. Andreasen, N.C. & D.W. Black. 2006. *Introductory Textbook of Psychiatry*. 4th edn. American Psychiatric Publishing. Arlington, VA.

22. Nestler, E.J., S.E. Hyman & R.C. Malenka. 2008. *Molecular Neuropharmacology: A Foundation for Clinical Neuroscience*. 2nd edn. McGraw-Hill Professional. Columbus, OH.

23. Sadock, B., V. Sadock & P. Ruiz, Eds. 2009. *Kaplan and Sadock's Comprehensive Textbook of Psychiatry*. Vol. 2, 9th edn. Lippincott Williams & Wilkins. Philadelphia, PA.

24. Schatzberg, A.F. & C.B. Nemeroff, Eds. 2009. *The American Psychiatric Publishing Textbook of Psychopharmacology*. 4th edn. American Psychiatric Publishing, Inc. Arlington, VA.

25. Tasman, A., J. Kay, J.A. Lieberman, *et al*., Eds. 2008. *Psychiatry*. Vols. 1 and 2, 3rd edn. Wiley. Hoboken, NJ.

26. Thase, M.E. & T. Denko. 2008. Pharmacotherapy of mood disorders. *Annu. Rev. Clin. Psychol.* **4:** 53–91.

27. Hoge, C.W., J.L. Auchterlonie & C.S. Milliken. 2006. Mental health problems, use of mental health services, and attrition from military service after returning from deployment to Iraq or Afghanistan. *JAMA* **295:** 1023–1032.

28. 1990 Vet Population from 1990 Census Metropolitan Status by State. 1990. United States Census Bureau.

29. Veterans: 2000 Census Brief. May 2003. US Census Bureau, US Department of Commerce, Economics and Statistics Adm.

30. Beckert, C.B., C. Zayfert & E. Anderson. 2004. A survey of psychologists' attitudes towards and utilization of exposure therapy for PTSD. *Behav. Res. Ther.* **42:** 277–292.

31. Cahill, S.P., E.B. Foa & E.A. Hembree. 2006. Dissemination of exposure therapy in the treatment of posttraumatic stress disorder. [Review]. *J. Trauma. Stress* **19:** 597–610.

32. Rees, C.S. & S. Stone. 2005. Therapeutic alliance in face-to-face versus videoconferenced psychotherapy. *Prof. Psychol.: Res. Pract.* **36:** 649–653.

33. Wray, B.T. & C.S. Rees. 2003. Is there a role for videoconferencing in cognitive behvioral therapy? Paper presented at the *Australian Association for Cognitive and Behaviour Therapy State Conference*, Perth, Western Australia, Australia.

34. Barry, J.M. 2004. *The Great Influenza: The Epic Story of the Deadliest Plague in History*. Viking Adult. New York.

Ann. N.Y. Acad. Sci. ISSN 0077-8923

ANNALS OF THE NEW YORK ACADEMY OF SCIENCES
Issue: *Psychiatric and Neurologic Aspects of War*

Recent advances in preventing mass violence

David A. Hamburg

DeWitt Wallace Distinguished Scholar, Weill Cornell Medical College, President Emeritus, Carnegie Corporation of New York, New York, New York

Address for correspondence: David A. Hamburg, M.D., DeWitt Wallace Distinguished Scholar, Weill Cornell Medical College, Department of Psychiatry, 525 East 68th Street, Box 171, New York, New York 10065. dah2013@med.cornell.edu

Since his presidency of the Carnegie Corporation of New York and co-chairmanship of the Carnegie Commission on Preventing Deadly Conflict, David Hamburg has been actively engaged in projects related to the prevention of genocide and other mass violence. In these remarks to the Association for Research in Nervous and Mental Disease, he describes the significance of preventing mass violence in the 21st century. In particular, he discusses the danger of nuclear and other highly lethal weapons, emphasizing examples of prevention drawn from the Cold War and subsequent period. He delineates practical steps that can be taken to prevent war and genocide, including restraints on weaponry, preventive diplomacy, fostering indigenous democracy, fostering equitable socioeconomic development, education for human survival, and international justice in relation to human rights. Training and support in preventive diplomacy are highlighted as crucially important, particularly in the context of the United Nations, using the novel Mediation Support Unit based out of the Department of Political Affairs as a key example. He concludes that the creation of international centers for the prevention of mass atrocities could provide a crucial resource in preventing mass violence.

Keywords: conflict prevention; genocide; nuclear weapons; preventive diplomacy; democracy; development; education; international justice; human rights; international cooperation; United Nations; European Union

Introduction: danger and opportunities

During the past several years at Cornell, I have led an intensive set of activities, a culmination of efforts over several decades to help prevent genocide and other mass violence. This newest phase on genocide includes (1) writing, editing, and dissemination of a book, *Preventing Genocide: Practical Steps toward Early Detection and Effective Action*,[1] the newly released updated edition,[2] and two related books: *No More Killing Fields*[3] and *Learning to Live Together*;[4] (2) the creation of an unprecedented unit on prevention of genocide at the United Nations (UN); (3) the creation of a parallel unit on prevention of genocide at the European Union (EU); (4) the preparation of an educational documentary based on the book;[5] and (5) the creation of a collection of filmed interviews with world leaders and eminent scholars on pioneering approaches to prevention of mass violence.[5]

I want to delineate practical steps that can be taken to prevent war and genocide including restraints on weaponry as well as promotion of democracy, fostering equitable socioeconomic development, and other pillars of prevention. There are new and exceptional efforts of international cooperation to reduce the nuclear danger drastically. All of this will take a long and winding path, but its importance is surely worth the efforts. Scholars of the Association for Research in Nervous and Mental Disease (ARNMD) caliber can be helpful in such innovations through their teaching, scholarship, creative thinking, and effective advocacy.

Highly lethal weapons have an intoxicating effect on political demagogues, religious fanatics, and ethnic haters. There is a recent and exceedingly dangerous movement toward proliferation of nuclear and other highly lethal weapons in the context of hateful, ruthless, even fanatical leadership.

We have reached a point in human history in which all populations, states, and regions are vulnerable to large-scale casualties from such leaders if they have full control of a state or powerful group. The threat is one that already involves many

doi: 10.1111/j.1749-6632.2010.05792.x

 Ann. N.Y. Acad. Sci. 1208 (2010) 10–14 © 2010 Association for Research in Nervous and Mental Disease.

countries, and, in principle, could involve all. This should stimulate the building of internationally cooperative efforts to overcome the problem of mass atrocities. As a practical matter, the problem simply can not be overcome without a high degree of international cooperation—pooling strengths and sharing burdens.

Some programs have been remarkably successful in reducing the risk of nuclear proliferation and terrorism. For example, the Nunn-Lugar initiative for cooperative threat reduction, in concert with other measures, has already been responsible for the dismantling of well over 5,000 nuclear warheads and the complete elimination of nuclear weapons in Ukraine, Kazakhstan, and Belarus. We must strengthen these proven programs, especially by extending the fruitful Nunn-Lugar efforts to include tactical nuclear weapons (which are particularly dangerous in the context of terrorism because they are readily portable, more affordable, and more easily guided to specific, short-range targets).

Since the whole world is in jeopardy, global cooperation should become feasible if there is sufficient understanding and fear. There must be a broad alliance of nations that will cooperate in identifying, accounting for, and rigorously safeguarding all the nuclear stocks in the world. The strongest countries (and many others) should offer security assurances to nations that voluntarily forgo nuclear weapons and join a common effort to build a robust international antiproliferation system. Strong countries can offer economic and trade benefits, especially in the area of energy supplies. They can supplement economic incentives with measures that enhance security in various ways—far more so than the possession of nuclear weapons.

Learning from the Cold War nuclear danger

As the years since the end of the Cold War have passed, much less has been done about diminishing the nuclear danger than most people had assumed. This was especially true since the overthrow of President Gorbachev. Indeed, he and President Reagan at their Reykjavik summit in 1986 had proposed steps toward the elimination of nuclear weapons altogether. This was not political palaver. It was a deep commitment on the part of both men to rid the world of incomparably deadly weapons that could serve no useful purpose, military or otherwise. They were inhibited by hard-line advisers and by constraints of domestic politics in each country and so their dream was not fulfilled.

Twenty years later, honoring the memory of that historic summit and their extraordinary vision, a group of distinguished scientists, scholars, and political leaders decided to revive the concept and begin a serious effort —necessarily extending over many years—to reduce nuclear weapons to zero. In order to do so, they recognized that it would be essential to formulate a step-by-step process in which deep analytical work would address the technical and political obstacles standing in the way of such progress.

The rationale for this very formidable venture is the recognition that steps being taken now are inadequate to face the fact that we are at a nuclear tipping point. The chance of nuclear weapons falling into utterly irresponsible and fanatically violent hands is a very real possibility. Deterrence is decreasingly effective in a world involving visions of paradise in case of nuclear retaliation and the growing acceptance of mass suicide. Astoundingly, many of the Cold War nuclear weapons are still on hair-trigger alert.

The analytical papers prepared on this subject during the past 2 years exceed any previous work in clarifying what obstacles would have to be overcome and how this exceedingly hard feat could be achieved.[6]

There are near-term steps that may well be taken by the United States and Russia, who have special obligation to demonstrate leadership, since most nuclear weapons are still in these two countries. Yet this U.S.–Russia dialogue must broaden on an international scale, including nonnuclear and nuclear nations. An international consensus on priorities should be achieved since people everywhere are at great risk.

We must make the goal of a world without nuclear weapons into a practical enterprise among nations, by building a strong political constituency for an international consensus on priorities—and pressing leaders to take advantage of these opportunities.

It is heartening, despite all the obstacles, that so many distinguished leaders in many fields and many countries are facing up to the dangers and applying their formidable abilities with great dedication. No one ever thought it would be easy. But neither is it beyond human capacities.

Categories for preventive action

There is much more to preventing mass violence than formulating agreed-upon rules for arms control. Indeed, pillars of prevention can be built to diminish greatly the risks of weaponry and mass atrocities. This will also require a high level of international cooperation above all among the established democracies on a worldwide basis. What are the pillars?

Proactive help to troubled countries and hostile groups, especially preventive diplomacy

Preventive actions cover a wide span of activities. The most rapid are proactive help in preventing mass violence, through preventive diplomacy and beyond. They require organizations, such as the UN, the EU, various regional organizations, and the established democracies to keep in close touch with all regions of the world so as to respond with empathy and concern in offering help promptly with early, ongoing action to prevent mass violence—for example, in mediation of conflict and helping to build internal capacity for nonviolent problem solving: in effect, helping people to see the mutual benefit of learning to live together.

Fostering indigenous democracy

Democracies thrive by finding ways to deal fairly with conflicts and resolve them below the threshold of mass violence. They develop ongoing mechanisms for settling disagreements. That is why, they are so important in preventing mass violence. This requires the growing spread of democracy and the application of democratic principles to intergroup and international conflicts. People who live in pluralistic democracies become accustomed to diverse needs and learn the art of working out compromises that are satisfactory to all groups. This does not mean democracy imposed by force, nor does it mean that a single, premature election will lead to peace and prosperity. But it does mean that patiently constructed democracies, based on fair processes of mutual accommodation, offer the best chance for nonviolent conflict resolution.

Fostering equitable socioeconomic development ("human development")

This is a much more practical goal today than it was a few decades ago, even though a long-rugged path still lies ahead. Investment in human and social capital is now generally accepted as a central part of development, especially in the form of promoting the health and education of girls and boys (and women and men) alike—to build a vigorous, dynamic population that is well-informed, capable, fair-minded, open-minded, and mutually supportive in times of personal and social stress; also social support networks in communities tackling their local problems constructively. The essential features of development—knowledge, skills, freedom, and health—can be achieved by sustained international cooperation that draws upon the unprecedented advances of modern science and technology.

Education for human survival

One of the fundamental underpinnings of successful socioeconomic development is comprehensive prosocial education, from preschool through graduate school. This must include women on an equal basis, not only as a matter of equity but also as a matter of economic stimulus. A crucial and badly neglected function is education for violence prevention, conflict resolution, and mutual accommodation. There is a substantial body of research to support such education.[7]

International institutions to reduce human rights abuses

Prevention of deadly conflict starts with the recognition of the immense dangers of egregious, pervasive human rights violations, typically enforced in repressive states. Such violations lead toward ethnic, religious, and international wars as well as genocide. Sooner or later, these atrocities must be prevented, and bad outcomes averted, by promoting democracy, equitable economies, and the creation of strong civil institutions that protect human rights. Prevention is not simply smoothing over a rough spot in intergroup or international relations—it requires creating a durable basis for peaceful conditions of living together, especially by protecting the human rights of all the people through clear norms and effective, humane institutions.

Training and support in preventive diplomacy

International organizations and democratic governments need staff trained in knowledge and skills to prevent serious conflict—to diminish violent inclinations, wherever they occur. To be effective, diplomats must be aware of the range and relative value of the options open to them. To carry out preventive diplomacy they also need a solid understanding of major causes of conflict, actions likely to lead to conflict escalation or de-escalation, and a variety of strategies that have proved successful in resolving conflicts and diminishing the contagion of hatred.[8] Thus, they need substantial training in negotiation and mediation that moves disputing parties toward a mutually acceptable resolution of their problems. To address these problems and bridge the gap between theory and practice, Connie Peck initiated training and research that evolved into the United Nations Institute for Training and Research Program in Peacemaking and Preventive Diplomacy. This program has become increasingly influential in recent years, especially in regard to the high-level mediators representing the UN Secretary-General or his EU counterpart.

The agenda of the mediator must include the important grievances and positions of all sides; these grievances and positions must be expressed in neutral terms. Mediators must also assume a problem-solving manner that recognizes the interests—concerns, fears, and aspirations.

One of the mediator's jobs is to alert the stronger party to the long-term negative consequences of continuing the conflict, both in domestic destruction of lives, resources, and infrastructure, and also in loss of status and opportunities in the region and the larger world community.

Mediation support unit: a promising innovation in preventive diplomacy

In a recent report to the General Assembly, Secretary-General Ban Ki-moon emphasized, "Now focus must be put on the Organization's capacity to prevent and resolve conflict—a better investment than dealing with the costly aftermath of war and a critical investment to ensure the billions of dollars spent on development by Member States, the international financial institutions and the United Nations itself are not wasted when armed conflict or war erupts" (p. 3).[9] This is strongly in the pathway of the Carnegie Commission on Preventing Deadly Conflict that I co-chaired with Cyrus Vance.[10]

Francis Deng, the distinguished Under-Secretary-General for Prevention of Genocide, has emerged as a world leader in the prevention of mass violence; his unit has made substantial progress in the field

and works closely with worldwide UN professionals. It is unprecedented in the history of the UN.

A crucial part of this opportunity is third-party mediation, among the UN's best tools to prevent and resolve dangerous conflicts everywhere—providing it builds on its present momentum in this direction. In October 2006, a continually upgraded databank for professional mediators was established as a reference.[11] This databank received a UN-wide award in 2008, since it offers access to peace agreements, peace agreement summaries, literature on peace-making issues, a substantial legal library applicable to peacemaking, and links to other useful websites.

Even the most talented and persuasive mediators can not get far without resources that include a practical and professional support staff with knowledge specific to the occasion. Military means may be useful in the short term for checking a particular conflict, but only political solutions achieved through negotiations offer hope of putting a definitive end to a conflict—and to do so without an intervening disaster.

The Mediation Support Unit (MSU) in the United Nations Department of Political Affairs (DPA) has emerged during the past few years due to the need for professional support for preventive diplomacy in various forms.

The MSU is designed to be a locus of expertise and best practice on mediation-related activities worldwide. It serves the UN as a whole, regional, and subregional organizations, as well as other peacemaking bodies. It draws on the world's experiences—no matter where they arise—to develop guidelines, operational tools and training opportunities; and it manages the online databank of peace agreements and peacemaking experience. It supports ongoing mediation efforts in two main ways: (1) country/region-specific operational support and (2) institutional and capacity-building support.

The support takes a variety of forms, including:

- researching and advising on substantive and technical issues, for example, border demarcation, structuring cessation of hostilities agreements, civil society participation, minority rights, confidence-building measures, and natural resource sharing;
- participating in peace talks in an advisory capacity, on a short-notice stand-by basis if necessary;

- organizing dialogue, workshops and training for parties in conflict; and
- identifying, deploying and funding external experts.

The MSU innovation offers the possibility over the next decade of creating a worldwide cadre of expert mediators who can intervene early and constructively in an emerging conflict.

International centers for the prevention of mass atrocities

Focal points associated with great international organizations and major democracies could provide an extremely valuable reservoir of knowledge and skills, as well as a home base for mobilization of many different institutions and organizations that could make good use of this information. Such centers could stimulate worldwide cooperative efforts in the next few decades to greatly reduce the occurrence of mass atrocities. They would stimulate new ideas, new research, new education, and new modes of cooperation among diverse entities that can contribute to prevention. Thus, I have concentrated much effort in the past 5 years on institutional innovations and have been enormously grateful for the cooperation of Kofi Annan and Ban Ki-moon at the UN and Javier Solana at the EU.

Concluding comment

The remarkable improvements in the human condition that have occurred during my lifetime suggest that prevention of genocide is also within reach in this century. We have seen the end of colonialism and imperialism; unprecedented advances in health and reduction of poverty; the worldwide spread of human rights, including the success of the U.S. civil rights movement of the 1960s; the end of fascist and communist totalitarianism; the end of the Cold War; the end of apartheid and the emergence of democracy in South Africa—indeed, the spread of democracy throughout much of the world; and the end of slavery. All of these advances have limits and periodic setbacks, but they represent great changes for the better. These are strong expressions of emerging human decency; yet, we need constant vigilance to mobilize human capacities for fully learning to live together in personal dignity and shared human-

ity. Those of us here today can do a lot to stimulate interest in this great mission, to disseminate ideas of the kind delineated here, and generate better ideas so that our children and grandchildren will move us into a world of decent human relations at last.

Acknowledgments

This research effort was facilitated by the extraordinary, indeed unique encouragement, stimulation, and inspiration from Dr. Jack Barchas, a great leader in psychiatry and medicine and a dear friend for half a century. His leadership of the ARNMD in the past 10 years has been outstanding. Funding for these activities was received from the DeWitt Wallace Fund of Weill Cornell Medical College.

Conflicts of interest

The author declares no conflicts of interest.

References

1. Hamburg, D.A. 2008. *Preventing Genocide: Practical Steps Toward Early Detection and Effective Action.* Paradigm Publishers. Boulder, CO.
2. Hamburg, D.A. 2009. *Revised and Updated: Preventing Genocide: Practical Steps Toward Early Detection and Effective Action.* Paradigm Publishers. Boulder, CO.
3. Hamburg, D.A. 2002. *No More Killing Fields: Preventing Deadly Conflict.* Rowman & Littlefield Publishers. New York.
4. Hamburg, D.A. & B.A. Hamburg. 2004. *Learning to Live Together: Preventing Hatred and Violence in Child and Adolescent Development.* Oxford University Press. New York.
5. Documentary and related set of filmed interviews are available at: http://lib.stanford.edu/pg (accessed September 24, 2010).
6. SeeDrell, S.D. & J.E. Goodby. 2009. *A World Without Nuclear Weapons: End State Issues.* Hoover Institution Press. Stanford, CA.
7. Hamburg, D.A. & B.A. Hamburg. 2004. *Learning to Live Together: Preventing Hatred and Violence in Child and Adolescent Development.* Oxford University Press. New York.
8. Hayner, P. 2009. Negotiating Justice: Guidance for Mediators. Henry Dunant Centre for Humanitarian Dialogue. New York.
9. Ki-moon, B. November 2, 2007. Report to the 62nd Session of the UN General Assembly, United Nations A/62/521. United Nations. New York.
10. See Carnegie Commission on Preventing Deadly Conflict. 1997. Final Report: Carnegie Commission on Preventing Deadly Conflict. Carnegie Corporation of New York. New York.
11. Available at: www.un.org/peacemaker (accessed April 29, 2010).

Ann. N.Y. Acad. Sci. ISSN 0077-8923

ANNALS OF THE NEW YORK ACADEMY OF SCIENCES
Issue: *Psychiatric and Neurologic Aspects of War*

"When hatred is bred in the bone:" the social psychology of terrorism

Jerrold M. Post

The George Washington University, Washington, DC

Address for correspondence: Jerrold M. Post, M.D., Elliott School of International Affairs, 1957 E Street, NW, Suite 600F, Washington, DC 20052. jpost@gwu.edu

Terrorists are not crazed fanatics. Indeed, terrorist groups screen out emotionally unstable individuals—they would be a security risk. Rather it is group, organizational, and social psychology, with particular emphasis on collective identity that motivates terrorist behavior. There is a diverse spectrum of terrorist psychologies and motivations. In terms of generational provenance, nationalist–separatist terrorists are carrying on the mission of their parents—they are loyal to families who have been damaged by the regime. In contrast, social–revolutionary terrorists are disloyal to families who are loyal to the regime. Religious fundamentalist terrorists are "killing in the name of God." Suicide, proscribed by the Koran, has been reframed as martyrdom, which is highly valued. The new media, especially the Internet, have played an increasingly prominent role in radicalizing individuals, creating a virtual community of hatred. Understanding terrorist psychology is crucial to formulating effective counter-terrorist strategy. Key elements include inhibiting potential terrorists from joining the group, creating tension within the group, facilitating exit from the group, reducing support for the group, and delegitimating its leader.

Keywords: suicide terrorism; martyrdom; terrorist psychology; radicalization; counterterrorism

It is widely assumed that terrorists who kill innocents for a cause and are willing to give their lives for that cause are crazed fanatics. But in fact, terrorism scholars have concluded that as individuals terrorists are psychologically normal. Martha Crenshaw has observed that, "The outstanding common characteristic of terrorists is their normality" (p. 390).[1] John Horgan has emphasized in his book on the psychology of terrorists that there are no individual psychological traits that distinguish terrorists from the general population.[2] In contrast, Post has called attention to the powerful effect of group dynamics on terrorist psychology and behavior.[3]

The consensus document prepared by the Committee on the Psychological Roots of Terrorism for the International Summit on Democracy, Terrorism and Security in Madrid, 2005 concluded that[4]:

1. Explanations of terrorism at the level of individual psychology are insufficient in trying to understand why people become involved in terrorism. Indeed, it is not going too far to assert that terrorists are psychologically "normal" in the sense of not being clinically psychotic. They are neither depressed, severely emotionally disturbed, nor are they crazed fanatics. Indeed, terrorist groups and organizations screen out emotionally unstable individuals. They represent a security risk. There is a multiplicity of individual motivations. For some it is to give a sense of power to the powerless; for others, revenge is a primary motivation; for still others, to gain a sense of significance. Within each group there will be motivational differences among the members, each of whom will be motivated to different degrees by group interest versus self-serving actions as well as those inspired by ideology.

2. It is not individual psychology, but group, organizational, and social psychology, with a particular emphasis on "collective identity," that provides the most powerful lens to understand terrorist psychology and behavior. For some groups, especially nationalist/terrorist groups, this collective identity is established extremely early, so that "hatred is bred in the

doi: 10.1111/j.1749-6632.2010.05694.x

bone." The importance of collective identity and the processes of forming and transforming collective identities can not be overemphasized. This in turn emphasizes the sociocultural context, which determines the balance between collective identity and individual identity. A clear consensus exists that it is not understanding individual psychopathology but group, organizational, and social psychology, which provides the greatest analytic power in understanding this complex phenomenon, a phenomenon where collective identity is paramount. Terrorists have subordinated their individual identity to the collective identity, so that what serves the group, organization, or network is of primary importance.

To better understand how psychologically normal individuals can righteously pursue such violent extremism, it is useful to consider their generational provenance. The following diagram conveys the manner in which generational transmission of hatred shapes terrorist identity for two major types of terrorists: social–revolutionary terrorists and nationalist–separatist terrorists.[5]

As Figure 1 conveys, in many ways, the generational dynamics of social–revolutionary terrorists and nationalist–separatist terrorists are mirror images.[6] The social–revolutionary terrorists, whose generational dynamics are represented in the lower left cell, are striking out against the generation of their parents who are loyal to the regime. Their acts of terrorism are acts of revenge for hurts, real and imagined, against the generation of their parents. A member of the German terrorist group, Red Army Faction, declared, "These are the corrupt old men who gave us Auschwitz and Hiroshima."

Since the implosion of the Soviet Union, these groups, which were steeped in Marxist-Leninist doctrine, such as the Red Army Faction in Germany and the Red Brigades in Italy, have largely disappeared. But it is interesting to consider that these are the dynamics of Osama bin Laden, the founding leader of al-Qaeda. When he lashed out at the Saudi royal family for their apostasy in providing shelter to U.S. military bases in "the land of the two cities," (Saudi Arabia, referring to the holy shrines of Mecca and Medina) he was striking out verbally at the Saudi leadership that had enriched his family. For his trouble, bin Laden was deprived of his Saudi passport and citizenship and his family, whose economic interests were threatened, turned their back on their brother. So bin Laden is not merely an Islamist fundamentalist terrorist, he has the classic generational dynamics of the social revolutionary, and can be considered as the revolutionary leader of radical Islam, seeking to propagate its message through violence against the modernizing West.

In contrast, the nationalist–separatist terrorists, represented in the upper right hand cell, are loyal to parents and grandparents who are disloyal to the regime, were damaged by the regime. They are carrying on the mission of their parents and grandparents, who are dissident to the regime. Whether in the pubs of Northern Ireland or the coffee houses in Gaza and the occupied territories, and they have

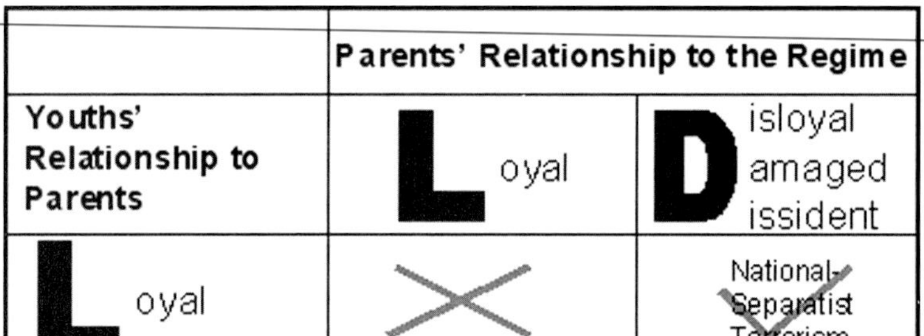

Figure 1. The manner in which generational transmission of hatred shapes terrorist identity for two major types of terrorists: social–revolutionary terrorists and nationalist–separatist terrorists.

heard of the social injustice visited upon their parents and grandparents, and they have heard their parents complaining of the lands stolen from them and their economic hardships. They have been raised on this bitter gruel of victimhood; their hatred has been "bred in the bone."

Carrying on the mission of his parents: Omar Rezaq of the Abu Nidal Organization[7]

This is well illustrated by the life story of Omar Rezaq whom I interviewed for 3 days in the spring of 1996 in connection with his trial in federal district court in Washington, DC, for the federal crime of skyjacking.[7] It was Rezaq, a member of the Abu Nidal group, who played a central role in seizing the EgyptAir plane, which was forced down in Malta in 1985. Rezaq shot five hostages, two Israeli women and three Americans—before the botched SWAT team attack by Egyptian forces led to more than 50 casualties. Convicted of murder in a Malta court, after 7 years Rezaq was given amnesty and released. But subsequently, he was arrested by FBI agents for the crime of skyjacking.

Rezaq's mother was 8 years old in 1948 at the time of the 1948 Arab Israeli War (called the war of Independence by Israel, the "Catastrophe" by Arab nations.) Forced to flee their home in Jaffa, an Arab suburb of Tel Aviv, she and her parents fled to her grandfather's farm on the West Bank. There they lived a comfortable life until 1967, when, ironically, the defendant Omar Rezaq was 8 years old. As a consequence of the 1967 war, they were forced to flee the West Bank, ending up in a refugee camp in Jordan. The mother bitterly exclaimed to her son, "This is the second time this has happened to me, being forced to flee from my home."

Rezaq was educated in a school in the refugee camp supported by UNESCO funds. His teacher was a member of the Palestinian Liberation Organization (PLO) and a member of Fatah, the secular Palestinian group. In 1968, the battle of Karameh occurred, in which Arafat led a group of Palestinian guerrillas who fought a 12-h battle against a superior Israeli force, galvanizing the previously dispirited Palestinian population. The spirit of the revolution was everywhere, especially in the camps, and the PLO became a rallying point. In Rezaq's words, "the revolution was the only hope."

His teacher told young Rezaq and his classmates that the only way to become a man was to become a soldier of the revolution and fight for the lands stolen from their parents and grandparents. In the mornings, he learned reading, writing, and arithmetic; in the afternoons, he was trained to be a soldier in the revolution, learning small weapons handling, booby traps, explosives, and training on obstacle courses. This was preparation for a role of which he was intensely proud—he was preparing to become a fighter for the cause. He had been imbued with the narrative of victimization since early childhood, and had been taught that it was the occupying enemy, Israel, that was the cause of all of their family's hardships.

The statement, "It's not us; it's *them; they* are responsible for our problems" provides a psychologically satisfying explanation for what has gone wrong in the lives of those who become terrorists. And it is therefore not only not immoral, it becomes a moral imperative to strike out at *them*, to remove the source of the problems.

After finishing intermediate school, Rezaq went on to technical school under UN auspices. There were branches of the revolution in this school; each group tried to recruit the new students. Rezaq became more deeply involved in politics. He was taught that the only way to get back his country was if the PLO would fight against Israel. And he was increasingly determined to join that fight.

Two years of obligatory service in the Jordanian army were required. At 1977, at age 19, Rezaq was sent to a camp near Iraq for military training. The Palestinians were treated as second-class citizens. After only 3 months in the Jordanian army, Rezaq went AWOL and joined Fatah. He went to a military camp where he was given a military uniform and was trained in the use of machine guns, pistols, and hand grenades. He also received intense political indoctrination. Now he was energized, fully committed, at last in a fighting revolutionary organization. He wanted "to work, wanted to fight. There was only one way to regain Palestine and that was to fight Israel in order to regain all of Palestine, from the sea to the river."

He moved from group to group, initially enthused, then disillusioned, each group more militant than the preceding. When he was next involved in guerilla action, he had pride in what he was doing as a soldier for the revolution. "I started dreaming that one day we will have a country, have an identity, [be] our own citizens." After attacking an Israeli patrol, his morale took a major boost. "This was for my country." He felt this was the right way, the path for him to follow. He felt a sense of excitement in the danger.

As a result of U.S.-brokered negotiations, Arafat and the PLO were to leave Lebanon. Disillusioned with Arafat and the mainstream PLO, Rezaq decided to stay on in Lebanon to fight. He ultimately made his way to the most violent of the Palestinian terrorist groups, the Abu Nidal group.

After intense training, he was given an important mission. He was told the mission was to hijack an airliner in order to obtain the release of antigovernment Egyptians in prison in Egypt. He felt good about the mission. He now had a purpose. This is what he had been preparing for since boyhood.

The operation

In describing the operation, Rezaq related the entire episode in a cool, matter of fact manner—logical, detailed, calm, not emotionally overwrought—the professional military man reporting on a military action.

After the terrorists took over the plane, in accordance with the plan, they forced it down in Malta in order to refuel before the final leg. The control tower said they would not provide petrol until the hostages were released. Rezaq informed the control tower they would not release the hostages until the plane was refueled. Malta control refused, insisting that the hijackers release all of the hostages or there would be no petrol.

As Rezaq explained, it was an impasse. And they had been told that it was important to begin killing the hostages in order to demonstrate their credibility and give them leverage. He remembered the mission instructions concerning the Israelis and Americans. If there were Israelis in the plane, he was told he must kill them directly, for they were enemies of Palestine. Since America supported Israel, Americans should then be used as leverage, and should be killed if no petrol was provided. Rezaq now went through the passports, and found passports of two Israeli women and three Americans. Having given an ultimatum to the control tower that he would begin killing hostages unless they refueled the plane, when they did not provide petrol, he told the stewardess to bring him an Israeli. It was a woman. He described in a cool detached manner, demonstrating, grabbing her hair with his left hand and placing the

revolver to her forehead and then blowing her brains out.

When I asked him about his emotional state at the time of the killings, and how he reacted to killing a person at close range, he looked at me with perplexity, and responded as if it should be self-evident, that it was what he had been instructed to do, it was the plan for the mission.

Having demonstrated that they should take him seriously, he gave a second ultimatum. But by now he was hungry, so he had some lunch. The calm, matter of fact manner in which he described being hungry, and eating his lunch was indistinguishable from the manner in which he described shooting the Israeli woman in the head. In the same matter of fact way, he then told of shooting the second Israeli woman in the head. As to the impact of killing a woman, he responded to my question concerning how it felt to shoot a woman, that there was no difference. He had been told that both Israeli men and women served in the army, so both were the enemy, and both deserved to die.

The Maltese authorities still had not provided petrol, so Rezaq then ordered the air crew to bring him the Americans. The first American was shot. Because there was still no petrol, he then had them bring the second American and shot him as well.

The storming of the plane followed.

This case in many ways epitomizes the generational transmission of hated, and also emphasizes the dehumanization of the enemy, which facilitates killing the enemy in the name of the cause. Like his fellow terrorists, he believed that his actions were justified, were not wrongful but were righteous acts in the service of the Palestinian revolution. He had been socialized to blame all of his and his people's difficulties on the enemy and that violent actions against the enemy were justified. He rationalized that the injustices against the Palestinian people justified his violent acts.

When one has been nursed on the mother's milk of hatred and bitterness, the need for vengeance is "bred in the bone." In ethnic/nationalist conflicts, hatred has been transmitted generationally, and the psychopolitics of hatred are deeply rooted.

Interviews with incarcerated Middle East terrorists

Over an 18-month period prior to the most recent outbreak of violence that erupted after the failure of the Camp David talks of the fall of 2000, interviews were conducted with 31 Palestinian terrorists and three Hizballah members.[8] Subjects represented both secular and Islamist groups. The interviewers were trained in developing a comfortable interpersonal situation, which was not coercive or threatening. The interviews focused on issues of socialization and personal experience as opposed to operational and tactical procedures, and interviewers were trained to avoid questions that could be considered interrogation aiming at eliciting tactical intelligence. Since many of the prisoners were serving multiple life sentences, the interviewers were instructed to play to their egos and help the subjects find a "sense making" explanation for their actions.

Secular terrorists in their own words

Like Omar Rezaq, the secular terrorists had been steeped in hatred from early in their lives. The hatred socialized toward the Israeli was remarkable, especially given that few reported any contact with Israelis.

> You Israelis are Nazis in your souls and in your conduct. In your occupation you never distinguish between men and women, or between old people and children. You adopted methods of collective punishment; you uprooted people from their homeland and from their homes and chased them into exile. You fired live ammunition at women and children. You smashed the skulls of defenseless civilians. You set up detention camps for thousands of people in subhuman conditions. You destroyed homes and turned children into orphans. You prevented people from making a living, you stole their property, you trampled on their honor. Given that kind of conduct, there is no choice but to strike at you without mercy in every possible way.

While most Fatah members reported their families had good social standing, their status and experience as refugees was paramount in their development of self-identity.

> I belong to the generation of occupation. My family are refugees from the 1967 war. The war and my refugee status were the seminal events that formed my political consciousness, and provided the incentive for doing all I could to help regain our legitimate rights in our occupied country.

For the secular terrorists, enlistment was a natural step.

> Enlistment was for me the natural and done thing . . . in a way, it can be compared to a young Israeli from a nationalist Zionist family who wants to fulfill himself through army service.
> My motivation in joining Fatah was both ideological and personal. It was a question of self-fulfillment, of honor and a feeling of independence . . . the goal of every young Palestinian was to be a fighter.
> After recruitment, my social status was greatly enhanced. I got a lot of respect from my acquaintances, and from the young people in the village.

View of armed attacks

Armed attacks are viewed as essential to the operation of the organization. There is no question about the necessity of these types of attacks to the success of the cause.

> You have to understand that armed attacks are an integral part of the organization's struggle against the Zionist occupier. There is no other way to redeem the land of Palestine and expel the occupier. Our goals can only be achieved through force, but force is the means, not the end. History shows that without force it will be impossible to achieve independence. Those who carry out the attacks are doing Allah's work. . .
> The more an attack hurts the enemy, the more important it is. That is the measure. The mass killings, especially the martyrdom operations, were the biggest threat to the Israeli public and so most effort was devoted to these. The extent of the damage and the number of casualties are of primary importance.

In addition to causing as many casualties as possible, armed action provided a sense of control or power for Palestinians in a society that had stripped them of it. Inflicting pain on the enemy was paramount in the early days of the Fatah movement.

> I regarded armed actions to be essential, it is the very basis of my organization and I am sure that was the case in the other Palestinian organizations. **An armed action proclaims that I am here, I exist, I am strong, I am in control, I am in the field, I am on the map.** An armed action against soldiers was the most admired. . . .the armed actions and their results were a major tool for penetrating the public consciousness.

The sentence in bold face emphasizes how difficult it is to leave the revered role of fighter for the cause, and how difficult it is to end these nationalist–separatist conflicts. Whether in Northern Ireland, Sri Lanka, or Palestine, occupying the role of the freedom fighter may well be the high point of the young man's life, giving it purpose and significance, and to return to a mediocre job on an assembly line would pale by comparison.

Islamic extremists in their own words

For both secular and Islamist terrorists, but especially for the latter, the shaping influence of the mosque was regularly emphasized.

> I came from a religious family which used to observe all the Islamic traditions. My initial political awareness came during the prayers at the mosque. That's where I was also asked to join religious classes. In the context of these studies, the sheik used to inject some historical background in which he would tell us how we were effectively evicted from Palestine.

> The sheik also used to explain to us the significance of the fact that there was an IDF military outpost in the heart of the camp. He compared it to a cancer in the human body, which was threatening its very existence.

> At the age of 16 I developed an interest in religion. I was exposed to the Moslem brotherhood and I began to pray in a mosque and to study Islam. The Koran and my religious studies were the tools that shaped my political consciousness. The mosque and the religious clerics in my village provided the focal point of my social life.

> Major actions become the subject of sermons in the mosque, glorifying the attack and the attackers.

Community support was important to the families of the fighters as well:

> Families of terrorists who were wounded, killed or captured enjoyed a great deal of economic aid and attention. And that strengthened popular support for the attacks.

> Perpetrators of armed attacks were seen as heroes, their families got a great deal of material assistance, including the construction of new homes to replace those destroyed by the Israeli authorities as punishment for terrorist acts.

Joining Hamas or Fatah increased social standing:

> Recruits were treated with great respect. A youngster who belonged to Hamas or Fatah was regarded more highly than one who didn't belong to a group, and got better treatment than unaffiliated kids.

> Anyone who didn't enlist during that period (intifada) would have been ostracized.

The justification of suicide bombings

The Islamist terrorists, in particular, provided the religious basis for what the West has called suicide terrorism as the most valued technique of jihad, distinguishing this from suicide, which is proscribed in the Koran. One suicide bomb commander in fact became quite angry when the term was used in our question, angrily exclaiming:

> This is not suicide. Suicide is selfish, it is weak, it is mentally disturbed. This is istishhad (martyrdom or self-sacrifice in the service of Allah).

Several of the Islamist terrorist commanders interviewed called the suicide bomber holy warriors who were carrying out the highest level of jihad.

> A martyrdom operation is the highest level of jihad, and highlights the depth of our faith. The bombers are holy fighters who carry out one of the more important articles of faith.[a]

> It is attacks when their member gives his life that earn the most respect and elevate the bombers to the highest possible level of martyrdom.

> I asked Halil what is was all about and he told me that he had been on the watch list for a long time and did not want to get caught without realizing his dream of being a martyrdom operation bomber. He was completely calm and explained to the other two bombers, Yusuf and Beshar, how to detonate the bombs, exactly the way he had explained things to the bombers in the Mahane Yehuda attack. I remember that besides the tremendous respect I had for Halil, and the fact that I was jealous of him, I also felt slighted that he had not asked me to be the third martyrdom operation bomber. I understood that my role in the movement had not come to an end and the act that I was not on the wanted list and could operate relatively freely could be very advantageous to the movement in the future.[b]

---

[a]Hassan Salame, responsible for the wave of suicide bombings in Israel in 1996, in which 46 were killed. He is now serving 46 consecutive life sentences.
[b]Quote from prisoner sentenced to 26 life terms for role in several suicide-bombing campaigns.

Sense of remorse/moral red lines

When it came to moral considerations, we believed in the justice of our cause and in our leaders. . . . I don't recall every being troubled by moral questions.

The organization had no red lines or moral constraints in actions against Jews. Any killing of a Jew was considered a success, and the more the better.

The lack of remorse or moral considerations was particularly striking in the military wing of Hamas, Izz al-Din al-Qassam. There is a deep sense of righteousness in their discussion of their actions and the legitimacy of action undertaken by the action in the fight for their cause. There is also a sense that the actions of the Israeli Security Forces provide justification for any action they might take. The language becomes more forceful in this section as the Israelis are referred to as "the enemy" and "foreign occupiers"—the Israelis are depicted as "them," not as people living within the same community.

The organization has no moral red lines. We must do everything to force the enemy to retreat from out lands. Nothing is illegitimate in achieving this. As for the organization's moral red lines, there were none. We considered every attack on the occupier legitimate. The more you hurt the enemy, the more he understands.

In a jihad, there are no red lines.

Ariel Merari, an Israeli expert on terrorism who teaches at Harvard each fall, remarked ironically to me that "teenagers are the same the world around."[9] He observed the teenagers in Harvard Square, talking over pizza about their team, the (then) super bowl bound New England Patriots, the stars they worshipped on the team, talking about their dreams of becoming a National Football League star when they grew up. It was just the same, Merari remarked ironically, for Palestinian teenagers in the refugee camps, only their favorite team was Hamas, the stars they worshipped were the latest *shahids* (martyrs) and they hoped to become a *shahid* when they grew up, *which they wouldn't.* Indeed, they have martyr trading cards in the camps, just like baseball or football cards. He has described the shaping of Palestinian suicide bombers as a "suicide terrorist assembly line." He sees this as a phenomenon of social psychology, not individual psychopathology. First, they are recruited or volunteer, agreeing to be trained to become a suicide bomber. Then they are identified as "living martyrs," gaining prestige in the community, and finally they make the video, talking about their motivation for their mission. These tapes, which are used for recruitment, are a crucial last step, a public declaration. After this sequence, Merari notes it is almost impossible for the suicide bomber to back down, for the shame would be unbearable. Thus it is much more a phenomenon of social psychology than individual psychopathology.

Comparison of Palestinian and al-Qaeda suicide terrorists

Mohammad Hafez has emphasized that three conditions are necessary to support suicide terrorism: a culture that values martyrdom, an organization that chooses this strategy as forwarding their goals, and individuals in a recruitment pool who are alienated and despairing and psychologically available to pursue this course.[10,11]

It is useful to contrast the suicide bombers of Hamas and Islamic Jihad, whose commanders were interviewed in the study from which the above quotes were drawn, with the suicidal hijackers of 9/11. Psychological autopsies of 93 Palestinian suicide bombers have been conducted by Israeli authorities. Aged 17-22, these young men were unemployed, uneducated, and unmarried. Unformed youth, when they were recruited, or volunteered to become a martyrdom operation bomber, they were informed by the suicide bomb commanders, who were very skillful at manipulating them, that they had a wretched life to look forward to (the unemployment rate in the Palestinian camps was running 40%, more so for those with no education), they could do something significant with their lives, they would enter the hall of martyrs, their parents would be proud of them, and would gain prestige and financial benefit. From the moment they entered the safe house, they were never left alone. On the night before the operation, someone would sleep in the same room, to ensure that they did not backslide. On the day of the action, they would be physically escorted to the pizza parlor or disco.

In vivid contrast, the suicidal hijackers of 9/11 were older, 28–33, had higher education, and came from comfortable middle class homes in Saudi Arabia or Egypt. Mohamed Atta, the commander, was 33, and he and two of his colleagues were in masters' degree programs at the technological university in Hamburg, Germany. They were fully formed adults, who had subordinated their individuality to the group, and uncritically accepted the dictates of their destructive charismatic leader, Osama bin Laden. Their major identification was as members of the al-Qaeda organization, and if the action required brought benefit to the organization, they would give their lives for the cause. Most interesting, they had been on their own in the West for upward of 7 years, blending in with society, while keeping like a laser beam within them their mission to give of their lives while claiming the lives of thousands of victims, all of this in the name of Allah.

The virtual community of hatred

The impact of the communication revolution upon radicalization and terrorism can not be overstated. In particular, 24/7 cable news and the Internet have played major roles in the socialization of extremism and in forming what may be called a virtual community of hatred. Hezbollah uses television to broadcast its message and propaganda to its supporters, both locally and internationally. Al-Manar (the Beacon) TV switched to satellite broadcasts in 2000, disseminating an anti-Israel and anti-American messaged to a large Muslim audience. A typical Al-Manar broadcast, for example, televised a statement in favor of acts of suicide terrorism, reframed as martyrdom, as a method for anti-Israel resistance.

> "In the culture of resistance, the culmination of humanity and human dignity is the decision to perform istishhad [martyrdom] in order to grant life to one's people and dignity to one's nation and homeland."[12]

It is interesting to observe that while decrying the evils of modernization, terrorist organizations fully exploit modern communications technology in disseminating their extremist messages. The Internet in particular has been a powerful medium. The military wing of Hamas created a "Military Academy" that runs online courses for bomb making, featuring a 14-lesson course. In 1996, the Hamas website posted *The Mujahideen Poisons Handbook*, a 23-page handbook on preparing poisons and toxins.[13]

Consider this message concerning their Internet strategy, posted on an al-Qaeda website, addressed to Muslim Internet professionals.

> Due to the advances of modern technology, it is easy to spread news, information, articles and other information over the Internet. We strongly urge Muslim Internet professionals to spread and disseminate news and information about the Jihad through e-mail lists, discussion groups, and their own websites. If you fail to do this, and our site closes down before you have done this, be held you to account before Allah on the Day of Judgment
> ... This way, even if our sites are closed down, the material will live on with the Grace of Allah.

More pointedly, the following message appeared in an al-Qaeda site 4 months before the Madrid train station bombing of March, 2004.

> In order to force the Spanish government to withdraw from Iraq, the resistance should deal painful blows to its forces. . . It is necessary to make the utmost use of the upcoming general election in March next year. We think that the Spanish government could not tolerate more than two, maximum three blows, after which it will have to withdraw as a result of popular pressure. If its troops remain in Iraq after these blows, the victory of the Socialist Party is almost secured, and the withdrawal of the Spanish forces will be on its electoral program.[14]

In the event, in fact the Spanish government remained in Iraq, withdrawal of the forces became a pillar of the Socialist party platform, and the Socialist party did secure victory, withdrawing its forces from Iraq shortly after coming to power.

Weimann, in *Terror on the Internet*, speaks of the proliferation of radical Islamist websites, estimating 4,800 radical Islamist websites.[15] In *Digital Diasporas*, Brinkerhoff addresses the manner in which the Internet can provide a coherent function for alienated émigrés.[16] But if in so doing, the cohering messages are anti-establishment, extolling the values of extremism, they can consolidate a radical group identity. An isolated, alienated individual may have had no face to face contact with other individuals, but through the magic of the Internet can feel that he belongs to a powerful movement and may be moved from increasingly radical thought to violent action in support of that movement. This is true for right wing extremism as well.

Implications for counterterrorism

Terrorism is a vicious species of psychological warfare, waged through the media. It is a war for hearts and minds. If one accepts this premise, then "the war against terrorism" will not be won with smart bombs and missiles. One does not counter psychological warfare with high-tech weapons. In fact, military retaliation can be counter-productive. The way to counter psychological warfare is with psychological warfare. This is to emphasize that psychological operations should be *the primary weapon* in the war against terrorism, a tool that has been insufficiently used in countering terrorism.[17]

Four major elements of a psychological program designed to counter terrorism are to:

1. "Inhibit" potential terrorists from joining terrorist groups and organizations;
2. "Produce dissention" within the groups;
3. "Facilitate exit" from the groups; and
4. "Reduce support" for the groups and "Delegitimize" their leaders.

These elements are components of a strategic psychological operations program that must be conducted over decades. For when hatred is "bred in the bone," these attitudes are not easily changed. It was Lenin who memorably conveyed, "The goal of terrorism is to terrorize." This suggests a fifth requisite element of a sustained campaign of strategic psychological operations, namely

5. "Insulating the target audience," the public, from the intended goals of the terrorist to terrorize.

Conflicts of interest

The author declares no conflicts of interest.

References

1. Crenshaw, M. 1981. The causes of terrorism. *Comp. Polit.* **13:** 379–399.
2. Horgan, J. 2005. *The Psychology of Terrorism.* Routledge. New York.
3. Post, J.M. 1986. Hostilité, conformité, fraternité: the group dynamics of terrorist behavior. *Int. J. Group Psychother.* **36:** 211–224. (See also Post, J.M. 1987. It's us against them: the group dynamics of terrorist behavior. *Terrorism* **10:** 23–36.)
4. Post, J.M. 2005. The psychological roots of terrorism. *Addressing the Causes of Terrorism, The Club de Madrid Series on Democracy and Terrorism* **Vol. 1:** 7–12.
5. This generational matrix was first introduced by the author

in Post, J.M. 1984. Notes on a psychodynamic theory of terrorism. *Terrorism: Int. J.* **7:** 241–256.
6. Expanded discussion of the generational provenance of terrorist groups will be found in Post, J.M. 2005. When hatred is bred in the bone: psychocultural foundations of contemporary terrorism. *Pol. Psychol.* **26:** 615–636. (See also Post, J.M. 2006. The psychological dynamics of terrorism. In *The Roots of Terrorism.* L. Richardson, Ed.: 17–28. Routledge. New York and Post, J.M. 2007. *The Mind of the Terrorist: The Psychology of Terrorism from the IRA to al-Qaeda.* Palgrave Macmillan. New York.)
7. This discussion is drawn from Post, J.M. 2000. Murder in a political context: profile of an Abu Nidal terrorist. *Bull. Acad. Psychiatry Law* **28:** 171–178.
8. Post, J.M., E. Sprinzak & L. Denny. 2003. The terrorists in their own words: interviews with 35 incarcerated Middle Eastern terrorists. *Terrorism Pol. Violence* **15:** 171–184.
9. Personal communication with Ariel Merari, 2003.
10. For a detailed comparison of Palestinian and Al-Qaeda suicide terrorism, see Post, J.M. 2007. Section III Religious extremist terrorism: killing in the name of God. In *The Mind of the Terrorist: The Psychology of Terrorism from the IRA to Al-Qaeda.* Palgrave Macmillan. New York, pp. 161–216 and Post, J.M., F. Ali, S.W. Henderson, *et al.* 2009. The psychology of suicide terrorism. *Psychiatry: Interpersonal Biol. Process.* **72:** 13–30. Emphasis is given to the reframing of suicide, which is prohibited by the Koran, as martyrdom, which is given an elevated status.
11. Hafez, M. 2003. *Manufacturing Human Bombs: The Making of Palestinian Suicide Bombers.* United States Institute of Peace Press. Washington, DC.
12. "Hezbollah" Special Information Report. June 2003. *Intelligence and Terrorism Information Center at the Center for Special Studies.* http://www.terrorism-info.org.il/malam_multimedia/ENGLISH/IRAN/PDF/JUNE_03. PDF (accessed March 1, 2010).
13. Weimann, G. 2006. Virtual training camps: terrorists' use of the Internet. In *Teaching Terror: Strategic and Tactical Learning in the Terrorist World.* J. Forest, Ed.: 110–132. Rowman and Littlefield. Lanham, MD.
14. Jihadi Iraq, hopes and dangers. Part of Al-Qaeda manual, published online through *Global Islamic Media,* December 2003. http://www.mil.no/felles/ffi/start/article.jhtml?articleID=71589 (accessed April 28, 2010).
15. Weimann, G. 2006. *Terror on the Internet: The New Arena, the New Challenges.* The United States Institute of Peace Press. Washington, DC.
16. Brinkerhoff, J. 2009. *Digital Diasporas: Identity and Transnational Engagement.* Cambridge University Press. Cambridge, MA.
17. A detailed analysis of the role of strategic information operations in countering terrorism will be found in Post, J.M. 2005. Psychological operations and counter terrorism. *Joint Force Quart.* **27:** 105–110.

Ann. N.Y. Acad. Sci. ISSN 0077-8923

A trauma-like model of political extremism: psycho-political fault lines in Israel

Nathaniel Laor,[1,2,3,4] Alma Yanay-Shani,[1,2] Leo Wolmer,[1,2] and Oula Khoury[1,2]

[1]Tel-Aviv Community Mental Health Center, Tel-Aviv, Israel. [2]Cohen-Harris Center for Trauma and Disaster Intervention, Tel-Aviv, Israel. [3]Sackler School of Medicine, Tel-Aviv University, Tel-Aviv, Israel. [4]Yale Child Study Center, New Haven, Connecticut

Address for correspondence: Nathaniel Laor, M.D., Ph.D., Tel-Aviv Community Mental Health Center, 9 Hatzvi Street, Tel-Aviv 67197, Israel. nlaor@netvision.net.il

This study examines a trauma-like model of potentially violent political extremism among Jewish Israelis. We study the psychosocial characteristics of political extremists that may lie at the root of sociopolitical instability and assess personal (gender, stressful life events, Holocaust family background, and political activism) and psychological parameters (self- and political transcendence, perceived political threats, in/out-group identification ratio) that may predict readiness to engage in destructive political behavior. We examine the ideological zeal of various political groups, the relationship between the latter and perceived political threats, and the predictors of extreme political activism. Results showed that the extreme political poles displayed high level of ideological and morbid transcendence. Right extremists displayed higher perceived threats to physical existence and national identity. Left extremists scored highest on perceived moral integrity threat. Higher perceived threats to national identity and moral integrity, risk, and self-transcendence statistically explain morbid transcendence. When fear conjures up extremely skewed sociopolitical identifications across political boundaries, morbid transcendence may manifest itself in destructive political activity.

Keywords: trauma; political extremism; transcendence; threats; fault line conflict; Jewish-Arab conflict

Introduction

Fault line political conflicts are characterized by struggles between identity groups for control over territory or people with the aim of occupying this territory and freeing it from the control of "nongroup" members. Such struggles may lead to outbursts of extreme violence.[1] This study examines the Israeli scene against the backdrop of the second Intifada, exploring within a trauma-like model the factors that have driven Jewish-Israeli extremists to implement aggressive orientations politically.

On the basis of attitudes toward issues of moral, existential, and national identity as well as of aggression and reconciliation, Bar-Tal[2–4] defined the construct "ethos of conflict": in Jewish Israelis, conflict triggers traumatic historical schemata (e.g., the Holocaust) that give rise to processes of cross-national identification and demonization.

Feeling threatened increases ethnocentrism and xenophobia,[5] promotes intolerance,[6] increases willingness to take risks,[7] and is a fundamental cause of prejudice.[8] Conflicts breed perceived threat, in-group identification, and political intolerance.[9] They characterize three kinds of perceived threat: to security, democracy, and to Jewish identity.

Maslow's theory of the hierarchy of needs views the devotion to a cause beyond the self (self-transcendence) as a motivational step beyond self-actualization.[10] Researchers suggested enlisting the notion of self-transcendence to understand religious violence and terrorism.[11] Cloninger *et al.*[12] see self-transcendence as encompassing a sense of self-actualization, fulfillment, and direction in one's life, but do not refer to political transcendence, the experience that life is meaningless without the vibrancy of political ideals. Considering political ideals as more important than life itself and adhering to extreme political ideologies may lead to

doi: 10.1111/j.1749-6632.2010.05693.x

morbid intentions involving the annihilation of self and others.

This study examines personal (e.g., gender, life events, Holocaust background, political activism) and psychological (self- and political transcendence, perceived political threats, ethos of conflict, in-group, and out-group sociopolitical identification) parameters predicting readiness to engage in destructive political behavior. We investigate: (1) the level of ideological zeal characterizing various political groups; (2) the relationship between extreme political ideology and perceived political threats and their association with personal risk and vulnerability; (3) empathy of political factions with the conflicting groups; and (4) predictors of extreme political activism.

We postulate that (a) compared to political centrists, extremists will show higher levels of self-transcendence, ideology devotion, perceived political threat, morbid transcendence, and exposure to stressful events; (b) the extreme political right will be more sensitive to threats to physical existence and national identity, whereas the political left will be more challenged by threats to moral integrity; (c) the extreme left will be more empathetic toward the Palestinians than toward the Jewish Israelis and the settlers, whereas the extreme right will be more empathetic toward the settlers than toward the Jewish Israelis and the Palestinians; and (d) ideological and morbid political zeal, as well as the balance of empathy toward the in-group and the out-group predict extreme political activism.

Recent research proposed a stress-based model of political exclusionism. This paper extends the implications of the model for political extremism in general, emphasizing ideological and psychological parameters.[13]

Method

Subjects

The data were collected during the 3-month period preceding Israel's disengagement from the Gaza Strip (August 2005). The questionnaires were completed by a convenience sample of 245 Israeli-Jewish participants (44% male, mean age = 26.8, SD = 7.4): 99 university students (40.4%, mean age = 23.7, SD = 2.8), 93 West Bank settlers (38%, mean age = 24.7, SD = 5.3), and 53 left-wing activists (21.6%, mean age = 29.4, SD = 6.02).

Participants were ascribed to a political group on the basis of (a) their reported vote in the 2003 election, and (b) their political attitude on a scale ranging from "definite right" (5) to "definite left" (1). Participants who voted for a right-wing extremist party (e.g., "National Union") and defined themselves as "right" or "definite right" were classified as "extreme right." Settlers living on the West Bank who identified their political stance as "definite right" were also included in the "extreme right" group even if they voted for nonextremist parties (e.g., Likud) ($n = 82$). Participants who voted for a left-wing extremist party (e.g., National Democratic Alliance) and identified their political stance as "left" or "definite left" were classified as "extreme left" ($n = 41$). Participants who voted for nonextremist parties (e.g., Labor, Likud) and identified their political stance as indeterminate right or left were labeled "center" ($n = 92$). Thirty participants could not be classified according to this algorithm and were not included in the analysis.

Compared to the center and the left-wing participants, the right-wing participants being mainly orthodox nationalists, are mostly married (17%, 12%, and 57%, respectively; $\chi^2 = 78.15$, $df = 6$, $P < 0.001$) and have more children (0.37 ± 0.87, 0.22 ± 0.76, and 1.38 ± 1.89, respectively; $F[2, 209] = 16.02$, $P < 0.001$), despite being slightly younger (27.11 ± 8.6, 29.21 ± 6.32, and 24.47 ± 5.46, respectively; $F[2, 211] = 6.67$, $P < 0.005$).

Instruments

The following questionnaires were administered individually

A *demographic questionnaire* collected information concerning gender, age, religious identity, voting, political identification, and affect of the Holocaust to the individual and the family.

Political activism: This scale, developed for this study, describes three levels of political activism: low (complete indifference and avoidance of any political activity); moderate (participating in political debates, donating money for political causes, publicly expressing political opinions); or high (organizing demonstrations and violating the law to express political opinions).

Self-transcendence was measured by the three self-transcendence factors of Cloninger *et al.*'s.[14] *Temperament and Character Inventory* (TCI): *self-forgetful versus self-conscious experience* (e.g., "I often become so fascinated with what I'm doing I get lost in the moment, as if I'm detached from time and place"); *transpersonal identification versus self-isolation* (e.g., "I sometimes feel so connected to nature that everything seems to be part of one living organism"); *spiritual acceptance versus rational materialism* (e.g., "I seem to have a 'sixth sense' that sometimes allows me to know what is going to happen").

Political transcendence was measured by a 17-item scale developed for this study with scores ranging from (1) not at all to (5) strongly. A principal components factor analysis (Varimax rotation) revealed two factors (eigenvalues > 1): (a) Ideological Transcendence consisted of 10 items (e.g., "I devote my life to fulfilling my views") and (b) morbid Transcendence consisted of seven items (e.g., "I am willing to die to preserve the right of my people to live in this land"). The internal reliability coefficients (Cronbach's α) were 0.80 and 0.73, respectively.

Ethos of conflict: The short version[15] of Zafran's[16] questionnaire based on the concept "ethos of conflict" consists of 16 items describing various aspects of the Israeli-Arab conflict. A total score reflects right-wing hawkish ideology (Cronbach's α = 0.92).

Risk: This scale consists of 10 items covering stressful life events during the past year (e.g., divorce, death in the family, birth of a child, car accident, exposure to terrorist attacks, hospitalization). A risk index, a significant predictor of posttraumatic stress, was computed as the sum of the items checked.[17]

Sociopolitical identification: Participants rated their identification with and empathy toward the suffering of Israeli settlers, Palestinians living on

the West Bank, and Israeli citizens who are not settlers. Three variables reflecting the sociopolitical fault lines were computed as the ratios of identification with (1) Israelis over Palestinian (I/P), (2) settlers over Palestinians (S/P), and (3) settlers over Israelis (S/I).

Perceived political threat: A 13-item scale was developed to assess perceived political threat. Participants reported to what extent each item worried them on a daily basis, on a scale ranging from (0) not at all to (3) all the time. Factor analysis (Varimax rotation) yielded three factors (eigenvalues > 1; 5, 4, and 3 items, respectively): (1) moral integrity (e.g., "A deliberate discrimination policy will be carried out against Israeli Arabs"); (2) national identity (e.g., "Some of Israel's land will be returned to the Palestinians"); and (3) physical existence (e.g., "The State of Israel will be destroyed physically"). Internal reliability coefficients were 0.74, 0.81, and 0.68, respectively.

Procedure

Following the Institutional Review Board approval, trained experimenters administered the questionnaires anonymously and explained the project explores political and ideological viewpoints. To ensure cooperation, a trained key group member distributed the questionnaires to settlers and left-wing activists.

Results

Table 1 shows a positive correlations between the TCI and the newly developed ideological and morbid transcendence scales ($r = 0.439$ and 0.233, both $P < 0.01$, respectively) and between morbid and ideological transcendence ($r = 0.415$, $P < 0.01$). The

Table 1. Pearson correlations between transcendence categories, perceived threats, and risk ($n = 285$)

	Morbid transcendence	Ideological transcendence	Self-forgetful	Transpersonal identification	Spiritual acceptance	Total self-transcendence
Morbid transcendence	1	0.415[**]	0.121[*]	0.393[*]	0.173[**]	0.273[**]
Ideological transcendence	0.415[**]	1	0.330[**]	0.437[**]	0.295[**]	0.439[**]
Physical existence threat	0.247[**]	0.274[**]	−0.015	0.125[*]	0.263[**]	0.199[**]
Moral integrity threat	0.238[**]	0.195[**]	0.101	0.156[*]	−0.122[*]	0.061
National identity threat	0.144[*]	0.091	0.013	0.120	0.156[*]	0.142[*]
Risk	0.169[*]	0.253[*]	0.119[*]	0.228[**]	0.180[**]	0.233[**]

[*] $P < 0.05$.
[**] $P < 0.01$.

three perceived threats correlated positively with most transcendence scales, except moral integrity, which correlated negatively with the TCI spiritual acceptance scale (r range $= -0.122–0.274$).

The sociopolitical identification ratios (S/P, I/P, and S/I) correlated negatively to the threat to moral integrity ($r = -0.21. -0.25, -0.13$, respectively, $P < 0.001$ except for the last) and positively to threat to national identity ($r = 0.36, 0.28, 0.26$, respectively, all $P < 0.001$) and to physical existence ($r = 0.29, 0.28, 0.28$, respectively, all $P < 0.001$).

Gender differences

Multivariate analysis of variance (ANOVA) showed no main effect for gender and no significant gender $\times$ political group interaction for the three threats, TCI, ideological transcendence, sociopolitical identification, political involvement, and Holocaust influence (all $P > 0.05$). Males reported higher morbid transcendence than females (mean $\pm$ SD $= 2.77 \pm 0.79$ and 2.23 ± 0.81, respectively) ($F[1, 185] = 11.04$, $P < 0.001$). There were no significant gender $\times$ political group interactions for political activism and morbid transcendence ($P > 0.05$).

Political group and self-transcendence

Table 2 summarizes the mean levels of total self-transcendence and its subscales by political group. One-way ANOVAs followed by Bonferroni *post hoc* tests revealed that subjects on the extreme politi-

cal left and center reported significantly lower levels of total self-transcendence compared to subjects on the extreme right ($F[2, 206] = 11.4$, $P < 0.01$). Furthermore, extreme right participants reported higher levels of Spiritual Acceptance ($F[2, 206] = 19.8$, $P < 0.01$) compared to extreme left and center participants, and higher levels of Transpersonal Identification compared to the center ($F[2, 206] = 4.28$, $P < 0.01$). No significant differences emerged for the self-forgetful subscale ($F[2, 206] = 1.55$, $P > 0.05$).

Political group, Holocaust background, ideological and morbid transcendence

One-way ANOVA followed by Bonferroni *post hoc* tests indicated that extreme right and extreme left participants reported higher morbid ($F[2,206] = 16.22$, $P < 0.01$) and ideological ($F[2,206] = 8.52$, $P < 0.01$) transcendence compared to participants on the center (Table 2).

The distribution of the political groups according to political activism (low/moderate/high) shows the highest activism among extreme left participants (0%, 12%, 88%, respectively), lower in the extreme right group (12%, 61%, 27%, respectively), and lowest in the center group (66%, 32%, 2%, respectively) ($\chi^2 = 147.2$, $df = 4$, $P < 0.001$).

Only among extreme left participants significant positive associations appeared between perceived

Table 2. Risk, transcendence subscales, and perceived threats by political group

	Extreme left		Center		Extreme right		
	M	SD	M	SD	M	SD	$F(2, 206)$
Risk	1.83	1.59	1.48[a]	1.39	2.27[a]	1.34	6.57[**]
Morbid transcendence	2.64[a]	0.66	2.13[ab]	0.77	2.87[b]	0.75	16.22[**]
Ideological transcendence	3.25[a]	0.65	2.87[ab]	0.76	3.40[b]	0.66	8.52[**]
Total self-transcendence	13.62[a]	6.89	14.97[b]	6.09	18.69[ab]	4.86	11.40[**]
Self-forgetful	5.17	2.48	5.52	2.59	5.54	2.35	1.55
Transpersonal identification	3.22	2.15	2.93[a]	2.25	4.10[a]	1.96	4.28[**]
Spiritual acceptance	4.80[ab]	3.47	6.53[ac]	2.97	9.14[bc]	2.45	19.87[**]
Moral integrity threat	9.80[ab]	3.25	5.47[a]	3.12	5.33[b]	3.64	27.84[**]
National identity threat	6.05[a]	2.94	5.61[b]	2.74	8.73[ab]	3.36	23.99[**]
Physical existence threat	1.88[ab]	1.11	2.49[a]	0.25	2.91[b]	0.33	18.18[**]
Ethos of conflict	1.55[ab]	0.24	2.83[ac]	0.58	3.82[bc]	0.38	248.6[***]

Groups with the same superscript letter are significantly different according to Bonferroni *post hoc* test ($P < 0.05$).
[**] $P < 0.01$.
[***] $P < 0.001$.

impact of the Holocaust on their life and morbid transcendence as well as between their perceived feelings of hurt by the Holocaust and their sociopolitical identification with Palestinians (both $r = 0.35$, $P < 0.05$). The proportion of individuals reporting their families were Holocaust survivors was greater among extreme left participants than among extreme right ones (66% and 42%, respectively, $\chi^2 = 21.59$, $df = 6$, $P < 0.001$). However, a greater proportion of extreme right participants reported feeling personally hurt by the Holocaust to a moderate or high degree compared to those on the extreme left (62% and 34%, respectively; $\chi^2 = 14.35$, $df = 6$, $P < 0.05$).

Political group, risk, ethos of conflict, and perceived threat

The three political groups differed significantly on the risk index ($F[2, 212] = 6.57$, $P < 0.005$). Bonferroni *post hoc* test revealed increased risk among extreme right participants compared to those at the political center.

The analysis of the three perceived threats according to political group showed that extreme left participants scored highest on the moral integrity threat ($F[2, 206] = 27.8$, $P < 0.001$) and lowest on the physical existence threat ($F[2, 207] = 18.2$, $P < 0.001$), whereas those on the extreme right scored highest on the national identity threat ($F[2, 206] = 24.0$, $P < 0.001$) (Table 2).

Extreme right participants reported the highest ethos of conflict score and those on the extreme left the lowest ($F[2, 206] = 248.6$, $P < 0.001$). Ethos of conflict was associated positively with threats to national identity and physical existence, and negatively with moral threat ($rs = 0.29, 0.44$, and -0.37, respectively, all $P < 0.001$). Also, ethos of conflict was positively associated with morbid but not with ideological transcendence ($r = 0.40$, $P < 0.001$ and $r = 0.0$, $P > 0.05$, respectively).

Sociopolitical identification

A one-way ANOVA showed that the three political groups differed in their sociopolitical identification with Israelis (extreme left < extreme right) ($F[2, 176] = 3.6$, $P < 0.05$), settlers (extreme left < center < extreme right) ($F[2, 177] = 97.2$, $P < 0.001$), and Palestinians (extreme left > center > extreme right) ($F[2, 177] = 118.9$, $P < 0.001$).

Extreme left participants identified more strongly with Palestinians than with Israelis ($t[33] = 2.28$,

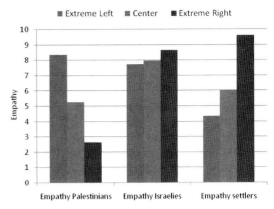

Figure 1. Empathy toward self and others by political group. (In color in *Annals* online.)

$P < 0.05$), and more strongly with Israelis than with settlers ($t[33] = 10.79$, $P < 0.001$). Extreme right participants identified significantly more strongly with settlers than with Israelis ($t[57] = 4.83$, $P < 0.001$) (Fig. 1).

Prediction of morbid transcendence and I/P and S/P ratios

According to stepwise multiple regression analyses, higher national identity and moral integrity threats, risk, and total self-transcendence contributed to the statistical explanation of morbid transcendence ($F[4, 182] = 9.86$, $P < 0.001$). Lower perceived threat to moral integrity, and higher perceived threat to both national identity and physical existence, as well as of total self-transcendence, predicted the I/P and the S/P ratios ($F[4, 159] = 15.51$, $P < 0.001$; and $F[4, 161] = 25.67$, $P < 0.001$, respectively).

Discussion

This study proposes a trauma-like model of sociopolitical destructive instability propagated by violent adherence to extreme ideologies within the context of the Israeli-Arab conflict in a period of ongoing polarization. Canetti-Nisim *et al.* recently attempted the same objective with a different methodology.[13] In their study, a telephone survey of a representative sample of Israeli Jews found that exclusionist attitudes toward Palestinian Israeli citizens were directly predicted by perceived threat from them, and indirectly by psychological distress associated with exposure to terrorist attacks. Our study included individuals in the center and extreme poles of the political spectrum and conceptualized specific threats for each pole. The fact that these two studies performed almost simultaneously reach similar conclusions strengthens the validity of the findings.

Our first hypothesis, that both extreme political poles display higher self-transcendence and political zeal compared to the center was supported almost completely. Both extreme poles displayed a high level of ideological and morbid transcendence. This result is in line with Van Hiel *et al.*, who found high levels of authoritarian aggression among activists of extremist left-wing parties in Belgium.[18] Contrary to our hypothesis, the extreme right was the highest on self-transcendence, whereas the extreme left did not differ significantly from the center. Extreme right participants also reported the highest risk. These findings can be explained by the low score of the left and the high score of the right extreme groups on the spiritual acceptance subscale of self-transcendence. The demographic characteristics of the extreme right group, which comprised mainly religious settlers, living on the Intifada-ridden West Bank, may explain their high score on spiritual acceptance.

The analyses also confirmed our second hypothesis that extreme groups differ in their perceived political threats. Extreme right participants scored higher than extreme left participants on perceived threats to physical existence and to national identity. The extreme left scored highest on perceived threat to moral integrity. Although the political center and the extreme left did not differ on perceived threat to national identity, the extreme left scored lowest on perceived threat to physical existence. This could be viewed in line with Shamir and Sagiv-Schifter who stated that the Zionist ideology may make it difficult for its adherents, in our case, particularly the extreme ones, to distinguish realistic threats from symbolic ones.[9]

The associations between ethos of conflict and the extreme groups' characteristic threats as well as with their level of morbid transcendence support Bar-Tal *et al.*'s[19] findings and may validate our political subgroups classification. Volkan labeled an entrenched collective painful memory as a "chosen trauma," or "a large-group's mental representation of a historic event that resulted in collective feelings of helplessness, victimization, shame, and humiliation at the hands of 'others'. . .." It becomes a significant element in the contemporary identity and is activated in the face of danger from the "other" "to enhance the group's identity and strengthen it to face the threat" (pp. 173–174).[20]

We propose that the "chosen trauma" of the extreme right may be diametrically opposed to that of the extreme left. The former counter-identifies with the historical experience as victim, revealing fears regarding existence and national identity. The latter counter-identifies with the victimizer, therefore expressing moral fears over becoming one. The fact that perceived threats to national identity and moral integrity together with cumulative risk and self-transcendence explained a significant proportion of morbid transcendence may support a "trauma-like" model of destructive political transcendence.

We also confirmed our third hypothesis that the extreme left identify more strongly with Palestinians than with Jewish Israelis and settlers, whereas the extreme right would identify more strongly with settlers than with Jewish Israelis and Palestinians. The tensions among the various sociopolitical identifications within each of the extreme groups may be formulated as constitutive of psychopolitical fault lines. The logic of historically chosen trauma is accompanied by vacillation between the poles of "identification with the aggressor or with the victim." Right-wing extremists seem to consider the aggressor's position, while left-wingers consider that of the victim. Beyond this regressive logic, one may claim that right-wing extremists are least empathic toward the "object-group" whereas left-wing extremists are least concerned about the threat to the physical safety of the "self-group." Interestingly, the level of morbid transcendence was predicted by the two perceived threats characterizing the extreme groups (i.e., national identity and moral integrity) against a background of stressful life events and self-transcendence. Hence, both extreme groups may be partially distorting reality, whether of "the self" or of "the object."

Indeed, within the extreme left group, perceived Holocaust influence was positively associated with their level identification with Palestinians, and feeling hurt by the Holocaust was positively correlated with morbid transcendence. These findings stand out in stark comparison to the extreme right group. Despite the greater proportion of extreme right families who reported to be Holocaust survivors, this family history had no association with morbid transcendence and empathy toward the other.

Furthermore, by partially disavowing considerations of self-safety, left-wing extremists can construct an idealized position, whose values may appear to belong within the Jewish history of moral self-sacrifice as well as within the universal community. By partially disavowing empathy toward the other, right-wing extremists can create an idealized position rooted in their commitment to values of existence and culture. Both extreme groups may use disavowal and idealization to avert the healing process over death-fear and of mourning over historical and current trauma. Destructive political action is conjured up in their place.

Finally, to our fourth hypothesis, that ideological and morbid political zeal as well as the ratio between in- and out-group sociopolitical identification predict extreme political activism. As with morbid transcendence, the I/P and S/P ratios were also significantly explained by low perceived threat to moral integrity, and high perceived threat to national identity and physical existence, as well as total self-transcendence. Perhaps the ratio between in- and out-group sociopolitical identification could serve as touchstone for dehumanization. If this is the case, our data support the notion that dehumanization inhibits guilt feelings and distress about the harm inflicted to the other and thus may operate as an important obstacle in creating support for reparation policies.[3]

We showed the important role played by perceived threats in determining sociopolitical attitudes and identification. Contrary to Altemeyer,[21] who found that conservatives perceive the world as more threatening than do liberals, we showed that both political extremes reported threat, though their type and content differed.

In conclusion, fault line wars may raise real and perceived threats to physical existence, group identity, and moral integrity. These, in turn, may reinforce conflicts in sociopolitical identification, which may find their expression in political ideology. A combination of psychosocial underpinnings may be at the root of violent political involvement. Within a political conflict situation that takes place against the backdrop of collective historical trauma, given personal risk, individuals with sensitivity to various types of threats may respond with high ideological transcendence. Ideology may serve an adaptive function but, at times, may get derailed and distort reality, transforming symbolic threats into con-

cretely perceived ones. These may invite immediacy and forcefulness. When fear conjures up skewed sociopolitical identifications, morbid transcendence may manifest in destructive political activity. Future research with larger representative samples could validate the model implied by our findings.

Limitations

This study has several limitations. First, the sample was not representative of the Jewish-Israeli population, but rather a convenience sample recruited to include individuals from the extreme left, extreme right, and center of the political spectrum. Because extremists are often involved in social protest and law infractions, their recruitment presented an objective difficulty reflected in their relatively smaller group size.

Second, several scales were developed for the study. Although the results provide initial validation, more meticulous attention should be given to their psychometric parameters.

Third, we did not measure participants' psychological distress and sociopolitical identification with Arab-Israeli citizens.

Fourth, we defined nine degrees of political involvement. Nevertheless, right-wing extremists living in unauthorized settlements may exhibit an extreme kind of political involvement akin to illegal activity.

Finally, we explored morbid attitudes and behavioral intentions rather than actual destructive behavior. The literature recognizes the partial relationship between behavioral intentions and actual behavior.[22]

Conflicts of interest

The authors declare no conflicts of interest.

References

1. Huntington, S.P. 1996. *The Clash of Civilizations and the Remaking of World Order*. Simon & Schuster. New York.
2. Bar-Tal, D. 1998. Societal beliefs in times of intractable conflict: the Israeli case. *Int. J. Confl. Manage* **9**: 22–50.
3. Bar-Tal, D. 2000. *Shared Beliefs in a Society: Social Psychological Analysis*. Sage. Thousand Oaks, CA.
4. Bar-Tal, D. 2007. *Living with the Conflict: Socio-Psychological Analysis of the Israeli-Jewish Society*. Carmel (Hebrew). Jerusalem.
5. Struch, N. & S.H. Schwartz. 1989. Intergroup aggression: its predictors and distinctness from in-group bias. *J. Pers. Soc. Psychol.* **56**: 364–373.

6. Marcus, G., J. Sullivan, E. Theiss-Morse & S. Wood. 1995. *With Malice Toward Some: How People Make Civil Liberties Judgments.* Cambridge University. New York.

7. Kahneman, D. & A. Tversky. 1979. Prospect theory: an analysis of decisions under risk. *Econometrica* **47:** 263–291.

8. Stephan, W.G. & C.W. Stephan. 2000. An integrated threat theory of prejudice. In *Reducing Prejudice and Discrimination.* S. Oskamp, Ed.: 23–46. Erlbaum. Mahwah, NJ.

9. Shamir, M. & T. Sagiv-Schifter. 2006. Conflict, identity, and tolerance: Israel in the Al-Aqsa Intifada. *Polit. Psychol.* **27:** 569–595.

10. Maslow, A.H. 1969. Toward a humanistic biology. *Am. Psychol.* **24:** 724–735.

11. Kfir, N. 2002. Understanding suicidal terror through humanistic and existential psychology. In *The Psychology of Terrorism: Public Understanding, Vol. 1.* C.E. Stout, Ed.: 143–157. Praeger Press. Westport, CT.

12. Cloninger, C.R., D.M. Svrakic & T.R. Przybeck. 1993. A psychobiological model of temperament and character. *Arch. Gen. Psychiat.* **50:** 975–990.

13. Canetti-Nisim, D., E. Halperin, K. Sharvit & S.E. Hobfoll. 2009. A new stress-based model of political extremism. *J. Confl. Resolut.* **53:** 363–389.

14. Cloninger, C.R., T.R. Przybeck, D.M. Svrakic & R.D. Wetzel. 1994. *The Temperament and Character Inventory (TCI). A Guide to its Development and Use.* Center for Psychobiology of Personality, Washington University. St. Louis, MO.

15. Wolff, V. 2004. The Relation Between the Escapism Phenomenon in Israel and the Extent of Adherence to the Conflict Ethos. Unpublished master's thesis, Tel-Aviv University (Hebrew).

16. Zafran, A. 2002. Measuring Israeli Ethos of Conflict: Antecedents and Outcomes. Unpublished master's thesis, Tel Aviv University (Hebrew).

17. Wolmer, L., N. Laor & Y. Yazgan. 2003. School reactivation programs after disaster: could teachers serve as clinical mediators? *Child. Adol. Psych. Clin. North Am.* **12:** 363–381.

18. Van Hiel, A., B. Duriez & M. Kossowska. 2006. The presence of left-win authoritarianism in Western Europe and its relationship with conservative ideology. *Polit. Psychol.* **27:** 769–793.

19. Bar-Tal, Y., D. Bar-Tal & E. Cohen-Hendeles. 2006. The influence of context and political identification on Israeli Jews' views of Palestinians. *Peace Conflict: J. Peace Psychol.* **12:** 229–250.

20. Volkan, V. 1997. *Blood Lines: From Ethnic Pride to Ethnic Terrorism.* Westview Press. Boulder, CO.

21. Altemeyer, B. 1998. The other "authoritarian personality." *Adv. Exp. Soc. Psychol.* **30:** 47–92.

22. Sheppard, B.H., J. Hartwick & P.R. Warshaw. 1988. The theory of reasoned action: a meta-analysis of past research with recommendations for modifications and future research. *J. Consum. Res.* **15:** 325–343.

Ann. N.Y. Acad. Sci. ISSN 0077-8923

From an unlicensed philosopher: reflections on brain, mind, society, culture—each other's environments with equal "ontologic standing"

Jonathan Shay

Newton, Massachusetts

Address for correspondence: Jonathan Shay, M.D., Ph.D., 31 Jefferson St. Newton, Massachusetts 02458.
jshayinma@comcast.net

Philosophic conclusions drawn from work with psychologically and morally injured combat veterans include that brain, mind, society, and culture "co-evolved." The four encompass the complete human phenomenon, but not all are reducible to the physical brain. None of the four are "ontologically prior" to the others, when viewed over the entire lifecycle. All four are what I call "each other's environments," with obligatory cross-boundary flows—each with each in both directions. Rigorous, but nonreductionist interdisciplinary research, in the vein of "evo-devo" in embryology, is called for in the study of the human phenomena. On the basis of these conclusions, I offer a few practical comments on clinical work with psychologically and morally injured combat veterans.

Keywords: veterans; interdisciplinary; philosophy; character; "moral injury;" thumos

I come before you as an unlicensed philosopher who aspires to understand the human being as a whole. This "flyover" may be a bit vertiginous, zooming in and out with my own personal lens, first taking in the whole, then focusing down to the mind, and finally within mind to character.

Dumb luck has been very kind to me. Twenty-two years ago I went to work for the Veterans Administration, intending to restart my laboratory research career in the neurosciences, and the veterans "kidnapped me." They redirected my life and I thank them for it. But as Louis Pasteur famously said, "Chance favors prepared minds" (*"Dans les champs de l'observation, le hazard ne favorise que les esprits préparés"*). Talcott Parsons, whose name is not widely heard any more, had prepared my mind, and his personal example had prepared me to venture into fields new to me. More dumb luck, I stumbled into saying some useful new things about Homer's *Iliad* and *Odyssey,* two navigation lights of our culture.

For the last 45 years, since my intensive 2-year contact with Talcott Parsons,[a] I have regarded these four human realizations—brain, mind, so-ciety, culture—as each other's obligatory environments, the principle subsystems of the "human critter," as Parsons did. None of these four have ontologic priority, being really, really, *really* real, with the others mere epiphenomena, Platonic shadows on the wall or shining bubbles on the "real" stream.

Often, we contribute knowledge because we have spotted a particularly rich experimental model or research site: *Escherichia coli,* the worm *Caenorhabditis elegans,* the fruit fly, and the isolated rabbit retina have been such in the life sciences, as the

---

[a] 1961–1963. Parsons laid out his own attempt at such a grand synthesis at the end of his life in "A Paradigm of the Human Condition," in *Action Theory and the Human Condition.*[1] This volume also contains a complete bibliography of Parsons's published writings. His ambition to see the human as a whole was quite evident a decade and a half earlier when he was my senior tutor. Some of what he wrote in this chapter rings as excessively impressed with ways of thinking that enjoyed great prestige during his lifetime; but that will justly be said of anyone, including myself.

doi: 10.1111/j.1749-6632.2010.05797.x

Burgess shale is in paleontology, pulsars in astronomy. My work with psychologically and morally injured combat veterans persuaded me that the ways a person's character is changed by bad experience is a particularly rich site to reveal the interactions between brain, mind, society, and culture.

I want to pay tribute to an all-too-rare quality that I experienced in Parsons: he was more interested in helping others become airborne than in recruiting disciples to fly behind him in formation. He *had* studied briefly with Karl Jaspers at Heidelberg in the 1920s. Encouraging the philosophic flights of his students rather than recruiting disciples was one of Jaspers's leading traits. Parsons never murmured a word or look of criticism when I blithely told him that I didn't like his terminology "action system" because it was far too kinetic, thus excluding sessile organisms, such as trees, which are no less action systems. Pretty brash for a young pup with the great man in Harvard's Emerson Hall. I preferred then, and still prefer, the more descriptive "conditionally autonomous systems."

Parsons is of course remembered as the leading sociologist of the middle third of the last century, not as a philosopher. But sociology had emerged as a discipline out of philosophy only a generation before him. His intellectual ambitions were never contained by disciplinary boundaries. I found his conceptual machinery congenial—very physiological and embryological in its workings; today, we might say it was very evo-devo.

Here is my summary of what has stayed with me over the years as a broadly applicable set of abstractions about the kind of system we ourselves are, and, in a fractal sort of way, it encompasses many subsystems that have the same (abstract) characteristics:

- bounded with respect to environment[s]—inside/outside always significant (Parsons's "pattern maintenance" functional requirement);
- obligatory exchanges across boundary with environments—what the system needs to get *from* the environments and eject *into* the environments (Parsons's "goal attainment" functional requirement);
- conflicting requirements are always possible, giving rise to the requirement to rank, com-

promise, or subsume conflicts (Parsons's integrative functional requirement); and
- variability in environments' capacities to provide and accept gives rise to internal generalized resources to buffer adverse environments (Parsons's adaptive functional requirement).

Systems can be extremely complex, possess many interactions among the parts, and manifest positive or negative feedback among the parts and still not be a conditionally autonomous system or action system. To be an action system, it must have an actively maintained and monitored boundary and have *obligatory* input/output requirements with its environment, *but be capable of temporary, conditional autonomy from environmental variation.* So by this definition, an entire watershed, or giant kelp bed may be an ecosystem with highly complex interactions within it [and indeed many action systems within it—the living organisms] and many feedback loops, but not itself be an action system. We are animals with absolute requirements to take in oxygen and to excrete CO_2, to take in and excrete water. The not-entirely-predictable-nor-controllable environment must be able to provide and to accept, but in the face of external variation or threat, we can hold our breath and our water for limited times. We are *conditionally* autonomous with respect to these inputs from the environment(s) and outputs to the environment(s). Parsons termed the simplest form of these a *single interchange*.

When inputs and outputs to varying environments persist over a long time, Parsons identified another broadly applicable abstract feature: that a second input–output pair arises, the functional significance of which is primarily *information* about the state of the environment with respect to the obligatory inputs/outputs. He termed the most highly developed of these *abstract media of exchange*, betraying the origins of this concept in his studies of economies in relation to other parts of social systems.

Parsons's view, from the orbit of Mars, so to speak, was that brain, mind, society, and culture were each other's environments, each having obligatory inputs from and outputs to every other, if they were to develop (epigenesis!—Parsons apparently read some Waddington on the prompting of psychoanalytic theorists) and maintain structure.

The human *is* a conditionally autonomous system, and, like other phenomena of life, is part of nature, evolved through natural selection. It emerged in its present form roughly 150k–50k years ago with our current brain, mind, society, and culture appearing simultaneously, having *co-evolved* during the hundred thousand years or so. Fuzziness about the timeline comes from the extreme poverty of the physical record. My assertion is this: When the fully modern human brain first appeared, mind, society, and culture were also fully formed—there has never been a neurologically intact adult *homo sapien* with a half a language, a third of a mind, or a quarter of a social system. During the prior million or so years, these four had co-evolved.

We are in the habit of seeing the material brain and the body carrying it as being really real, in the sense that mind, society, and culture are contingent on live humans to carry and enact them. In some sense, we have *made* them. But they have surely made *us*. After a worldwide neutron bomb annihilation of all human life, the well-preserved human artifacts would be incapable of regenerating living humans. Conceptually, this is not much different than a termite's nest being incapable of regenerating the living termites if all have been killed. The more interesting cases are the reverse: if all of the termites are spared, but their nest is completely obliterated, can the survivors regenerate the nest and raise up a new generation of termites? The answer is, of course, that it depends—upon the species, what stage of the reproductive cycle the colony is in, and so forth, when destroyed. If the nest destruction is persistent and comprehensive enough, the current generation can not reproduce another lifecycle. It may be cutely true that the nest is a gene's way of making another gene, but it is equally true that a gene is a nest's way of making another nest. Brain, mind, society, and culture mutually create each other during lifecycles. A fascinating thought-experiment runs this with humans: If all of the artifacts of human mind (memory wipe!), society, and culture (Biblical legends of Babel and of Lamech apply!) were destroyed, completely sparing the physical human bodies, vegetative, and brain function, what would these humans recreate?

So there's nothing at all biologically unusual about humans evolving in relation to the environments that they themselves have created.

I agree with Parsons's placement of culture in the "pattern-maintenance" role with its pervasive task of boundary definition, maintenance, and policing. *Language* is central to culture. We are accustomed to the idea that humans evolved a "language organ" that made its learning and production possible. As far back as Aristotle, this has been seen as a species marker. However, every neurologically intact human has the capacity to acquire any human language. We are all biologically wired to do this—so, why is there not a single universally intelligible Humanspeak?[b]

To broaden the speculation further, the normative codes of "what's right"—every society has them, even though the content of these codes varies as much as the grammars and vocabularies of languages vary—these codes have language-like properties, with one prominent difference: the moral intelligibility or unintelligibility of another person's acts are registered in the realm of the emotions. Moral intelligibility or unintelligibility evokes "strong evaluation," the realm of blame and praise. By contrast, imagine yourself by the radio in some cosmopolitan center—think Vienna—tuning from station to station in different languages that you don't know—they are all unintelligible, and you may have historical associations or esthetic preferences for the sound of one over another, but the reaction is probably not viscerally emotional, neither *nemesis* nor *kharis*. The capacity to acquire language and to inhabit the social and emotional code of "what's right" evolved together.[2–6] Together they mark and police the boundaries of the human action system.

The emergence of the human action system is properly and legitimately one of the "major transitions in evolution,"[7] which number less than a dozen. Some notable earlier ones reveal the biological justification for this all-too-human narcissistic claim: first, the enclosure of replicating molecules by a membrane, creating a boundary and imposing a common fate on the cell's different replicators (genes) both by enclosing them all and by linking them all in a single chromosome. Simple modern bacteria still have this character. Second, the enclosure of the replicators in a further membrane, the nuclear membrane and the possibly

---

[b]Here is a conjecture I invite you to chew on: that the mutual *unintelligibility* of different languages is itself an active process and an evolved product of natural selection related to the boundary function of culture.

simultaneous development of complex communities of mitochondria or chloroplasts within single cells—apparently starting as parasites, but became intracellular symbionts. How natural selection solved pattern maintenance in such a situation is a fascinating story, but that's for another time. Then, between 500 and 1,000 million years ago the emergence of metazoans—multicellular animals—established a boundary and imposed a common fate on the multitude of same and different cell types.

Jumping a few transitions to the human action system, culture encloses a society in a membrane of language and *nomos* (the *very* broad-gauged word beloved by the Athenian tragic poets, for which my English is "what's right") creating shared fates. Even the huge human action systems of the modern world have multiple environments, but in our ancestral setting in the last quarter million years the most important environment has been that of *other* human action systems. From Charles Darwin through Jane Goodall,[8] other humans and particularly other human groups are the single most important evolutionary forcing function—the most important "hostile force of nature" in our ancestral environment. I have argued elsewhere[9] that ancestral warfare in the Upper Paleolithic drove this explosive brain growth in the blink of an evolutionary eye. Evidence for evolutionary forcing can be seen in the over-stretched vascular anatomy of the human brain. The blood vessels of the human brain remind me of the water and sewer infrastructure of a Third World capital, with infrastructure built for a half-million population, but now bursting or shutting down, under the load of 10,000,000. Our extreme human susceptibility to strokes, is the product of this outrun infrastructure, particularly strokes arising from the arteries penetrating the basal ganglia from the arterial roundabout at the base of the brain, called the Circle of Willis, and from nearby runs of the main cerebral arteries.

At the beginning of this piece, I alluded to some of the insights that I believe I have glimpsed in the course of my work with psychologically and morally injured combat veterans.

Betrayal of "what's right" (as locally, culturally defined) by someone holding legitimate authority (squarely in the social system) in a high-stakes situation (in the mind of the person injured) is coded by the brain as physical attack, mobilizing the body for danger and for flight, preemption, or counter-attack. I have used the term "moral injury" for this whole constellation. When these three conditions are present, the body reacts massively in the same ways it reacts to physical threat, physical attack. You can see that the whole human critter—brain, mind, society, and culture—is caught up in this concept of "moral injury."

When things are good, rather than bad, the same are in play: good-enough fulfillment of "what's right" by legitimate power holders is an essential input to the mind to shape and maintain the stability of *thumos,* of character—the adult mind's pattern-maintenance subsystem. This is the sum-total of a person's ideals, ambitions, and attachments, plus an added term for the amount of motivational energy infusing them.[c] Character is shaped and reshaped throughout life, mainly by how power is used in social interaction. Character is energetic; it is dynamic and highly emotional. This is why I prefer to use the juicy Homeric word *thumos* interchangeably with character. In classical, democratic Athens, *thumos* meant "the energy of spirited honor,"[d] which gives some flavor to what I am trying to get at here.

---

[c]Forty-five years ago, "Action Theory and Ego Psychology: A Model of the Personality." Harvard College Senior Honors Thesis in Social Relations (#839), 1963. Parsons's theorizing about conditionally autonomous systems ("action systems") had a kind of fractal character, where the same four functional problems demanded solutions *within* subsystems. So if the unitary human critter was simultaneously brain, mind, society, culture, corresponding to his infamous formalism AGIL, each of these subsystems, in turn, faced the same functional requirements based on their nature as action systems. Parsons and his colleagues spent decades filling out this analysis for the social system. If anyone is curious, my four-function model of the mind ("personality" in those days)—much beholden to psychoanalytic ego psychology—fell out as follows: [L] narcissistic system (for which I now like the Homeric word *thumos,* because *narcissism* has been killed off as a neutral scientific term—and as much as it makes us squirm, character *is* a narcissistic structure); [I] system of ego identifications; [G] object system; [A] preconscious (cognitive, expressive, and linguistic) facilities. Currently, along with Francis Fukuyama and others, I am trying to put *thumos* back into circulation as a more neutral and nonpathologized word for the same body of phenomena and functions as *narcissism.*

[d]Professor Amelie Rorty, personal communication.

American psychiatry has hugged to itself a particular philosophical position on the invulnerability of adult character to traumatically bad experience. This position has a long and brilliant philosophic pedigree. Earliest known to us from Plato, it says: if you make it out of childhood with BOTH good breeding (today we would say, "good genes") AND good upbringing, your good character will set like stone, unbreakable by *any* bad experience. The pedigree runs through the Stoics, Kant, and Freud.

The current American diagnostic system does a pretty good job ("PTSD") of capturing the persistence of physiological and psychological adaptations to physical danger after the danger has passed, but has a blind spot with regard to moral injury and "social death." In particular, American psychiatry rejects the idea that bad experience of *any* kind can deform adult good character, explicitly rejecting the WHO diagnosis, "Persistent Personality Change after Catastrophic Experience," and rejecting diagnostic recognition for the predictable deformities of character, emotional dysregulation, and liquefaction of identity that occur in conditions of captivity and torture—whether official torture, or private torture, such as domestic battering, kidnapping, prostitution, incest, and other conditions of enslavement. The slave systems that exist in so many U.S. prisons—where the more brutal prisoners literally buy and sell the bodies of the weaker ones, in a Devil's Bargain with the under staffed guards—spews social and psychiatric toxicity into the society of a magnitude that we would never stand for, as if it were a factory or mine spewing neurotoxicity! American psychiatry has blinded, disabled, and disqualified itself, mainly, in my opinion, because of its embrace of Plato's brilliantly bad idea.[e]

There are several problems with this philosophic position, despite its pedigree. Mainly, it is factually wrong. If the conditions of moral injury are

[e]This was proposed to the American Psychiatric Association under the cumbersome tag, Disorders of Extreme Stress, Not Otherwise Specified, but is essentially the same as the better known formulation by Judith Herman, "complex PTSD." I invite the reader to compare the characteristics of the conditions of "coercive control"—pathogenic for complex PTSD—described by Herman with Orlando Patterson's classic description of the social processes of enslavement. I submit that these are identical. James Gilligan, *Violence*,[10] describes the prison slave systems.

bad enough, even the noblest character can be wrecked. For the molecular genetics reductionists, whose promissory notes about future brain science breakthroughs have flooded us chest-deep, there is no problem with Plato's formulation, only that the molecular genetic neuroscience is not quite here YET. A generation ago we nearly drowned in promissory notes from the early-childhood-experience reductionists. The molecular genetics reductionists will be no more able to redeem their promises of future conclusive, usable knowledge in this territory than the early-childhood-experience reductionists.

Finally, I want to bring damage to *thumos* from moral injury down out of the abstract clouds to the level of clinical practice: thumotic disturbances make patients difficult to deal with in a number of important ways:

- Oscillations between extremes of self-respect, from godlike grandiosity and godlike wrath to inert, almost lifeless collapse of self-care, aboulia, the state that was first medicalized by the Swiss, Johannes Hofer, in the 18th century, under the name *nostalgia*.
- Destruction of the capacity for "social trust." This means that morally injured veterans will not trust you on the basis of your credentials and institutional position. For many clinicians this is taken as a personal affront.
- When social trust is destroyed, it is replaced by an active expectancy of harm, humiliation, and exploitation.
- Together, these often win the patient a paranoid psychosis or personality diagnosis. Stay close to the phenomenology. We learn nothing additional about this human being by applying the word *paranoid*.
- Stable and trustworthy face-to-face community among psychologically injured combat veterans promotes recovery from these injuries. Credentialed mental health professionals should regard fostering and protecting this in the clinic as a key task.
- Stable and trustworthy face-to-face community among clinicians in the mental health workplace is both a critical success factor in working with such veterans, but is also the key to occupational health and safety for the clinicians.

- A small handful of pharmaceuticals provide palpable benefits to psychologically and morally injured veterans in conjunction with psychological and social treatments.

Once a clinician has gained equanimity in the face of vocal denials of trustworthiness, two enormous challenges remain: coping with one's own reactions to the atrocious trauma narratives, and the manifold tests of trust that morally injured trauma survivors invent. Nobody can safely do this clinical work alone, nor have to. The characteristics of the mental health workplace—in particular, the social practices of the clinical team—prove critical both to clinical success with these patients and to protecting the clinicians themselves from "secondary traumatic stress" injuries.[11–14,f]

Conflicts of interest

The author declares no conflicts of interest.

---

[f] Someone interested in seeing what I did with [did to?] Homer's *Iliad* and *Odyssey* and learning more about combat trauma can look at Shay.[12,13] For Athenian tragic theater and the relationship between the "pathogen load" of war trauma and that society's capacity for democratic process, see Shay.[14] For evolutionary speculations, see Ref. 9. For military writings and talks, such as *Secretary of the Navy's Guest Lecture* and the *Commandant of the Marine Corps Trust Study,* they are available electronically by email from the author at jshayinma@comcast.net.

References

1. Parsons, T. 1978. *Action Theory and the Human Condition.* Free Press. New York, NY.
2. Dunbar, R. 1996. *Grooming, Gossip, and the Evolution of Language.* Harvard University Press. Cambridge, MA.
3. Leakey, R. 1994. *The Origin of Humankind.* Basic Books. New York.
4. Sober, E. & D.S. Wilson. 1998. *Unto Others: The Evolution and Psychology of Unselfish Behavior.* Harvard University Press. Cambridge, MA.
5. Williams, G.C. 1966. *Adaptation and Natural Selection.* Princeton University Press. Princeton, NJ.
6. Wilson, D.S. 2002. *Darwin's Cathedral: Evolution, Religion, and the Nature of Society.* University of Chicago Press. Chicago, IL.
7. Maynard-Smith, J. & Eörs Szathmáry. 1998. *The Major Transitions in Evolution.* Oxford University Press. New York.
8. Goodall, J. 1986. *The Chimpanzees of Gombe: Patterns of Behavior.* Harvard University Press. Cambridge, MA.
9. Shay, J. 2000. Killing rage: physis or nomos—or both? In *War and Violence in Ancient Greece.* Hans van Wees, Ed.: 31–56. Duckworth and the Classical Press of Wales. London.
10. Gilligan, J. 1997. *Violence: Reflections on a National Epidemic.* Vintage Books. New York, NY.
11. Shay, J. & J. Munroe. 1999. Group and milieu therapy of veterans with complex PTSD. In *Posttraumatic Stress Disorder: A Comprehensive Text.* P.A. Saigh & J.D. Bremner, Eds.: 391–413. Allyn & Bacon. Boston, MA.
12. Shay, J. 1995. *Achilles in Vietnam: Combat Trauma and the Undoing of Character.* Atheneum. New York; and paperback, 1995. Simon & Schuster, Touchstone. New York.
13. Shay, J. 2002. *Odysseus in America: Combat Trauma and the Trials of Homecoming.* Scribner. New York.
14. Shay, J. 1995. The birth of tragedy—out of the needs of democracy. *Didaskalia: Ancient Theater Today* [Online journal] Vol. 2 No. 2. April, 1995. www:http://www.didaskalia.net/issues/vol2no2/shay.html (accessed September 22, 2010).

Ann. N.Y. Acad. Sci. ISSN 0077-8923

ANNALS OF THE NEW YORK ACADEMY OF SCIENCES

Issue: *Psychiatric and Neurologic Aspects of War*

Military traumatic brain injury: an examination of important differences[a]

Louis M. French

Defense and Veterans Brain Injury Center, Walter Reed Army Medical Center, Washington, DC. Department of Orthopaedics and Rehabilitation, Walter Reed Army Medical Center and National Naval Medical Center, Washington, DC. Department of Neurology, Uniformed Services University of the Health Sciences, Bethesda, Maryland

Address for correspondence: Louis M. French, Psy.D., Walter Reed Army Medical Center, Department of Orthopaedics and Rehabilitation, MATC Bldg. 2A, Room 203, 6900 Georgia Ave, NW, Washington DC 20307. louis.french@us.army.mil

Traumatic brain injury, especially mild traumatic brain injury, is a common consequence of modern warfare. In the current conflicts in Iraq and Afghanistan, much attention has been devoted to blast as a "new" mechanism of brain injury. While the evidence for primary blast effects upon the central nervous system is limited and controversial, there are a number of aspects of blast-induced brain injury that may be different. These include high rates of sensory impairment, pain issues, and polytrauma. In addition, the emotional context in which the injury occurred must also be considered in understanding the clinical presentation of these patients. Successful treatment of these individuals must use a multidisciplinary approach focused on the varied conditions that occur in those injured.

Keywords: military TBI; mild TBI; blast injury; war trauma

Introduction

Traumatic brain injury (TBI) is likely as old as warfare. In modern military medicine much of the focus has been on the effects of bullets and metallic fragments upon the brain. In World War I, for example, the English neurologist Sir Gordon Holmes detailed his observations on over 2,000 cases of head injury, including a detailed analysis of 23 cases involving penetrating injury to the visual cortex.[1] Much of that work was influenced by the work of the Japanese ophthalmologist Tatsuji Inouye who created the first relatively accurate map of the primary visual cortex; the map was based on his correlational observations of visual field defects following penetrating injuries to the occipital cortex during the Russo-Japanese war of 1904.[2] In later years, Teuber made significant contributions to our understanding of the effects of penetrating brain injury in warfare by studying those injured in World War II.[3] Alexander Luria, whose work contributed much to the beginnings of what is now known as neuropsychology, also studied injured soldiers during World War II.[4,5] His rehabilitation work centered on focal brain injury and how it affected cognition, language, and motor functioning. In addition, the work of Grafman *et al.*[6,7] and Carey *et al.*[8] during the Vietnam era helped increase our understanding of both the acute effects and the late neurobehavioral changes of brain injuries. These contributions have allowed for further developments in modern military medicine and provided a strong foundation for our investigations today.

TBI in Iraq and Afghanistan

In the current conflicts in Iraq and Afghanistan, the focus on severe and penetrating brain injuries has shifted; the attention is now being placed on closed TBI and those brain injuries at the milder end of the spectrum, especially mild TBI (mTBI) or concussion, as it is also known. TBI severity is based on such measures as the Glasgow Coma Scale,[9] duration of loss of consciousness or coma, and duration of posttraumatic amnesia (see

[a]The views expressed in this paper are those of the author and do not reflect the official policy of the Department of Army, Department of Defense, or U.S. Government.

doi: 10.1111/j.1749-6632.2010.05696.x

Ann. N.Y. Acad. Sci. 1208 (2010) 38–45 © 2010 Association for Research in Nervous and Mental Disease.

Table 1. U.S. DoD TBI classification system

Classification	Duration of unconsciousness	Alteration of consciousness (AOC)	Posttraumatic amnesia
Mild	<30 min	A moment up to 24 h	<24 h
Moderate	30 min–24 h	If AOC > 24 h then severity based on other criteria	1–7 days
Severe	>24 h		>7 days

Table 1). Current United States Department of Defense (DoD) ICD-9 derived diagnoses of TBI in the DoD Health Care System show that for 2009, penetrating brain injury accounted for just 1.4% of the total brain injuries, while severe closed brain injury accounted for less than 1% of the total. Of the of 27,862 TBIs counted in the year 2009, about 78% (21,859) were classified as mild (available at http://www.dvbic.org/TBI-Numbers.aspx) (see Fig. 1). These percentages are consistent in the period 2003–2009, where a total of 134,476 brain injuries were reported. It should be noted that these numbers are limited to those that presented to the military health care system. There are likely others, largely mTBI, who never sought medical treatment or came to the attention of health care providers. Data suggest that during deployment as many as 20% or more may have suffered a concussion. Those with TBI during deployment are more likely to report postinjury and postdeployment somatic and/or neuropsychiatric symptoms than those without such an injury history.[10]

In Operation Iraqi Freedom (OIF) and Operation Enduring Freedom (OEF), from October 2001 to January 2005, the Joint Theater Trauma Registry reported that of those with battle injuries, a total of 1,566 combatants sustained 6,609 combat wounds. The wounds were to the head (8%), eyes (6%), ears (3%), face (10%), neck (3%), thorax (6%), abdomen (11%), and extremities (54%). The proportion of head and neck wounds from 2001 to 2005 was higher than the proportion suffered in World War II, Korea, and Vietnam wars. Furthermore, while gunshot wounds accounted for 18% of the injuries from 2001 to 2005, those sustained from explosions accounted for 78% of the injuries, the highest proportion seen in any large-scale conflict.[11]

Blast injury—the "newest" mechanism of injury

As a result of OIF/OEF, injury due to blast has received significant attention,[12–15] leading one to believe that this is a "new" injury mechanism. However, the effects of explosions on the brain were described as early as 1916 in the medical literature.[16] Explosions were also a significant source of injury in World War I and World War II, accounting for 35–73% of the injuries, respectively.[11] The cluster of symptoms that became known as "shell shock" was originally thought to be related to blast exposure, although the idea was controversial even during World War I and in the years after.[17]

The results of the meta-analysis[18] published by the World Health Organization collaborating center task force on mTBI suggest that the vast majority of adults have good outcomes following uncomplicated mTBI, typically recovering in full within months. In terms of cognition, any decrements that are apparent in neuropsychological functioning after mTBI typically resolve in 1–3 months.[19] While this suggests that the majority of those sustaining mTBI, even under combat conditions, will have good recovery over the longer term, even transient symptoms may have military operational consequences. Slowed reaction time, headache, dizziness, or inattention may have implications for combat readiness or troop welfare. Even among military personnel that are not injured, there is recognition that combat operations may have cognitive consequences due to stress, sleep deprivation, or other factors.[20,21] Troop commanders are increasingly aware of these issues and have been supportive of the military's effort to screen for mTBI on the battlefield, including use of the Military Acute Concussion Evaluation (MACE)[22] and standardized DoD

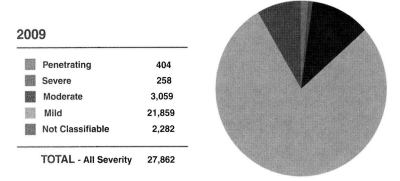

2009

Penetrating	404
Severe	258
Moderate	3,059
Mild	21,859
Not Classifiable	2,282
TOTAL - All Severity	27,862

Figure 1. ICD-9 derived diagnoses of TBI in the DoD health care system. (In color in *Annals* online.)

clinical practice guidelines around management of mTBI.

Outcome studies in mTBI have typically described civilian populations, but there may be differences in the military population or in mTBI acquired under combat conditions. Even in those without TBI, military deployment can result in increased emotional distress or overt psychiatric disorders.[23,24] In one military sample (prior to the current conflict), increased behavioral problems were shown in a group with TBI, as compared to their uninjured peers.[25] In that sample, the relative risk for behavioral discharge was 1.8 times greater for those with mTBI, and discharge for alcoholism or drug use was 2.6 times greater for mTBI. We have very limited knowledge about longer-term outcomes in those diagnosed with TBI in the current conflicts. However, one recent study[26] examining psychiatric outcomes of service members with TBI reported lower rates of posttraumatic stress disorder (PTSD) and mood/anxiety disorders among those with both mild and moderate-severe TBI, about 22–27 months following injury. Their study relied on provider diagnosis as opposed to self-report measures, however. This may partly explain the contradictory findings, as not everyone may seek out the help of a health care provider. In service members severely injured enough to require transport to a large military medical center in the United States, even mTBI has been noted to have important implications for the rehabilitation process.[27]

Blast, as a mechanism of injury for TBI, may play a role in symptom presentation and recovery of those injured. In the military injured, blast as a mechanism of injury has been used to guide treatment and structure treatment teams.[28] In one sample seen in the Department of Veterans Affairs (VA) polytrauma system, the pattern of injuries was different among those with injuries due to blasts versus other mechanisms. Injuries to the face (including eye, ear, oral, and maxillofacial), penetrating brain injuries, symptoms of posttraumatic stress, and auditory impairments were more common in blast-injured patients than in those with war injuries of other etiologies.[29] Another sample in the VA polytrauma system showed that service members injured by blast had a broader spectrum of physical injuries, higher levels of admission and discharge opioid analgesic use, reduced improvement in pain intensity following treatment, and much higher rates of PTSD and other psychiatric diagnoses than those injured in combat via motor vehicle collisions, falls, or other mechanisms.[30] This is also consistent with what has been observed in civilian victims of terror attacks, with those injured in blast having more body regions injured than those injured through other mechanisms, and being more severely injured overall.[31] In a sample at Walter Reed Army Medical Center (WRAMC), those with TBI related to blast were significantly more likely to have had a skull fracture, seizure, or lower limb amputation than those not injured in a blast. They also were more likely to have acute stress symptoms than those who suffered TBI through other mechanisms.[32]

Blast-related comorbidities

A polytrauma "triad" has been reported[33] with rates of chronic pain, PTSD, and persistent postconcussive symptoms (PPCS) present in 81.5%, 68.2%, and 66.8% of one sample, respectively. From this study, only 3.5% of the individuals seen were without chronic pain, PTSD, or PPCS, and 42.1% of the sample were diagnosed as having all three conditions concurrently. In the polytrauma population this introduces significant challenges for care and requires a multidisciplinary, integrated approach for success to be achieved.[34] The prevalence of polytrauma in the blast population may complicate the recovery for those who, under the best of circumstances, would otherwise have an uneventful recovery from their mTBI. Polytrauma patients, even without brain injury, have high rates of neurobehavioral symptoms including memory difficulties, irritability, mood swings, suspiciousness, amotivation, and guilt.[35] Some pain conditions, namely headache, also occur frequently in the TBI population.[36]

In a civilian population, minimal extracranial injuries and low pain have been shown to predict better outcomes for return to work after mTBI.[37] In one group who sustained mTBI and who also suffered extracranial injuries, 44% of the patients with additional injuries were still in treatment at 6 months after injury, compared to just 14% of the patients with isolated mTBI. They also had resumed work less frequently and reported more limitations in their physical functioning. Those that required continued rehabilitative treatments also reported significantly more severe postconcussive symptoms.

Individuals with traumatic limb amputations require extensive rehabilitation, and their recovery is influenced by a variety of medical, emotional, and social issues.[38,39] In a review of military service members injured in 2001–2006 (87% of these by explosive device), 5.2% of all serious injuries and 7.4% of major limb injuries underwent amputation. This rate is similar to that of previous conflicts (e.g., 8.3% in Vietnam).[40] Overall, amputation rates have markedly fallen with less than seven per month for 2009, contrasted to a high of 17 per month in 2007. Blast-induced limb loss with resulting loss of blood, as well as with high numbers of individuals that have sustained penetrating bodily injuries with at least some degree of hemorrhage, have raised concerns around some aspects of the trauma and its potential effects on outcome. Over 80% of the patients treated by one U.S. marine forward resuscitation surgical unit were in hemorrhagic shock.[41] With significant loss there is the possibility of hemorrhagic or hypoxemic posttraumatic insults on the central nervous system. It has been shown[42] that inadequate cerebral blood flow can contribute to

increased morbidity after TBI. It has been reported that hypotension is a significant risk factor for death following trauma, even in the absence of a TBI.[43] Following TBI, the brain appears to be especially vulnerable to posttraumatic hypoxemia.[42] However, the long-term effects of severe hemorrhage (with or without co-occurring TBI) on cognition, emotion, or other neurobehavioral symptoms are largely unknown.

Sensory difficulties are another concern. Despite excellent protective wear, service members still suffer injuries to the eyes and ears.[44,45] In a group of polytrauma patients injured by blast,[46] the rates of visual impairment were more than double compared to other causes of polytrauma. Overall, the rate of visual impairment in blast-related injury was 52% compared with 20% for all other sources of injury. In a group of patients with TBI and co-morbid combat ocular trauma at WRAMC,[47] explosive fragmentary munitions accounted for 79% of TBI-associated combat ocular trauma. Severe TBI was more frequently associated with combat ocular trauma than milder TBI. Overall, TBI occurred in two-thirds of all combat ocular trauma, and ocular trauma was a common finding in all TBI cases. In another sample of Iraq and Afghanistan veterans treated in a VA polytrauma center and injured by blast, 62% complained of hearing loss and 38% reported tinnitus. This compares to rates of 44% with hearing loss and 18% with tinnitus in those injured through some mechanism other than blast.[48] For those with impairments in both hearing and vision, the difficulties may be even more significant. Dual sensory impairment has been associated with increased rates of depression,[49] and lower overall health-related quality of life.[50] Lew et al.[51] describe a VA sample in which hearing impairment was identified in 19% of the sample, visual impairment in 34% of the sample, and dual sensory impairment in 32% of the sample. Surprisingly, only 15% of the patients were without sensory impairments in either the auditory or the visual modality. Those with dual sensory impairment had difficulties participating in the rehabilitation process, and showed an overall reduction in both total and motor functional independence measure scores at discharge.

Other difficulties that may hamper recovery following blast injury may include vestibular dysfunction/dizziness and blast effects on cognition. With regards to cognition, severity of injury is more predictive of neuropsychological functioning than is mechanism of injury; analysis of neuropsychological test measures suggest there are no differences in patterns of cognitive test performance in those that suffered TBI related to blast versus other mechanisms.[52] Many U.S. military service members who have been exposed to blasts and who are returning from Iraq and Afghanistan also complain of vertigo, gaze instability, motion intolerance, and other symptoms consistent with peripheral vestibular pathology.[53] It has been suggested that blast exposure can induce vestibular disorders, and related symptoms are significantly different than those seen in blunt head trauma, with the vestibular characteristics and objective tests of vestibular function significantly worsening in blast exposed patients as a function of time between injury and presentation.[54]

In the deployed combat environment, everyday experience involves exposure to potentially emotionally traumatic situations. A survey of U.S. combat infantry units following combat duty in Iraq or Afghanistan showed high rates of potentially traumatic combat experiences.[23] The rate of mental disorders after deployment to Iraq was 27.9%. The rates of PTSD were also significantly associated with having been wounded, with those respondents having a greater than threefold increase. In anyone hospitalized for physical injury there is increased risk of PTSD. One study[55] of injured trauma survivors across the United States showed that 22% of the injury survivors had symptoms consistent with the diagnosis of PTSD 12 months after hospitalization. High levels of postinjury emotional distress, as well as physical pain, were associated with an increased risk of PTSD symptoms. In one military survey, the rates of PTSD and depression among soldiers who were seriously injured and required medical evacuation and hospitalization at a tertiary military medical care center was about 4% for PTSD and/or depression at 1 month following injury. These rates increased to 12.2% for PTSD and 8.9% for depression at 4 months, and were roughly the same at 7 months. High levels of self-reported physical problems at the 1-month point were significantly predictive of PTSD and depression at 7 months.[56] The relationship between PTSD and physical injury has been previously reported in Israeli war veterans, with odds of developing PTSD following traumatic injury approximately eight times greater than following injury-free emotional trauma.[57]

The relationship between PTSD and mTBI is complex, and not fully understood. It has been suggested[58] that damage to the prefrontal cortex in TBI results in disruption of neural networks involved in the regulation of anxiety, making the affected individual more vulnerable to the effects of an emotionally traumatic event. In a recent military sample[59] of 76 service members with burn injuries, the incidence rate of PTSD was 32% and mTBI was 41%. Eighteen percent screened positive for both conditions. Hoge et al.[60] have reported increasing rates of PTSD and depression in a military sample as they experienced an increasingly "threatening" type of injury. The uninjured sample rates of PTSD were about 9%. In those that were injured in a place other than the head, the rates were slightly over 16%. For those with mTBI with alteration of consciousness, the rates were just over 27%. In those with mTBI with loss of consciousness, the rates were over 43%. In a Vietnam era military sample with both TBI and PTSD, mTBI (even in its chronic state) was associated with increased rates of headaches, sleep problems, and memory difficulties. More importantly, TBI has been shown to complicate or prolong recovery from preexisting or comorbid conditions, such as PTSD.[61]

The frequent co-occurrence of both conditions and potential interactive effects have treatment implications for those injured. Postconcussive symptoms may actually increase the likelihood of developing PTSD, because these symptoms interfere with adequate adjustment to the event.[62] In addition, cognitive or neurobehavioral impairments associated with TBI may influence the efficacy of treatments for PTSD or other mental health conditions. Psychotherapeutic or educational strategies may require intact cognition to work maximally. Even subtle attentional or memory difficulties might affect learning or other aspects of the treatment process. Unfortunately, few psychological treatments for anxiety or PTSD have been studied in people with TBI. There is some evidence for the effectiveness of cognitive behavioral therapy (CBT) for treatment of acute stress following mTBI, and for CBT combined with neurorehabilitation for generalized anxiety in those who sustained TBI of mild to moderate severity. One study[63] examined a comprehensive outpatient neuropsychological rehabilitation program that targeted psychological dysfunction, emotional distress, and accompanying functional disabilities. The results suggested that intensive outpatient treatment consisting of both CBT and cognitive remediation was beneficial for the treatment of persistent emotional distress following mTBI and may have had some effect on related cognitive difficulties. There are also few studies of pharmacological treatments of mood and anxiety in TBI patients,[64,65] and benefits of medication may be complicated by sensitivity to drug-induced side effects.[66]

Conclusions

TBI, especially mTBI, is a common consequence of modern warfare. Following TBI, regardless of injury mechanism, there are significant issues that may affect recovery and cause significant distress. These include somatic symptoms, such as headache, sleep disturbance, and dizziness; emotional difficulties, such as irritability and mood change; and cognitive difficulties, such as attentional dysfunction, memory problems, or difficulties in communication. Typically, the frequency and duration of such symptoms is related to injury severity. However, continued expression of symptoms may, in part, be linked to emotional factors.[60,67]

In the current conflicts in Iraq and Afghanistan much attention has been devoted to explosive blast as an injury mechanism, especially brain injury. While the evidence for primary blast effects (effects of the blast "wave" itself) upon the central nervous system is limited,[68] and an area of active investigation,[69] there are a number of aspects of blast-induced brain injury that may be different from more "typical" injury mechanisms, such as motor vehicle accidents or falls. These include high rates of sensory impairment, pain issues, and polytrauma. In addition, the emotional context in which the injury occurred must also be considered in understanding the clinical presentation of these patients. Successful treatment of these individuals must use a multidisciplinary approach focused on the varied conditions that occur in those injured. A thorough assessment of all comorbid conditions must be undertaken and addressed. For some individuals this can be accomplished in the primary care setting. For others, especially those suffering polytrauma, a specialized program involving neurology, psychiatry, behavioral health, occupational therapy, physical therapy, pain medicine, and other relevant disciplines should be considered for successful treatment.

Conflicts of interest

The author declares no conflicts of interest.

References

1. McDonald, I. 2007. Gordon Holmes Lecture: Gordon Holmes and the neurological heritage. *Brain* **130:** 288–298.
2. Lanska, D.J. 2009. Historical perspective: neurological advances from studies of war injuries and illnesses. *Ann. Neurol.* **66:** 444–459.
3. Semmes, J., S. Weinstein, L. Ghent, *et al.* 1954. Performance on complex tactual tasks after brain injury in man: analyses by locus of lesion. *Am. J. Psychol.* **67:** 220–240.
4. Luria, A.R. 1976. *The Working Brain: An Introduction to Neuropsychology*. Basic Books. New York.
5. Luria, A.R. 2004. *The Man with a Shattered World: The History of a Brain Wound*. Harvard Press. Boston.
6. Grafman, J., B.S. Jonas, A. Martin, *et al.* 1988. Intellectual function following penetrating head injury in Vietnam veterans. *Brain* **111:** 169–184.
7. Raymont, V., A. Greathouse, K. Reding, *et al.* 2008. Demographic, structural and genetic predictors of late cognitive decline after penetrating head injury. *Brain* **131:** 543–558.
8. Carey, M.E., W. Sacco & J. Merkler. 1982. An analysis of fatal and non-fatal head wounds incurred during combat in Vietnam by U.S. forces. *Acta Chir. Scand.* **508:** 351–356.
9. Teasdale, G. & B. Jennett. 1974. Assessment of coma and impaired consciousness. A practical scale. *Lancet* **2:** 81–84.
10. Terrio, H., L.A. Brenner, B.J. Ivins, *et al.* 2009. Traumatic brain injury screening: preliminary findings in a US Army Brigade Combat Team. *J. Head Trauma Rehabil.* **24:** 14–23.
11. Owens, B.D., J.F. Kragh, Jr., J. C. Wenke, *et al.* 2008. Combat wounds in operation iraqi freedom and operation enduring freedom. *J. Trauma* **64:** 295–299.
12. Martin, E.M., W.C. Lu, K. Helmick, *et al.* 2008. Traumatic brain injuries sustained in the Afghanistan and Iraq wars. *J. Trauma Nurs.* **15:** 94–99, quiz 100–101.
13. Ritenour, A.E. & T.W. Baskin. 2008. Primary blast injury: update on diagnosis and treatment. *Crit. Care Med.* **36:** S311–S317.
14. Wolf, S.J., V.S. Bebarta, C.J. Bonnett, *et al.* 2009. Blast injuries. *Lancet* **374:** 405–415.
15. Okie, S. 2005. Traumatic brain injury in the war zone. *N. Engl. J. Med.* **352:** 2043–2047.
16. Mott, F.W. 1916. The Lettsomian Lectures: on the effects of high explosives on the central nervous system. *Lancet* **187:** 545–553.
17. Jones, E., N.T. Fear & S. Wessely. 2007. Shell shock and mild traumatic brain injury: a historical review. *Am. J. Psychiatry* **164:** 1641–1645.
18. Carroll, L.J., J.D. Cassidy, P.M. Peloso, *et al.* 2004. Prognosis for mild traumatic brain injury: results of the WHO Collaborating Centre Task Force on mild traumatic brain injury. *J. Rehabil. Med.* **43:** S84–S105.

19. Schretlen, D.J. & A.M. Shapiro. 2003. A quantitative review of the effects of traumatic brain injury on cognitive functioning. *Int. Rev. Psychiatry* **15:** 341–349.

20. Lieberman, H.R., G.P. Bathalon, C.M. Falco, *et al.* 2005. Severe decrements in cognition function and mood induced by sleep loss, heat, dehydration, and undernutrition during simulated combat. *Biol. Psychiatry* **57:** 422–429.

21. Lieberman, H.R., G.P. Bathalon, C.M. Falco, *et al.* 2005. The fog of war: decrements in cognitive performance and mood associated with combat-like stress. *Aviat. Space Environ. Med.* **76:** C7–C14.

22. French, L.M., M. McCrea & M. Baggett. 2008. The Military Acute Concussion Evaluation (MACE). *J. Spec Oper. Med.* **8:** 77–83.

23. Hoge, C.W., C.A. Castro, S.C. Messer, *et al.* 2004. Combat duty in Iraq and Afghanistan, mental health problems, and barriers to care. *N. Engl. J. Med.* **351:** 13–22.

24. Polusny, M.A., C.R. Erbes, P.A. Arbisi, *et al.* 2009. Impact of prior Operation Enduring Freedom/Operation Iraqi Freedom combat duty on mental health in a predeployment cohort of National Guard soldiers. *Mil. Med.* **174:** 353–357.

25. Ommaya, A.K., A.M. Salazar, A.L. Dannenberg, *et al.* 1996. Outcome after traumatic brain injury in the U.S. military medical system. *J. Trauma* **41:** 972–975.

26. MacGregor, A.J., R.A. Shaffer, A.L. Dougherty, *et al.* 2010. Prevalence and psychological correlates of traumatic brain injury in Operation Iraqi Freedom. *J. Head Trauma Rehabil.* **25:** 1–8.

27. French, L.M. & G.W. Parkinson. 2008. Assessing and treating veterans with traumatic brain injury. *J. Clin. Psychol.* **64:** 1004–1013.

28. Scott, S.G., H.G. Belanger, R.D. Vanderploeg, *et al.* 2006. Mechanism-of-injury approach to evaluating patients with blast-related polytrauma. *J. Am. Osteopath. Assoc.* **106:** 265–270.

29. Sayer, N.A., C.E. Chiros, B. Sigford, *et al.* 2008. Characteristics and rehabilitation outcomes among patients with blast and other injuries sustained during the Global War on Terror. *Arch. Phys. Med. Rehabil.* **89:** 163–170.

30. Clark, M.E., R.L. Walker, R.J. Gironda, *et al.* 2009. Comparison of pain and emotional symptoms in soldiers with polytrauma: unique aspects of blast exposure. *Pain Med.* **10:** 447–455.

31. Peleg, K., L. Aharonson-Daniel, M. Michael, *et al.* 2003. Patterns of injury in hospitalized terrorist victims. *Am. J. Emerg. Med.* **21:** 258–262.

32. Warden, D. 2006. Military TBI during the Iraq and Afghanistan wars. *J. Head Trauma Rehabil.* **21:** 398–402.

33. Lew, H.L., J.D. Otis, C. Tun, *et al.* 2009. Prevalence of chronic pain, posttraumatic stress disorder, and persistent postconcussive symptoms in OIF/OEF veterans: polytrauma clinical triad. *J. Rehabil. Res. Dev.* **46:** 697–702.

34. Gironda, R.J., M.E. Clark, R.L. Ruff, *et al.* 2009. Traumatic brain injury, polytrauma, and pain: challenges and treatment strategies for the polytrauma rehabilitation. *Rehabil. Psychol.* **54:** 247–258.

35. Frenisy, M.-C., H. Benony, K. Chahraoui, *et al.* 2006. Brain injured patients versus multiple trauma patients: some neurobehavioral and psychopathological aspects. *J. Trauma* **60:** 1018–1026.

36. Packard, R.C. 2008. Chronic post-traumatic headache: associations with mild traumatic brain injury, concussion, and post-concussive disorder. *Curr. Pain Headache Rep.* **12:** 67–73.

37. Stulemeijer, M., S.P. Van Der Werf, B. Jacobs, *et al.* 2006. Impact of additional extracranial injuries on outcome after mild traumatic brain injury. *J. Neurotrauma* **23:** 1561–1569.

38. Pasquina, P.F., J.W. Tsao, D.M. Collins, *et al.* 2008. Quality of medical care provided to service members with combat-related limb amputations: report of patient satisfaction. *J. Rehabil. Res. Dev.* **45:** 953–960.

39. Messinger, S.D. 2009. Incorporating the prosthetic: traumatic, limb-loss, rehabilitation and refigured military bodies. *Disabil. Rehabil.* **31:** 2130–2134.

40. Stansbury, L.G., S.J. Lalliss, J.G. Branstetter, *et al.* 2008. Amputations in U.S. military personnel in the current conflicts in Afghanistan and Iraq. *J. Orthop. Trauma* **22:** 43–46.

41. Chambers, L.W., P. Rhee, B.C. Baker, *et al.* 2005. Initial experience of US Marine Corps forward resuscitative surgical system during Operation Iraqi Freedom. *Arch. Surg.* **140:** 26–32.

42. DeWitt, D.S. & D.S. Prough. 2009. Blast-induced brain injury and posttraumatic hypotension and hypoxemia. *J. Neurotrauma* **26:** 877–887.

43. Shafi, S. & L. Gentilello. 2005. Hypotension does not increase mortality in brain-injured patients more than it does in non-brain-injured patients. *J. Trauma* **59:** 830–835.

44. Helfer, T.M., M. Canham-Chervak, S. Canada, *et al.* 2010. Epidemiology of hearing impairment and noise-induced hearing injury among U.S. military personnel, 2003–2005. *Am. J. Prev. Med.* **38:** S71–S77.

45. Hilber, D., T.A. Mitchener, J. Stout, *et al.* 2009. Eye injury surveillance in the U.S. Department of Defense, 1996–2005. *Am. J. Prev. Med.* **38:** S78–S85.

46. Goodrich, G.L., J. Kirby, G. Cockerham, *et al.* 2007. Visual function in patients of a polytrauma rehabilitation center: a descriptive study. *J. Rehabil. Res. Dev.* **44:** 929–936.

47. Weichel, E.D., M.H. Colyer, C. Bautista, *et al.* 2009. Traumatic brain injury associated with combat ocular trauma. *J. Head Trauma Rehabil.* **24:** 41–50.

48. Lew, H.L., J.F. Jerger, S.B. Guillory, *et al.* 2007. Auditory dysfunction in traumatic brain injury. *J. Rehabil. Res. Dev.* **44:** 921–928.

49. Capella-McDonnall, M.E. 2005. The effects of single and dual sensory loss on symptoms of depression in the elderly. *Int. J. Geriatr. Psychiatry* **20:** 855–861.

50. Chia, E.M., P. Mitchell, E. Rochtchina, *et al.* 2006. Association between vision and hearing impairments and their combined effects on quality of life. *Arch. Ophthalmol.* **124:** 1465–1470.

51. Lew, H.L., D.W. Garvert, T.K. Pogoda, *et al.* 2009. Auditory and visual impairments in patients with blast-related traumatic brain injury: effect of dual sensory impairment on functional independence measure. *J. Rehabil. Res. Dev.* **46:** 819–826.

52. Belanger, H.G., T. Kretzmer, R. Yoash-Gantz, *et al.* 2009. Cognitive sequelae of blast-related versus other mechanisms of brain trauma. *J. Int. Neuropsychol. Soc.* **15:** 1–8.

53. Scherer, M.R. & M.C. Schubert. 2009. Traumatic brain injury and vestibular pathology as a comorbidity after blast exposure. *Phys. Ther.* **89:** 980–992.

54. Hoffer, M.E., C. Balaban, K. Gottshall, *et al.* 2010. Blast exposure: vestibular consequences and associated characteristics. *Otol. Neurotol* **31:** 232–236.

55. Zatzick, D.F., F.P. Rivara, A.B. Nathens, *et al.* 2007. A nationwide US study of post-traumatic stress after hospitalization for physical injury. *Psychol. Med.* **37:** 1469–1480.

56. Grieger, T.A., S.J. Cozza, R.J. Ursano, *et al.* 2006. Posttraumatic stress disorder and depression in battle-injured soldiers. *Am. J. Psychiatry* **163:** 1777–1783, quiz 860.

57. Koren, D., D. Norman, A. Cohen, *et al.* 2005. Increased PTSD risk with combat-related injury: a matched comparison study of injured and uninjured soldiers experiencing the same combat events. *Am. J. Psychiatry* **162:** 276–282.

58. Kennedy, J.E., M.S. Jaffee, G.A. Leskin, *et al.* 2007. Posttraumatic stress disorder and posttraumatic stress disorder-like symptoms and mild traumatic brain injury. *J. Rehabil. Res. Dev.* **44:** 895–920.

59. Gaylord, K.M., D.B. Cooper, J.M. Mercado, *et al.* 2008. Incidence of posttraumatic stress disorder and mild traumatic brain injury in burned service members: preliminary report. *J. Trauma* **64:** S200–S206.

60. Hoge, C.W., D. McGurk, J.L. Thomas, *et al.* 2008. Mild traumatic brain injury in U.S. soldiers returning from Iraq. *N. Engl. J. Med.* **358:** 453–463.

61. Vanderploeg, R.D., H.B. Belanger & G. Curtiss. 2009. Mild traumatic brain injury and posttraumatic stress disorder and their associations with health symptoms. *Arch. Phys. Med. Rehabil.* **90:** 1084–1093.

62. Meares, S., E.A. Shores, A.J. Taylor, *et al.* 2008. Mild traumatic brain injury does not predict acute postconcussion syndrome. *J. Neurol. Neurosurg. Psychiatry* **79:** 300–306.

63. Tiersky, L.A., V. Anselmi, M.V. Johnston, *et al.* 2005. A trial of neuropsychologic rehabilitation in mild-spectrum traumatic brain injury. *Arch. Phys. Med. Rehabil.* **86:** 1565–1574.

64. Warden, D.L., B. Gordon, T.W. McAllister, *et al.* 2006. Guidelines for the pharmacologic treatment of neurobehavioral sequelae of traumatic brain injury. *J. Neurotrauma* **23:** 1468–1501.

65. Lee, H.B., C.G. Lyketsos & V. Rao. 2003. Pharmacological management of the psychiatric aspects of traumatic brain injury. *Int. Rev. Psychiatry* **15:** 359–370.

66. Warden, D.L. & L.A. Labbate. 2005. Posttraumatic stress disorder and other anxiety disorders. In *Textbook of Traumatic Brain Injury*. J.M. Silver, T.W. McAllister & S.C. Yudofsky, Eds.: 231–243. American Psychiatric Publishing, Inc. Arlington.

67. Belanger, H.G., T. Kretzmer, R.D. Vanderploeg, *et al.* 2009. Symptom complaints following combat-related traumatic brain injury: relationship to traumatic brain injury severity and posttraumatic stress disorder. *J. Int. Neuropsychol. Soc.* **16:** 194–199.

68. Warden, D.L., L.M. French, L. Shupenko, *et al.* 2009. Case report of a soldier with primary blast brain injury. *Neuroimage* **47:** T152–T153.

69. Champion, H.R., J.B. Holcomb & L.A. Young. 2009. Injuries from explosions: physics, biophysics, pathology, and required research focus. *J. Trauma* **66:** 1468–1477.

Ann. N.Y. Acad. Sci. ISSN 0077-8923

ANNALS OF THE NEW YORK ACADEMY OF SCIENCES
Issue: *Psychiatric and Neurologic Aspects of War*

Effects of psychological and biomechanical trauma on brain and behavior

Thomas W. McAllister[1] and Murray B. Stein[2]

[1]Department of Psychiatry, Section of Neuropsychiatry, Dartmouth Medical School, Lebanon, New Hampshire. [2]Departments of Psychiatry, and Family and Preventive Medicine, University of California San Diego, La Jolla, California, and VA San Diego Healthcare System, San Diego, California

Address for correspondence: Thomas W. McAllister, M.D., Millennium Professor and Vice Chairman for Neuroscience Research, Director of Neuropsychiatry, Department of Psychiatry, Dartmouth Medical School, One Medical Center Drive, Lebanon, New Hampshire 03756. thomas.w.mcallister@dartmouth.edu

The current conflicts in Iraq and Afghanistan have resulted in a large cohort of military personnel exposed to combat-related psychological trauma as well as biomechanical trauma, including proximity to blast events. Historically, the long-term effects of both types of trauma have been viewed as having different neural substrates, with some controversy over the proper attribution of such symptoms evident after each of the major conflicts of the last century. Recently, great effort has been directed toward distinguishing which neuropsychiatric sequelae are due to which type of trauma. Of interest, however, is that the chronic effects of exposure to either process are associated with a significant overlap in clinical symptoms. Furthermore, similar brain regions are vulnerable to the effects of either psychological or biomechanical trauma, raising the possibility that shared mechanisms may underlie the clinically observed overlap in symptom profile. This paper reviews the literature on the neural substrate of biomechanical and psychological injury and discusses the implications for evaluation and treatment of the neuropsychiatric sequelae of these processes.

Keywords: traumatic brain injury (TBI); posttraumatic stress disorder (PTSD); psychological trauma; biomechanical trauma; behavior

Introduction

Traumatic brain injury (TBI) has received much attention as a frequent cause of injury and disability in the current conflicts in Iraq and Afghanistan.[1] Questions have been raised about whether the most common mechanism of TBI in these conflicts, blast concussive injury, results in different neuropsychiatric sequelae than those associated with more conventional contact or inertial forces.[2,3] Some investigators have suggested that the neuropsychiatric sequelae reported in military personnel returning from combat are better explained as the effects of exposure to psychological trauma with resultant depression or stress-related disorders (e.g., posttraumatic stress disorder [PTSD]).[4,5] The Department of Defense has underwritten an aggressive research program to address these questions, and much em-

phasis has been placed on the need to distinguish the effects of biomechanical and psychological trauma.

Investigators and clinicians new to this field might think that the neuropsychiatric effects of both biomechanical and psychological trauma have only recently been appreciated, but this is not the case.[6–8] In fact, debate about the relative roles of biomechanical and psychological trauma in symptom genesis have been taking place for well over 100 years.[6,9] Within a military context, these discussions first arose with the emergence of "shell shock" in World War I, a term supplanted by "postconcussional syndrome" (or some variation of that phrase) in World War II (see Jones *et al.*[6] for discussion). In each instance inordinate attention was placed on parsing out the neurologic/"organic" (biomechanical) contributions from the psychological/"psychoneurotic" contributions, with a reluctance to embrace the

doi: 10.1111/j.1749-6632.2010.05720.x

possibility that both forms of trauma might operate through overlapping and/or complementary mechanisms.

Older descriptions of military personnel with combat-related distress ring quite true with current clinical experience. For example, Cramer,[7] in describing the clinical picture of what he termed "cerebral blast concussion," wrote in 1949,

> . . . one or more nearby explosions, causing no overt or external harm to the skull, nevertheless render the subject unconscious. After this, he has a retrograde amnesia for all but the flash of the explosion, and thereafter anterograde amnesia for a variable period. During this time he may have great motor unrest and normal or exaggerated responses to stimuli. On regaining consciousness, he has intense and intractable headache, which later gives way to a milder, but constant, headache; tinnitus; intolerance of noises; tremors, and 'nervousness'. . . 'Anxiety' is manifest, and 'depression' and 'regression' are often employed to describe the dejection and muteness that characterize the behavior of the victim. Neurologic examination is, for the most part, 'negative' . . . the most frequent [symptoms are] the inability to tolerate loud noises or sudden movements; these stimuli sometimes precipitated strong startle responses . . . either spontaneous or in response to stimuli, such as the explosion of a shell or the passage of aircraft (p. 6).

Once again, there was great debate about the relative contributions of psychogenesis and physiogenesis. Lishman, in his study of World War II veterans with brain injury, posited that the initial insult had its basis in neural injury but psychological factors subsequently assumed greater importance in maintaining persistent symptoms, particularly after mild TBI (MTBI).[10–12]

Before the Diagnostic and Statistical Manual of Mental Disorders (3rd Edition) (DSM III) adopted the diagnostic category of PTSD, a variety of terms were used to describe behavior attributed to combat-related stress, including acute and chronic combat stress reaction, shell shock, and combat fatigue.[13] Thus, the interaction of psychological and biological trauma, particularly in a combat or military context, has a rich history that can inform our deliberations today. As a starting point for these considerations, this paper provides an update on

what is known about the neuropsychiatric sequelae of biomechanical and psychological trauma, as well as the effects of exposure to both. Clinical implications are also outlined.

Biomechanical aspects of brain injury

There are two broad categories of forces that result in brain injury: (1) contact or impact and (2) inertial acceleration or deceleration. Contact injuries result from the brain coming into contact with an object, which might include the skull or some external object.[14] The configuration of the external surface of the brain, how it is situated in the skull, and the uneven topography of the inner surface of certain skull regions are factors that result in heightened vulnerability to impact forces for certain brain regions.[15] Frequent sites of such injury are the anterior temporal poles, the lateral and inferior temporal cortices, the frontal poles, and the orbital frontal cortices.

Inertial injury results from rapid acceleration or deceleration of the brain with resultant shear, tensile, and compression forces. These forces have maximum impact on axons and blood vessels, resulting in axonal injury, tissue tears, and intracerebral hematomas. These mechanisms also produce more widespread or diffuse injury to white matter (known as diffuse axonal injury [DAI] or diffuse traumatic injury). Certain regions have a heightened vulnerability to this injury including the corpus callosum, the rostral brainstem, and the subfrontal white matter.[14] In addition, tissue-tear hemorrhages can occur. These are often small, ranging in size from miniscule petechiae to 1-cm lesions. They are characteristically located in the parasagittal portion of the brain, are associated with DAI, and are caused by acceleration-induced brain damage.[14]

Mechanical distortion of neurons at the time of injury is also associated with release of assorted neurotransmitters and subsequent triggering of complex excitotoxic injury cascades.[16] Although this probably occurs throughout the brain, the excitotoxic cascades and other forms of secondary injury, such as hypoxia and ischemia, have a disproportionate effect on certain brain regions, such as the hippocampus, even in the context of an otherwise fairly mild injury.[17]

The emergence of explosive devices, particularly "improvized explosive devices," as a primary method of attack in the conflicts in Iraq,

Afghanistan, and elsewhere, has called attention to "blast injury." Explosions generate a rapidly moving wave of over-heated expanding gases that compress surrounding air. The ongoing expansion of the heated gases eventually results in a drop in pressure with resulting reversal of the pressure wave. These fluctuations in pressure are associated with strain and shear forces (barotrauma) that can be particularly damaging to air and fluid-filled organs and cavities.[18] For example, the tympanic membrane can be ruptured with approximately a 30% increase in atmospheric pressure and is a useful, though not always, reliable indicator of blast exposure.[19] Blast can also be associated with significant brain injury.[20–24] At this time it is not clear if injury associated with blast is due to the high-pressure wave with distortion of vascular tissue, neural tissue or both, the inertial effects of buffeting by the alternating high- and low-pressure events, or some other mechanism. Additional mechanisms often come into play, including impact mechanisms from the head coming into contact with an object or penetrating injuries from fragments and debris (referred to as secondary blast injury), and rapid acceleration or deceleration of the brain causing inertial injury (tertiary injury), and exposure to toxic gas or chemicals as a result of the explosion (quaternary injury) debris.[19]

Animal models suggest that primary blast injury can be associated with neural injury, although the underlying mechanism is not clear.[25] For example, Cernak et al.[20,23] exposed rats to either whole body blast or localized pulmonary blast in which the brain was protected from the pressure wave with a steel plate. Both groups of animals showed hippocampal injury with neuronal swelling, cytoplasmic vacuolization, and loss of myelin integrity. These changes were associated with poorer performance on an active avoidance response task learned prior to the injury. This group has postulated that one potential mechanism is transmission of the pressure wave through cerebral vasculature, with subsequent injury to perivascular neural tissue, axonal stretching, release of neurotransmitters, and precipitation of the usual excitotoxic cascades,[20,23,26] although this is not yet firmly established.

Thus, the typical profile of injury involves a combination of focal and diffuse injury. There are certain brain regions that are particularly vulnerable to injury, including the frontal cortex and sub-frontal white matter; the deeper midline structures including the basal ganglia, the rostral brainstem; and the temporal lobes including the hippocampi. Certain neurotransmitter systems, particularly the catecholaminergic[27] and cholinergic systems,[28] are altered in TBI. Both of these systems play critical roles in a variety of domains important in behavioral homeostasis including arousal, cognition, reward behavior, and mood regulation. This profile of structural injury and neurochemical dysregulation plays a direct role in the common neurobehavioral sequelae associated with TBI including problems in cognition, emotional and behavioral regulation, and increased rates of psychiatric disorders.

The majority of brain injuries from the current conflicts fall into the mild category.[1,5] Thus, it is worth considering the evidence for neural injury associated with MTBI.

Animal models of brain injury using a variety of models across several species (fluid percussion, controlled cortical impact, combination models)[29,30] suggest that the neuropathology of brain injury occurs across a spectrum and injuries at the mild end of this spectrum are similar qualitatively to more severe injuries with axonal injury to subcortical white matter, hippocampus, thalamus, and cerebellum (e.g., Park et al.[31]). Axonal damage may range from stretching with associated poration that, if not severe, can seal over, to axotomy (see Farkas and Povlishock[32] for review) either at the time of injury if strain forces are sufficient, or that evolves over hours to days related to changes in the permeability of the axonal membrane and disruption of elements of the cytoskeleton, particularly axonal neurofilaments.

Assessing for neuropathological changes after MTBI in humans is limited to convenience samples of individuals who sustained an MTBI, died shortly thereafter of other causes and came to autopsy; however these studies also suggest that MTBI can be associated with neural damage.[33–35] For example, Blumbergs et al.,[34] using immunostaining for amyloid precursor protein as a marker for axonal injury, reported multifocal axonal injury in five individuals who had sustained very mild injuries with periods of unconsciousness as brief as 1 min. Bigler[33] described subtle neurocognitive and neuropathological abnormalities in a 47-year-old man who died 7 months after an MTBI of unrelated causes. In addition to the microscopic structural changes described above, both animal models and human studies suggest that MTBI can result in at least temporary alteration of the normal balance between cellular energy demand and energy supply (see Marcoux et al.[36]). Both animal and human studies have shown an increase in glucose utilization shortly after MTBI associated with a reduction in cerebral blood flow.[37–42]

The limitations inherent in obtaining human brain tissue after MTBI have driven interest in other avenues to detect neural injury, such as neuroimaging (see Levine et al.[43] and Belanger[44] for reviews). Although computed axial tomography scanning is most often used clinically, magnetic resonance imaging (MRI)-based methods are more sensitive in detecting the DAI and small hemorrhages that are generally believed to be the neuropathology associated with MTBI,[44,45] particularly using more recent image acquisition techniques, such as susceptibility-weighted imaging,[45] magnetoencephalography, and diffusion tensor imaging (DTI) (e.g., Refs. 46–48). It should be noted, however, that some recent studies using techniques, such as DTI, have failed to find evidence of white matter injury in patients with mild-to-moderate blast-related TBI,[49] underscoring the need for more research in this area. Functional imaging techniques, including single photon emission computed tomography, positron emission tomography, and functional MRI (fMRI), as well as magnetic resonance spectroscopy, also show some promise in clarifying the underlying pathophysiology of the sequelae of MTBI (see Refs. 50–53). It remains to be determined from future longitudinal imaging studies the extent to which detected abnormalities (if any) track with objective dysfunction and subjective complaints.

Psychological trauma and PTSD

PTSD prevalence has been estimated as approximately 17% among veterans of the current war in Iraq,[54] many of whom have also had a possible MTBI. Investigations into the pathophysiology of PTSD has focused on excessive activation of the amygdala by stimuli perceived to be threatening, and altered response to acute and chronic stress (see Refs. 55–57 for reviews). Amygdala activation produces outputs to a number of brain areas that mediate memory consolidation of emotional events and spatial learning (hippocampus), memory of emotional events and choice behaviors (orbital frontal cortex),

autonomic and fear reactions (locus coeruleus, thalamus, and hypothalamus), and instrumental approach or avoidance behavior (dorsal and ventral striatum).[58]

In PTSD, it is postulated that normal checks and balances on amygdala activation have been impaired so that the restraining influence of the medial prefrontal cortex (especially the anterior cingulate gyrus and orbitofrontal cortex) is disrupted.[59,60] Altered functional connectivity of the amygdala with other brain regions (e.g., Simmons et al.[61]) and resultant disinhibition of the amygdala may contribute to a vicious spiral of recurrent fear conditioning in which ambiguous stimuli are more likely to be appraised as threatening; mechanisms for extinguishing such responses are nullified, and key limbic nuclei are sensitized thereby lowering the threshold for fearful reactivity[60,62,63] (see Refs. 56, 64). A variety of neuroimaging studies (see Ref. 57) have confirmed that key nodal points in this circuitry do not function normally in individuals with PTSD.

Abnormal responses to acute and chronic stress may also play a role in PTSD. Abnormal hypothalamus–pituitary–adrenal (HPA) activity may have neurotoxic effects through activation of excitatory amino acids resulting in calcium influx into susceptible neurons.[65,66] Although excessive HPA system activity appears to be associated with trauma exposure and PTSD, the mechanism of its effect is not clearly worked out. For example, it may be expressed by elevated cortisol levels, as has been found in some PTSD patients and in children exposed to sexual trauma. Conversely, it may be expressed by reduced cortisol levels associated with supersensitivity of glucocorticoid receptors.[67–74]

Co-occurring biomechanical and psychological trauma

There was initially some controversy about the prevalence of comorbid TBI and PTSD (see Harvey et al.[75]). TBI is associated with partial or complete amnesia for the event, whereas a core symptom of PTSD is recurrent memory and reexperiencing of the event. Thus, at a theoretical level, some questioned the ability to have both conditions, particularly after MTBI.[76] Alternatively, if one allows for a partial or incomplete PTSD syndrome (i.e., without memory/reexperiencing of the event owing to neurogenic amnesia), others have argued that the two conditions can coexist. Warden et al.[77] found that none of the 47 military patients with TBI met full criteria for PTSD, because none had reexperiencing symptoms of the event. However, 13% of the patients did experience the avoidance and arousal symptom clusters of PTSD, suggesting that individuals can develop a form of PTSD without the reexperiencing symptoms.

The conflicts in Iraq and Afghanistan have spurred additional interest in the relationship between psychological and biomechanical trauma particularly in military populations (e.g., see Refs. 78–80). Although both conditions are quite prevalent in military personnel involved in the current conflict,[1] two recent studies highlight their complex interaction. Hoge et al.[5] found that 44% of Iraq war returnees reporting a TBI with loss of consciousness met criteria for PTSD, compared to 27% of those reporting altered mental status, 16% with other injuries, and 9% with no injury. Much of the variance observed in these groups with respect to physical health outcomes and symptoms could be accounted for by the presence of PTSD and/or depression. It is important to point out that participants were assessed 3–4 months after deployment and thus reflect individuals with persistent symptoms. Schneiderman et al.[81] found that combat-incurred MTBI approximately doubled the risk for PTSD and that a PTSD diagnosis was the strongest factor associated with persistent postconcussive symptoms. Belanger et al.[82] studied patients with mild and moderate-to-severe TBI and found that MTBI was associated with higher levels of postconcussion complaints approximately 2 years after injury. However, after adjusting for PTSD symptoms, these between group differences were no longer significant, leading the authors to conclude that much of the persistent symptoms after MTBI may be attributable to emotional distress.

These studies should not be construed as minimizing the effects of MTBI. Rather, they highlight the permissive or gateway effect that MTBI serves in increasing the relative risk for psychiatric disorders. The civilian literature has emphasized for a decade or more that one of the causes of persistent symptoms after MTBI (the issue the Hoge and Schneiderman papers address) is the development of a psychiatric disorder, such as depression or PTSD. As far back as 1973, Lishman,[11] in his review of the psychiatric sequelae of brain injury, refers to PTSD-like symptoms, including that "the circumstances of the accident may recur vividly in dreams, maintain states of anxiety, or become the focus for obsessional rumination or conversion hysteria" (p. 306). This suggests that it is important to distinguish a history of exposure to MTBI from attribution of current symptoms to that event. If one conceptualizes persistent symptoms as a postconcussive syndrome or "chronic TBI," one risks missing the diagnosis of a comorbid psychiatric disorder that could be quite responsive to appropriate treatment.[79]

Bryant and Harvey have reported a series of studies of individuals hospitalized after motor vehicle accidents, some with and some without MTBI. They have shown that rates of acute stress disorder 1 month after an accident are comparable in the two groups, and that acute stress disorder is a good predictor of those who go on to develop PTSD 6 months after injury.[83–86] For example, they studied 46 individuals admitted to a hospital after an MTBI (loss of consciousness [LOC] with posttraumatic amnesia <24 h) and 59 survivors of motor vehicle accidents without evidence of TBI 6 months after their accidents.[87,88] Twenty percent of the TBI group and 25% of the non-TBI group had PTSD. The TBI group had more postconcussive symptoms than did the non-TBI group. Furthermore, the TBI group with PTSD was significantly more symptomatic than the TBI without PTSD group. Recently, this group published results of a study of 1,167 traumatic accident survivors, 459 of whom had MTBI, the rest did not.[89] Three months after injury the MTBI group had higher rates of PTSD (11.8% versus 7.5%). Taken together, these studies suggest that TBI increases risk for PTSD, and that when present, PTSD can amplify postconcussive symptoms after an MTBI and complicate recovery. In their MTBI sample (LOC <15 min), Mayou et al. [90] found that an astonishing 48% of those with definite loss of consciousness had PTSD 3 months after injury, and one-third of their subjects with MTBI had PTSD 1 year after injury.

It is important to point out that much of the above discussion considers the question of the frequency of comorbid MTBI and PTSD from the same event and focuses primarily on the civilian population. Little is known about the comorbid condition in military populations and in those who may have PTSD from exposure to psychologically traumatic events experienced at time points unrelated to the TBI.

Interaction of psychological and biomechanical trauma

There are several issues that highlight the interaction between psychological and biomechanical trauma and suggest that it may make more sense to embrace these interactions rather than struggle to parse out the differences in the downstream effects of these processes.

Links between PTSD and injury in general

There is an interesting relationship between injury, including brain injury and PTSD. Several studies have suggested that physical injury in the context of a psychologically traumatic event is a risk factor for PTSD.[80,91] The link between TBI and subsequent PTSD appears particularly noteworthy (see Vasterling et al.[80] for discussion). For example, Mollica et al.[92] found that psychological trauma associated with brain injury in a civilian population was associated with higher rates of PTSD and depression than other types of injury. As noted earlier, studies by Hoge et al. have found higher rates of PTSD and depression in military personnel who may have had a TBI, particularly those who reported loss of consciousness,[5] and the Schneiderman et al. study[81] found that a probable TBI almost doubled the risk for PTSD; nor is this finding unique to the current conflicts. Vanderploeg et al.,[93] in a study of Vietnam era veterans, found that self-report of an MTBI was associated with an almost twofold increase in rate of PTSD even after controlling for a variety of other relevant variables; MTBI was also associated with a lower long-term likelihood of having recovered from PTSD. The mechanism for this relationship is not known but several factors may play a role.

Most recently, Bryant et al.[94] showed, using data from their prospective study of seriously injured trauma victims, that when an injury included MTBI, risk of new-onset PTSD was substantially higher than when the injury did not include MTBI. However, PTSD was not the only new-onset psychiatric disorder associated with MTBI; new cases of panic disorder, social phobia, and agoraphobia were also seen significantly more often in injured persons with MTBI than in those without MTBI. These data are consistent with the notion of the permissive or gateway effect that MTBI serves in increasing the relative risk for psychiatric disorders.

Common neural substrates

As described above, several brain regions at risk for injury from biomechanical trauma overlap with brain regions that appear to be dysfunctional, perhaps in a causative fashion, in PTSD.[15,78,95] For example, mesial temporal structures are vulnerable in TBI from both contact/impact forces, as well as increased sensitivity to excitotoxic injury. Hippocampal and amygdala injury are common. Both of these regions play key roles in PTSD as well, both in terms of contextual memory consolidation and fear conditioning. The hippocampus is also felt to be vulnerable to the effects of chronic stress, presumably through the mediating effects of the HPA axis. Thus biomechanical and neurochemically mediated damage could conceivably interact with neurohumoral dysregulation to create a milieu that lends itself to the development of PTSD. Orbitofrontal cortex is also vulnerable to TBI through impact forces as well as frontal subcortical axonal injury.

Neurocognitive factors

Both TBI and PTSD are associated with effects on cognition (see above). General intellectual function appears to play a role in determining risk for PTSD when exposed to psychological trauma.[96,97] Insofar as IQ may be a proxy for cognitive reserve and if a TBI reduces cognitive reserve, this could result in an increased association between TBI and PTSD. Vasterling et al.[80] have also suggested that processes, such as TBI, that might disrupt the processes of memory consolidation and integration and coherent processing and retrieval of emotional memories could put an individual at greater risk for development of PTSD.

Treatment implications

A full discussion of treatment approaches to TBI and PTSD is beyond the scope of this paper (see Refs. 79 and 98 for reviews), but several general points are worth making. Although there are evidence-based treatments for PTSD[98] and to a lesser extent TBI,[99–102] the approach to individuals with comorbid TBI and PTSD has not been studied to any great extent. We do not know at this point if treatments effective for PTSD are as effective if the individual has had a TBI; nor do we know if the efficacy of treatments that address symptoms attributable to TBI (e.g., cognitive complaints or deficits) are altered if the person also has PTSD. Most studies of PTSD treatment have excluded persons with a history of TBI, and studies of TBI sequelae typically have excluded persons with significant psychiatric illness including PTSD. Therefore, the generalizability of treatment approaches to the comorbid condition is unknown. Furthermore, the recent Institute of Medicine reports[98,100] on both conditions, were rather skeptical of the evidence supporting common practices in both conditions raising further questions about treatment efficacy.

Effect of TBI on treatment response

An important question is whether a history of TBI alters the response to standard pharmacological agents or cognitive behavioral treatments, and thus whether conventional treatment approaches require modification. There are some theoretical reasons to think that response to pharmacological agents might differ after a TBI. As described earlier, TBI is associated with dysregulation of several neurotransmitter systems integral to the homeostasis of mood, emotional control, and cognition (e.g., the catecholaminergic, serotonergic, and cholinergic systems), raising the possibility that medications that work through modulation of these neurotransmitters might behave differently after an injury. Insofar as a brain injury results in actual loss of neurons in brain regions modulating emotional control and cognition, there might be less substrate on which pharmacological agents can work and this might alter the side-effect profile. Alternatively, neurochemical dysregulation from the combination of both biomechanical and psychological trauma might create a milieu in which medication effects are more evident. It is also reasonable to ask whether individuals with cognitive complaints and/or deficits as experienced by many people with TBI will respond to cognitive processing therapy, prolonged exposure, or other cognitive behavioral interventions that are the standard of practice in the nonpharmacological treatment of PTSD.

Evaluation and attribution of effects of biomechanical and psychological trauma

As with any clinical condition, a proper evaluation is the foundation of a sound treatment plan. The overlap between the symptoms frequently endorsed by individuals with a history of TBI and those with a history of PTSD requires careful assessment of both conditions. For example, both groups may note problems in cognition (memory, attention), somatic concerns (headache), and affective dysregulation (impulsivity, irritability, anxiety), particularly in the time period shortly after the traumatic event (whether psychological, biomechanical, or both). Thus, accurate causal attribution of specific symptoms to a particular etiology may be difficult if not impossible. It is best in such situations for the clinician to keep an open mind about attribution, while at the same time establishing a clear etiological hypothesis in order to inform the therapeutic decision making. As a general rule, treatment trials should be initiated with one agent at a time, with a clear diagnostic formulation (e.g., "I am treating TBI related cognitive deficits" or "I am treating PTSD related sleep disturbance"). Both TBI and PTSD are associated with a heightened reactivity to environmental changes. Thus, the longer the treatment trial, the more confidence one has in assessing efficacy attributable to the specific intervention rather than to the nonspecific elements of treatment. There is also a strong sense among clinicians that the TBI population has a heightened sensitivity to medication side effects, necessitating lower starting doses and longer titration intervals. This also necessitates longer treatment trials.

Use of treatment algorithms for idiopathic psychiatric disorders as models

In the absence of a robust evidence base informing us about the treatment of behavioral disorders after TBI, most clinicians use treatment algorithms developed for idiopathic psychiatric disorders. This approach is supported by the limited available evidence[99] as well as expert opinion (e.g., Refs. 103, 104). Although a reasonable default position in the absence of a robust evidence base, this approach can have some pitfalls. It is particularly important to consider potential effects of a given agent or class of agent on the domains of cognition, arousal, sleep, and neurologic function, as these are domains on which standard psychotropic regimens can have adverse effects in one or both populations.

Cognition

Both TBI and PTSD are commonly associated with cognitive complaints and deficits.[95,105] Many of the medications commonly used in both conditions, such as antipsychotics, anticonvulsants, and some anxiolytics, can be associated with cognitive slowing and problems with memory and attention. Adrenergic agents can either enhance or impair cognition depending on their receptor agonist profile and their dose. Thus, particular care should be given to monitoring cognitive function when prescribing these agents.

As noted, cognitive behavioral therapies are a mainstay of PTSD treatment.[98] The impact that psychotropic medications may have on cognitive behavioral therapies shown to be effective in PTSD is unclear. Theoretically, medications known to impact attention and memory processes could alter the efficacy of psychotherapies that depend on intact cognitive processes in order to be effective.

Arousal

Individuals with TBI may complain of excessive fatigue or demonstrate reduced arousal or apathy. Conversely, those with PTSD typically have excessive arousal as a core component of the disorder, particularly in response to certain environmental contexts. Agents, such as central nervous stimulants that enhance catecholaminergic tone (e.g., methylphenidate), are commonly used to treat arousal and cognitive deficits in individuals with TBI but in theory (though this has yet to be proven in practice) could exacerbate core symptoms of PTSD.

Sleep

Disordered sleep is common in both individuals with TBI and those with PTSD.[106–108] Many of the psychotropics have complex effects on sleep, thus it is helpful for clinicians to familiarize themselves with these effects, discuss potential sleep changes with the patient, and monitor changes in sleep as the medication trial progresses.

Neurologic function

Individuals with a history of TBI have higher rates of seizures and may have problems with disequilibrium or balance, vision, and hearing,[109,110] as well as other neurologic concerns. Individuals with PTSD have less marked neurologic abnormalities as a general rule but have been reported to have higher rates of subtle neurologic abnormalities.[111] Many of the psychotropics can have adverse effects on sensory processing, gait, and balance, and are associated with increased rates of seizures. Thus, again, it is helpful for the clinician to bear these issues in mind when choosing a medication and to monitor for emergence or worsening of these symptoms during treatment.

Alterations in dosing

Related to the above concerns, most expert opinion suggests that conventional dosing strategies be altered in individuals with a history of TBI and ongoing sequelae.[95] Starting doses should be reduced and titration intervals prolonged. Clinicians should be alert to therapeutic responses at lower than expected doses and should not feel compelled to push through to higher "therapeutic" doses unless warranted by an incomplete response.

Summary

The literature reviewed suggests that the current conflicts in Iraq and Afghanistan are associated with a large cohort of military personnel exposed to episodes of biomechanical force sufficient to cause neurotrauma (sometimes multiple such exposures) and other physical injury, as well as episodes of combat and other forms of deployment-related psychological stress. Although such considerations have been associated with other periods of armed conflict, including the World Wars of the previous century, there is a growing appreciation that these different traumas overlap and interact in complex ways, and a better understanding of how common sequelae follow predictably from the profile of brain regions injured by both types of trauma.

From a neural perspective, several brain regions (hippocampus, amygdala, medial, and prefrontal cortex) vulnerable to biomechanical forces in the typical TBI, are the same regions implicated in the etiology of PTSD and other stress-related disorders, suggesting that although initiating events may differ, there may be a common etiological pathway resulting in the overlapping clinical symptoms. Furthermore, there appears to be a shared cognitive vulnerability. Those with lower cognitive reserve, or those who sustain a TBI, are at substantially greater risk for stress-related disorders. Although the mechanism is not clear yet, possibilities include the effects of decreased cognitive reserve with impaired coping capacity, as well as acute TBI-related disruption of the normal processing of emotional and psychologically traumatizing experiences with resultant heightened vulnerability to pathological emotional processing and emergence of stress-related disorders.

At this time, the treatment implications are not clearly established, but there are theoretical reasons to question whether the comorbid occurrence of both types of trauma might render conventional treatment approaches less effective or whether treatment approaches at least require some alterations. Further research should shed some light on this. In the meantime the use of conventional approaches, with modest common sense modifications to accommodate the clinical realities, is advised. These modifications include taking into account the effects of cognitive complaints and possible deficits on the pace of cognitive behavioral interventions, and the effects of psychotropic agents on cognition, arousal, sleep, and sensorimotor function.

Acknowledgments

Supported in part by grants NICHD R01 HD048176, 1R01HD047242, and 1R01HD48638; NINDS 1RO1NS055020; CDC R01/CE001254; DoD/CDMRP PT075446; NIMH K24MH64122; DoD/CDMRP W81XWH08-2-0159.

Conflicts of interest

The authors declare no conflicts of interest.

References

1. Tanielian, T. & L.H. Jaycox, Eds. 2008. *Invisible Wounds of War: Psychological and Cognitive Injuries, Their Consequences, and Services to Assist Recovery*. RAND Corporation. Washington, DC.

2. Sayer, N.A., C.E. Chiros, B. Sigford, *et al*. 2008. Characteristics and rehabilitation outcomes among patients with blast and other injuries sustained during the global war on terror. *Arch. Phys. Med. Rehabil*. **89:** 163–170.

3. Belanger, H., T. Kretzmer, R. Yoash-Gantz, *et al*. 2009. Cognitive sequelae of blast-related versus other mechanisms of brain trauma. *J. Int. Neuropsychol. Soc*. **15:** 1–8.

4. Hoge, C., H. Goldberg & C. Castro. 2009. Care of war veterans with mild traumatic brain injury: flawed perspectives. *N. Engl. J. Med*. **360:** 1588–1591.

5. Hoge, C., D. McGurk, J. Thomas, *et al*. 2008. Mild traumatic brain injury in U.S. Soldiers returning from iraq. *N. Engl. J. Med*. **358:** 453–463.

6. Jones, E., N. Fear & S. Wessely. 2007. Shell shock and mild traumatic brain injury: a historical review. *Am. J. Psychiatry* **164:** 1641–1645.

7. Cramer, F. 1949. Cerebral injuries due to explosion waves, cerebral blast concussion: a pathologic, clinical and electroencephalographic study. *Arch. Neurol. Psychiatry* **61:** 1–20.

8. Cramer, F. 1947. Cerebral injuries due to explosion waves: blast concussion. *J. Nerv. Ment. Dis*. **106:** 602–605.

9. Evans, R. 1994. The postconcussion syndrome: 130 years of controversy. *Semin. Neurol*. **14:** 32–39.

10. Lishman, W.A. 1968. Brain damage in relation to psychiatric disability after head injury. *Br. J. Psychiatry* **114:** 373–410.

11. Lishman, W.A. 1973. The psychiatric sequelae of head injury: a review. *Psychol. Med*. **3:** 304–318.

12. Lishman, W.A. 1988. Physiogenesis and psychogenesis in the "post-concussional syndrome." *Br. J. Psychiatry* **153:** 460–469.

13. Friedman, M.J., P.P. Schnurr & A. McDonagh-Coyle. 1994. Post-traumatic stress disorder in the military veteran. *Psychiatr. Clin. North Am*. **17:** 265–277.

14. Gennarelli, T. & D. Graham. 2005. Neuropathology. In *Textbook of Traumatic Brain Injury*. J. Silver, T. McAllister & S. Yudofsky, Eds.: 27–50. American Psychiatric Press. Washington, DC.

15. Bigler, E.D. 2007. Anterior and middle cranial fossa in traumatic brain injury: relevant neuroanatomy and neuropathology in the study of neuropsychological outcome. [review] [119 refs]. *Neuropsychology* **21:** 515–531.

16. Raghupathi, R., D.I. Graham & E. Al. 2000. Apoptosis after traumatic brain injury. *J. Neurotrauma* **17:** 927–938.

17. Umile, E.M., M.E. Sandel, A. Alavi, *et al*. 2002. Dynamic imaging in mild traumatic brain injury: support for the theory of medial temporal vulnerability. *Arch. Phys. Med. Rehabil*. **83:** 1506–1513.

18. Kocsis, J.D. & A. Tessler. 2009. Pathology of blast-related brain injury. *J. Rehabil. Res. Dev*. **46:** 667–672.

19. Depalma, R.G., D.G. Burris, H.R. Champion & M.J. Hodgson. 2005. Blast injuries. *N. Engl. J. Med*. **352:** 1335–1342.

20. Cernak, I., Z. Wang, J. Jiang, *et al*. 2001. Cognitive deficits following blast injury-induced neurotrauma: possible involvement of nitric oxide. *Brain Inj*. **15:** 593–612.

21. Cernak, I., J. Savic, Z. Malicevic, *et al*. 1996. Involvement of the central nervous system in the general response to pulmonary blast injury. *J. Trauma* **40:** S100–S104.

22. Mayorga, M.A. 1997. The pathology of primary blast overpressure injury. *Toxicology* **121:** 17–28.

23. Cernak, I., Z. Wang, J. Jiang, *et al*. 2001. Ultrastructural and functional characteristics of blast injury-induced neurotrauma. *J. Trauma* **50:** 695–706.

24. Warden, D. 2006. Military TBI during the Iraq and Afghanistan wars. *J. Head Trauma Rehabil*. **21:** 398–402.

25. Chen, Y., D.H. Smith & D.F. Meaney. 2009. In-vitro approaches for studying blast-induced traumatic brain injury. *J. Neurotrauma* **26:** 1–16.

26. Bhattacharjee, Y. 2008. Shell shock revisited: solving the puzzle of blast trauma. *Science* **319:** 406–408.

27. McAllister, T.W., L.A. Flashman, M.B. Sparling & A.J. Saykin. 2004. Working memory deficits after mild traumatic brain injury: catecholaminergic mechanisms and prospects for catecholaminergic treatment—a review. *Brain Inj*. **18:** 331–350.

28. Arciniegas, D.B. 2003. The cholinergic hypothesis of cognitive impairment caused by traumatic brain injury. *Curr. Psychiatry Rep*. **5:** 391–399.

29. Morales, D.M., N. Marklund, D. Lebold, *et al*. 2005. Experimental models of traumatic brain injury: do we really need to build a better mousetrap? *Neuroscience* **136:** 971–989.

30. Thompson, H., J. Lifshitz, N. Marklund, *et al*. 2005. Lateral fluid percussion brain injury: a 15-year review and evaluation. *J. Neurotrauma* **22:** 42–75.

31. Park, E., S. Mcknight, J. Ai & A. Baker. 2006. Purkinje cell vulnerability to mild and severe forebrain head trauma. *J. Neuropathol. Exp. Neurol.* **65:** 226–234.

32. Farkas, O. & J.T. Povlishock. 2007. Cellular and subcellular change evoked by diffuse traumatic brain injury: a complex web of change extending far beyond focal damage. *Prog. Brain Res.* **161:** 43–59.

33. Bigler, E. 2004. Neuropsychological results and neuropathological findings at autopsy in a case of mild traumatic brain injury. *J. Int. Neuropsychol. Soc.* **10:** 794–806.

34. Blumbergs, P.C., G. Scott, J. Manavis, *et al.* 1994. Staining of amyloid precursor protein to study axonal damage in mild head injury. *Lancet* **344:** 1055–1056.

35. Oppenheimer, D.R. 1968. Microscopic lesions in the brain following head injury. *J. Neurol. Neurosurg. Psychiatr.* **31:** 299–306.

36. Marcoux, J., D. McArthur, C. Miller, *et al.* 2008. Persistent metabolic crisis as measured by elevated cerebral microdialysis lactate-pyruvate ratio predicts chronic frontal lobe brain atrophy after traumatic brain injury. *Crit. Care Med.* **36:** 2871–2877.

37. Strebel, S., A.M. Lam, B.F. Matta & D.W. Newell. 1997. Impaired cerebral autoregulation after mild brain injury. *Surg. Neurol.* **47:** 128–131.

38. Junger, E.C., D.W. Newell, G.A. Grant, *et al.* 1997. Cerebral autoregulation following minor head injury. *J. Neurosurg.* **86:** 425–432.

39. Arvigo, F., M. Cossu, B. Fazio, *et al.* 1985. Cerebral blood flow in minor cerebral contusion. *Surg. Neurol.* **24:** 211–217.

40. Lee, S., M. Wong, A. Samii & D. Hovda. 1999. Evidence for energy failure following irreversible traumatic brain injury. *Ann. N.Y. Acad. Sci.* **893:** 337–340.

41. Giza, C. & D. Hovda. 2001. The neurometabolic cascade of concussion. *J. Athletic Training* **36:** 228–235.

42. Bergsneider, M., D. Hovda, S. Lee, *et al.* 2000. Dissociation of cerebral glucose metabolism and level of consciousness during the period of metabolic depression following human traumatic brain injury. *J. Neurotrauma* **17:** 389–401.

43. Levine, B., E. Fujiwara, C. O'Connor, *et al.* 2006. In vivo characterization of traumatic brain injury neuropathology with structural and functional neuroimaging. *J. Neurotrauma* **23:** 1396–1411.

44. Belanger, H., R. Vanderploeg, G. Curtiss & D. Warden. 2007. Recent neuroimaging techniques in mild traumatic brain injury. *J. Neuropsychiatry Clin. Neurosci.* **19:** 5–20.

45. Chastain, C.A., U. Oyoyo, M. Zipperman, *et al.* 2009. Predicting outcomes of traumatic brain injury by imaging modality and injury distribution. *J. Neurotrauma* **26:** 1183–1196.

46. Kraus, M.F., T. Susmaras, B.P. Caughlin, *et al.* 2007. White matter integrity and cognition in chronic traumatic brain injury: a diffusion tensor imaging study. *Brain* **130:** 2508–2519.

47. Niogi, S.N., P. Mukherjee, J. Ghajar, *et al.* 2008. Extent of microstructural white matter injury in postconcussive syndrome correlates with impaired cognitive reaction time: a 3t diffusion tensor imaging study of mild traumatic brain injury. *AJNR Am. J. Neuroradiol.* **29:** 967–973.

48. Huang, M., R.J. Theilmann, A. Robb, *et al.* 2009. Integrated imaging approach with MEG and DTI to detect mild traumatic brain injury in military and civilian patients. *J. Neurotrauma* **26:** 1213–1226.

49. Levin, H., E.A. Wilde, M. Troyanskaya, *et al.* 2010. Diffusion tensor imaging of mild to moderate blast related TBI and its sequelae. *J. Neurotrauma* **27:** 683–694.

50. Hattori, N., M. Swan, G. Stobbe, *et al.* 2009. Differential SPECT activation patterns associated with PASAT performance may indicate frontocerebellar functional dissociation in chronic mild traumatic brain injury. *J. Nucl. Med.* **50:** 1054–1061.

51. Alavi, A. & A.B. Newberg. 1996. Metabolic consequences of acute brain trauma: is there a role for pet? *J. Nucl. Med.* **37:** 1170–1172.

52. McAllister, T.W., L.A. Flashman, B.C. McDonald, *et al.* 2006. Mechanisms of working memory dysfunction after mild and moderate TBI: evidence from functional MRI and neurogenetics. *J. Neurotrauma* **23:** 1450–1467.

53. Gasparovic, C., R. Yao, M. Mannell, *et al.* 2009. Neurometabolite concentrations in gray and white matter in mild traumatic brain injury: an 1h-magnetic resonance spectroscopy study. *J. Neurotrauma* **26:** 1635–1643.

54. Hoge, C., C. Castro, S. Messer, *et al.* 2004. Combat duty in Iraq and Afghanistan, mental health problems, and barriers to care. *N. Engl. J. Med.* **351:** 13–22.

55. Neumeister, A., S. Wood, O. Bonne, *et al.* 2005. Reduced hippocampal volume in unmedicated, remitted patients with major depression versus control subjects. *Biol. Psychiatry* **57:** 935–937.

56. Friedman, M.J. & J.R.T. Davidson. 2007. Pharmacotherapy for PTSD. In *Handbook of PTSD: Science and Practice.* M.J. Friedman, T.M. Keane & P.A. Resick, Eds.: 376–405. Guilford Publications. New York.

57. Bremner, J.D. 2007. Functional neuroimaging in posttraumatic stress disorder. *Expert Rev. Neurother.* **7:** 393–405.

58. Davis, M. & P.J. Whalen. 2001. The amygdala: vigilance and emotion. *Mol. Psychiatry* **1:** 13–34.

59. Vermetten, E. & J.D. Bremner. 2002. Circuits and systems in stress. II. Applications to neurobiology and treatment in posttraumatic stress disorder. *Depress. Anxiety.* **16:** 14–38.

60. Charney, D.S. 2004. Psychobiological mechanisms of resilience and vulnerability: implications for successful adaptation to extreme stress. *Am. J. Psychiatry* **161:** 195–216.

61. Simmons, A., M. Paulus, S. Thorp, *et al.* 2008. Functional activation and neural networks in women with posttraumatic stress disorder related to intimate partner violence. *Biol. Psychiatry* **64:** 681–690.

62. Charney, D.S., A.Y. Deutch, J.H. Krystal, *et al.* 1993. Psychobiologic mechanisms of posttraumatic stress disorder. *Arch. Gen. Psychiatry* **50:** 295–305.

63. Friedman, M.J. 1994. Neurobiological sensitization models of post-traumatic stress disorder: their possible relevance to multiple chemical sensitivity syndrome. *Toxicol. Ind. Health* **10:** 449–462.

64. Southwick, S.M., L. Davis, D.E. Aikens, *et al.* 2007. Neurobiological alterations associated with PTSD. In *Handbook of PTSD: Science and Practice.* M.J. Friedman, T.M. Keane

& P.A. Resick, Eds.: 166–189. Guilford Publications. New York.

65. Sapolsky, R.M. 2000. The possibility of neurotoxicity in the hippocampus in major depression: a primer on neuron death. [comment]. *Biol. Psychiatry* **48:** 755–765.

66. Mcewen, B.S., J. Angulo, H. Cameron, *et al.* 1992. Paradoxical effects of adrenal steroids on the brain: protection versus degeneration. *Biol. Psychiatry* **31:** 177–199.

67. Debellis, M.D., G.P. Chrousos, L.D. Dorn, *et al.* 1994. Hypothalamic-pituitary-adrenal axis dysregulation in sexually abused girls. *J. Clin. Endocrinol. Metab.* **78:** 249–255.

68. Heim, C., J.D. Newport, R. Bonsall, *et al.* 2001. Altered pituitary-adrenal axis responses to provocative challenge tests in adult survivors of childhood abuse. *Am. J. Psychiatry* **158:** 575–581.

69. Lemieux, A.M. & C.L. Coe. 1995. Abuse-related posttraumatic stress disorder: evidence for chronic neuroendocrine activation in women. *Psychosom. Med.* **57:** 105–115.

70. Rasmusson, A.M., D.S. Lipschitz, S. Wang, *et al.* 2001. Increased pituitary and adrenal reactivity in premenopausal women with ptsd. *Biol. Psychiatry* **50:** 965–977.

71. Rasmusson, A.M. & M.J. Friedman. 2002. Gender issues in the neurobiology of PTSD. In *Gender and PTSD.* R. Kimerling, P.C. Ouimette & J. Wolfe, Eds.: 43–75. Guilford Press. New York.

72. Yehuda, R. 2002. Current status of cortisol findings in posttraumatic stress disorder. *Psychiatr. Clin. North Am.* **2:** 341–368.

73. Yehuda, R., D. Boisoneau, M.T. Lowy & E.L. Giller. 1995. Dose-response changes in plasma cortisol and lymphocyte glucocorticoid receptors following dexamethasone administration in combat veterans with and without posttraumatic stress disorder. *Arch. Gen. Psychiatry* **52:** 583–593.

74. Friedman, M.J., A.S. McDonagh-Coyle, J.E. Jalowiec, *et al.* 2001. Neurohormonal findings during treatment of women with ptsd due to childhood sexual abuse. In *Proceedings of the 17th Annual Meeting of the International Society for Traumatic Stress Studies.* New Orleans, LA.

75. Harvey, A., C. Brewin, C. Jones & M. Kopelman. 2003. Coexistence of posttraumatic stress disorder and traumatic brain injury: towards a resolution of the paradox. *J. Int. Neuropsychol. Soc.* **9:** 663–676.

76. Sbordone, R.J. & J.C. Liter. 1995. MTBI does not produce post-traumatic stress disorder. *Brain Inj.* **9:** 405–412.

77. Warden, D.C., L.A. Labbate, A.M. Salazar, *et al.* 1997. Posttraumatic stress disorder in patients with traumatic brain injury and amnestic for the event. *J. Neuropsychiatry Clin. Neurosci.* **9:** 18–22.

78. Stein, M.B. & T.W. McAllister. 2009. Exploring the convergence of post traumatic stress disorder and mild traumatic brain injury. *Am. J. Psychiatry* **166:** 768–776.

79. McAllister, T. 2009. Psychopharmacological issues in the treatment of TBI and PTSD. *Clin. Neuropsychol.* **23:** 1338–1367.

80. Vasterling, J.J., M. Verfaellie & K.D. Sullivan. 2009. Mild traumatic brain injury and posttraumatic stress disorder in returning veterans: perspectives from cognitive neuroscience. *Clin. Psychol. Rev.* **29:** 674–684.

81. Schneiderman, A., E. Braver & H. Kang. 2008. Understanding sequelae of injury mechanisms and mild traumatic brain injury incurred during the conflicts in Iraq and Afghanistan: persistent postconcussive symptoms and posttraumatic stress disorder. *Am. J. Epidemiol.* **167:** 1446–1452.

82. Belanger, H.G., T. Kretzmer, R.D. Vanderploeg & L.M. French. 2010. Symptom complaints following combat-related traumatic brain injury: relationship to traumatic brain injury severity and posttraumatic stress disorder. *J. Int. Neuropsychol. Soc.* **16:** 194–199.

83. Harvey, A.G. & R.A. Bryant. 1998. Acute stress disorder after mild traumatic brain injury. *J. Nerv. Ment. Dis.* **186:** 333–337.

84. Harvey, A.G. & R.A. Bryant. 1998. Predictors of acute stress following mild traumatic brain injury. *Brain Inj.* **12:** 147–154.

85. Bryant, R.A. & A.G. Harvey. 1998. Relationship between acute stress disorder and posttraumatic stress disorder following mild traumatic brain injury. *Am. J. Psychiatry* **155:** 625–629.

86. Broomhall, L.G., C.R. Clark, A.C. McFarlane, *et al.* 2009. Early stage assessment and course of acute stress disorder after mild traumatic brain injury. *J. Nerv. Ment. Dis.* **197:** 178–181.

87. Bryant, R.A. & A.G. Harvey. 1999. Postconcussive symptoms and posttraumatic stress disorder after mild traumatic brain injury. *J. Nerv. Ment. Dis.* **187:** 302–305.

88. Bryant, R.A. & A.G. Harvey. 1999. The influence of traumatic brain injury on acute stress disorder and posttraumatic stress disorder following motor vehicle accidents. *Brain Inj.* **13:** 15–22.

89. Bryant, R.A., M. Creamer, M. O'Donnell, *et al.* 2009. Posttraumatic amnesia and the nature of post-traumatic stress disorder after mild traumatic brain injury. *J. Int. Neuropsychol. Soc.* **15:** 862–867.

90. Mayou, R.A., J. Black & B. Bryant. 2000. Unconsciousness, amnesia and psychiatric symptoms following road traffic accident injury. *Br. J. Psychiatry* **177:** 540–545.

91. Koren, D., D. Norman, A. Cohen, *et al.* 2005. Increased PTSD risk with combat-related injury: a matched comparison study of injured and uninjured soldiers experiencing the same combat events. *Am. J. Psychiatry* **162:** 276–282.

92. Mollica, R.F., D.C. Henderson & S. Tor. 2002. Psychiatric effects of traumatic brain injury events in cambodian survivors of mass violence. *Br. J. Psychiatry* **181:** 339–347.

93. Vanderploeg, R., H. Belanger & G. Curtiss. 2009. Mild traumatic brain injury and posttraumatic stress disorder and their associations with health symptoms. *Arch. Phys. Med. Rehabil.* **90:** 1084–1093.

94. Bryant, R.A., M.L. O'Donnell, M. Creamer, *et al.* 2010. The psychiatric sequelae of traumatic injury. *Am. J. Psychiatry* **167:** 312–320.

95. McAllister, T. 2008. Neurobehavioral sequelae of traumatic brain injury: evaluation and treatment. *World Psychiatry* **7:** 3–10.

96. Breslau, N., V.C. Lucia & G.F. Alvarado. 2006. Intelligence and other predisposing factors in exposure to trauma and posttraumatic stress disorder: a follow-up study at age 17 years. *Arch. Gen. Psychiatry* **63:** 1238–1245.

97. Kremen, W.S., K.C. Koenen, C. Boake, *et al.* 2007. Pre-trauma cognitive ability and risk for posttraumatic stress disorder: a twin study. *Arch. Gen. Psychiatry* **64:** 361–368.

98. Committee on Treatment of Posttraumatic Stress Disorder, Institute of Medicine. 2008. *Treatment of Posttraumatic Stress Disorder: An Assessment of the Evidence.* The National Academies Press. Washington, DC.

99. Warden, D., B. Gordon, D. Katz, *et al.* 2006. Guidelines for the pharmacologic treatment of neurobehavioral sequelae of traumatic brain injury. *J. Neurotrauma* **23:** 1468–1501.

100. Institute of Medicine. 2009. *Gulf War and Health, Volume 7: Long-Term Consequences of Traumatic Brain Injury.* The National Academies Press. Washington, DC.

101. Cicerone, K., H. Levin, J. Malec, *et al.* 2006. Cognitive rehabilitation interventions for executive function: moving from bench to bedside in patients with traumatic brain injury. *J. Cogn. Neurosci.* **18:** 1212–1222.

102. Cicerone, K., C. Dahlberg, K. Kalmar, *et al.* 2000. Evidence-based cognitive rehabilitation: recommendations for clinical practice. *Arch. Phys. Med. Rehabil.* **81:** 1596–1615.

103. Alderfer, B.S., D.B. Arciniegas & J.M. Silver. 2005. Treatment of depression following traumatic brain injury. *J. Head Trauma Rehabil.* **20:** 544–562.

104. Silver, J., T. McAllister & D. Arciniegas. 2009. Depression and cognitive complaints following mild traumatic brain injury. *Am. J. Psychiatry* **166:** 653–661.

105. Vasterling, J.J., L.M. Duke, K. Brailey, *et al.* 2002. Attention, learning, and memory performances and intellectual resources in vietnam veterans: PTSD and no disorder comparisons. *Neuropsychology* **16:** 5–14.

106. Raskind, M., E. Peskind, D. Hoff, *et al.* 2007. A parallel group placebo controlled study of prazosin for trauma nightmares and sleep disturbance in combat veterans with post-traumatic stress disorder. [see comment]. *Biol. Psychiatry* **61:** 928–934.

107. Vaishnavi, S., V. Rao & J. Fann. 2009. Neuropsychiatric problems after traumatic brain injury: unraveling the silent epidemic. *Psychosomatics* **50:** 198–205.

108. Kraus, J., K. Schaffer, K. Ayers, *et al.* 2005. Physical complaints, medical service use, and social and employment changes following mild traumatic brain injury: a 6-month longitudinal study. *J. Head Trauma Rehabil.* **20:** 239–256.

109. Kapoor, N. & K. Ciuffreda. Vision problems. In *Textbook of Traumatic Brain Injury.* J. Silver, T. McAllister & S. Yudofsky, Eds.: American Psychiatric Publishing. Washington, DC. In press.

110. Cosetti, M. & A. Lalwani. Dizziness, imbalance and vestibular dysfunction after traumatic brain injury. In *Textbook of Traumatic Brain Injury.* J. Silver, T. McAllister & S. Yudofsky, Eds.: American Psychiatric Publishing. Washington, DC. In press.

111. Pitman, R.K., M.W. Gilbertson, T.V. Gurvits, *et al.* 2006. Clarifying the origin of biological abnormalities in PTSD through the study of identical twins discordant for combat exposure. *Ann. N.Y. Acad. Sci.* **1071:** 242–254.

Ann. N.Y. Acad. Sci. ISSN 0077-8923

ANNALS OF THE NEW YORK ACADEMY OF SCIENCES
Issue: *Psychiatric and Neurologic Aspects of War*

A unified science of concussion

Jun Maruta,[1] Stephanie W. Lee,[1] Emily F. Jacobs,[1] and Jamshid Ghajar[1,2]

[1]Brain Trauma Foundation, New York, New York. [2]Department of Neurological Surgery, Weill-Cornell Medical College, New York, New York

Address for correspondence: Jamshid Ghajar, Brain Trauma Foundation, 7 World Trade Center, 250 Greenwich Street, 34th Floor, New York, New York 10007. ghajar@braintrauma.org

The etiology, imaging, and behavioral assessment of mild traumatic brain injury (mTBI) are daunting fields, given the lack of a cohesive neurobiological explanation for the observed cognitive deficits seen following mTBI. Although subjective patient self-report is the leading method of diagnosing mTBI, current scientific evidence suggests that quantitative measures of predictive timing, such as visual tracking, could be a useful adjunct to guide the assessment of attention and to screen for advanced brain imaging. Magnetic resonance diffusion tensor imaging (DTI) has demonstrated that mTBI is associated with widespread microstructural changes that include those in the frontal white matter tracts. Deficits observed during predictive visual tracking correlate with DTI findings that show lesions localized in neural pathways subserving the cognitive functions often disrupted in mTBI. Unifying the anatomical and behavioral approaches, the emerging evidence supports an explanation for mTBI that the observed cognitive impairments are a result of predictive timing deficits caused by shearing injuries in the frontal white matter tracts.

Keywords: smooth pursuit; attention; prefrontal cortex; diffusion axonal injury (DAI); blast injury

Introduction

Cognitive sequelae from concussion, or mild traumatic brain injury (mTBI), are difficult to measure and often ascribed to the traumatic event or premorbid factors.[1,2] Because computer tomography (CT) images are normal for most mTBI patients,[3] little or no physical brain injury may be presumed[4]; however, the magnetic resonance imaging (MRI) technique of diffusion tensor imaging (DTI) can now detect microscopic brain white matter tract lesions.[5–8] These lesions are likely to be responsible for the postconcussive symptoms and may explain chronic difficulties experienced by some patients.

Considering the vulnerability of anterior white matter tracts to shearing and the involvement of these tracts in attention and moment-to-moment predictive timing, it may be timely to develop a unified approach to the prevention, diagnosis, and treatment of mTBI.

Incidence and definition

TBI has been referred to as the signature injury of the wars in Iraq and Afghanistan.[9,10] An estimated 320,000 service members deployed between 2001 and 2007 screened positive for a probable TBI.[10] Blast exposure has been indicated as the greatest source of injury accounting for the majority of TBIs sustained by service members.[11,12] TBI is graded in degree, from mild to severe, based on the acute effects of the injury on an individual's level of arousal and duration of amnesia. The Veterans Affairs/Department of Defense Clinical Practice Guideline classifies mTBI as a traumatically induced structural injury or physiological disruption of brain function as a result of an external force, with normal CT structural imaging, loss of consciousness <30 min, alteration of mental state <24 h, posttraumatic amnesia <1 day, and Glasgow Coma Score of 13–15.[13] A similar classification is used in the civilian population. The majority of TBIs sustained in both the military and civilian populations are classified as mild.[14,15]

Following mTBI, individuals can develop postconcussive syndrome (PCS): a constellation of symptoms that can be categorized as cognitive, affective, or somatic (Table 1).[16] PCS may lead to chronic disability.[17,18]

doi: 10.1111/j.1749-6632.2010.05695.x

 Ann. N.Y. Acad. Sci. 1208 (2010) 58–66 © 2010 Association for Research in Nervous and Mental Disease.

Table 1. Postconcussive symptoms

Cognitive	Somatic	Affective
• Memory difficulties	• Headache	• Irritability
• Decreased concentration	• Dizziness	• Depression
• Decreased processing speed	• Nausea	• Anxiety
	• Fatigue	
	• Sleep disturbances	
	• Blurred vision	
	• Tinnitus	
	• Hypersensitivity to light or noise	

Etiology and mechanism of injury

A common pathological feature of TBI includes distributed injuries to the subcortical white matter, or diffuse axonal injury (DAI), that may occur with or without a focal injury.[19–23] mTBI may involve DAI.[24] DAI presents, histologically, as microscopic lesions, myelin loss, axonal degeneration, or axonal swellings[19–23,25] but is difficult to detect with traditional CT and MRI scans.[5,26–29] In blunt closed-head injury, these diffuse axonal damages have been attributed to shear strain and tissue deformation caused by the rotational accelerations of the brain as an external force is applied to the head.[30,31] The shear strains and tissue deformations of the primary biomechanical injury and reactive edema represent the acute phase of TBI. Acute TBI may lead to axonal degeneration and neuronal cell death (secondary injury) that develops after the initial biomechanical incident, which represents the chronic phase of TBI. The rotational acceleration experienced by the brain can be produced by either a linear or angular acceleration of the head because the brain's motion is constrained by basal-frontal tethering.[31] It is of note that rotational acceleration of the brain, and thereby DAI, can be produced with or without a direct blow to the head as in cases of whiplash in a car accident.

Blast-related injuries can occur though a combination of four different mechanisms: primary (direct effects of the over- and under-pressure wave); secondary (effects of projectiles); tertiary (effects of wind, fragmentation of buildings and vehicles); and quaternary (burns, asphyxia, and exposure to toxic inhalants).[32] The pathophysiology of blast-related TBI is complex and not fully understood. Although

rotation-induced shearing is consistent with the secondary and tertiary effects, the primary effect alone is likely able to induce axonal injury.[33–35] Regardless, the functional deficits associated with blast-related mTBI do not appear different from non-blast-related mTBI.[36,37]

Current diagnostic methods in mTBI

Military mTBI screening methods

Because the severity of TBI is defined by the acute injury characteristics, the term "mild" should not be interpreted as an indicator of PCS symptom severity; PCS may develop in the days following concussion, and the extent of disability and treatment needs vary from patient to patient.[17,18,38,39] Currently, the method of mTBI diagnosis is highly dependent upon information obtained through patients' subjective self-report about the acute characteristics of their injury. Unlike moderate or severe TBI, which are more easily diagnosed acutely by decrements in arousal or abnormality in CT images, mTBI is much more ambiguous during the acute phases and may not be diagnosed until the affected individual complains of postconcussive symptoms or experiences difficulties in their social interactions or in job or school performance. Adding to the complexity, as a consequence of cognitive impairments that result from their injury, mTBI patients may have a reduced awareness of their deficits.[4,40] This is also the case with patients who have survived more severe TBIs.[41,42] Because of these challenges, the Department of Defense and the Department of Veterans Affairs have implemented system-wide multipoint screening and assessment procedures for detecting mTBI in service members engaged in and returning from the wars in Iraq and Afghanistan.[13,43–45]

During deployment, the military administers the Military Acute Concussion Evaluation (MACE), an adaptation of Standardized Assessment of Concussion,[46] as soon as possible following the injury. Postdeployment, the Brief Traumatic Brain Injury Survey (BTBIS)[47] included in the Warrior Administered Retrospective Casualty Assessment Tool (WARCAT) or the Post-Deployment Health Assessment (PDHA) is administered to the soldiers.[48] These screening measures are designed to be overly inclusive to reduce the risk of overlooking individuals with TBI;[44] any positive screen would need to be followed by a clinical interview and examination to either confirm or negate the diagnosis of mTBI. Evidence of structural brain damage is not part of the mTBI diagnostic criteria.[13]

Clinical assessments

Various methods exist to evaluate mTBI. Currently, neuropsychological testing is considered to be one of the most important assessment tools during both the acute and chronic phases of PCS. Typical neuropsychological batteries assess attention, working memory, and executive functions. One such battery, the Automated Neuropsychological Assessment Metric (ANAM), includes tasks like simple reaction time, code substitution, mathematical processing, and matching to sample.[49] ANAM is administered to every service member prior to deployment, and changes in cognitive functions after an injury may be identified or monitored using this assessment tool. Neuropsychological tests are sensitive to moderate to severe TBI[1,2] and may provide important insights into cognitive functioning during the acute phase of mTBI.[49,50] However, neuropsychological test performance seems to return to normal within several months in the mTBI population at large[1,2,50] and there is no association with number of lifetime TBIs, severity of TBI or number of postconcussive symptoms.[51] Underlying causes of persistent cognitive difficulties are not clear, but it is possible that deficits are too subtle or not detectable by traditional neuropsychological testing methods.[18,50]

CT plays a critical role in the clinical management of TBI owing to its wide availability and its speed and accuracy in the detection of skull fractures and intracranial hemorrhage.[3,24,52] CT is particularly useful for conditions that require immediate intervention and is indicated for moderate and severe TBI patients. However, CT performs poorly at detecting DAI,[5,26,27] and images often present as normal for most mTBI patients.[3]

Standard structural MRI outperforms CT in detecting DAI and secondary lesions,[21,26] and is often used in assessments of subacute and chronic TBI. However, DAI is still difficult to detect by conventional MRI,[5,27,28] and the presence of pathology may not be detected in cases of mTBI.[29,53] Neither CT nor MRI scans correlate well with the number of self-reported symptoms or performance on neuropsychological tests.[53–55]

Supplementing behavioral and structural assessment techniques, functional imaging can be used to evaluate the pathophysiological and functional sequelae of mTBI.[56] These methods include functional MRI, positron emission tomography (PET), single photon emission computed tomography (SPECT), electroencephalography (EEG), and magnetoencephalography (MEG). Functional MRI may be used to assess the degree of neural activation in TBI subjects carrying out cognitive tasks known to be disrupted by TBI.[57] Several PET studies show significant correlations between cognitive task performance and metabolic abnormalities[58–60]; however, the interpretations remain inconclusive regarding the types of metabolic changes in specific regions of interest across patients[59] and the relationship between global abnormalities and specific cognitive tasks.[60] SPECT may be able to predict neuropsychological test performance[61] but results are inconsistent.[62] Standard clinical EEG procedures used in hospitals detect abnormal activities caused by larger morphological changes like focal lesions and are therefore less useful in detecting the DAIs seen in mTBI; more specific measures of EEG associated with cognitive processes, such as event-related potentials, may be better at detecting the attention and memory deficits related to mTBI.[63] MEG, in conjunction with MRI, has also been shown to be useful in detecting abnormal activity in patients with PCS.[64]

Despite the multitude of available imaging and behavioral assessments of mTBI, there lacks a cohesive neurobiological explanation for the cognitive deficits observed. To understand the spectrum of mTBI outcome, we recommend an approach that unifies anatomical and behavioral assessments.

A unified approach to mTBI

Anatomy: diffusion tensor imaging

Unlike the traditional CT and MRI, DTI is an MRI modality that can provide quantitative characterization of intrinsic features of tissue microstructure and microdynamics.[65] DTI has provided a powerful new tool for detecting DAI and other microstructural changes in white matter associated with mTBI injury severity.[5–8] Although still considered experimental, the application of DTI shows great potential for the clinical diagnosis of mTBI.[52,66]

The three principle eigenvalues of the diffusion tensor matrix quantitatively describe the mobility of water molecules. Axial diffusivity is the largest of the eigenvalues and represents molecular mobility parallel to the local fiber tract direction; radial diffusivity is the average of the other two principle eigenvalues and represents mobility perpendicular to the fiber tract direction. Mean diffusivity serves as an index of water molecule mobility averaged over all directions. Changes in the axial and radial diffusivity indices may be used to specify the pathology that leads to changes in diffusion anisotropy, for example, myelin loss or axonal injury.[67]

Of the several quantitative parameters that can be derived from DTI,[65] fractional anisotropy (FA) is considered to be a robust indicator of white matter microstructural integrity.[5–8,27,53,68–70] In a parallel fiber arrangement of a white matter tract, the diffusion of water molecules is directionally constrained, resulting in a high FA value. The theoretical range of FA values is from 0 (isotropic) to 1 (completely anisotropic); the larger the value of the index, the larger the water molecule directionality. Either an increase above or decrease below the normal FA range likely indicates white matter abnormality.

Changes in axial diffusivity, radial diffusivity, and FA, may indicate different types of white matter abnormality, which may reflect different phases of progression of TBI.[66,71] Although there are still issues to be addressed, the DTI technology has so far demonstrated conclusively that mTBI is associated with wide-spread structural changes in cortical white matter tracts.[5–8,27,53,68–70,72] Also of note, the quantitative nature of DTI provides the opportunity to correlate injury severity with functional deficits measured by neuropsychological tests and other behavioral measures.[8,53,70,73]

Behavior: symptom assessment

The functional deficits associated with mTBI can be accounted by microstructural changes in the frontal white matter. Frequently, the outcome of DAI is strikingly similar to that of focal damage in the frontal lobe.[74] The cognitive symptoms of both types of injuries include deficits associated with concentration, memory, and high-level executive functions, such as planning and decision making.[54,57,74,75]

It has been suggested that preparatory neural activity, i.e., attention, enables the efficient integration of sensory information and goal-based representations.[76] This theoretical framework allows PCS to be grouped into primary and secondary symp-

Table 2. Attention-based categorization of postconcussive symptoms

Primary symptoms related to predictive timing deficit	Secondary symptoms related to PFC compensation and error signaling
• Decreased concentration	• Headache
• Memory difficulties	• Fatigue
• Decreased processing speed	• Sleep disturbances
• Decreased awareness	• Irritability
• Balance and coordination problems	• Depression
• Blurred vision	• Anxiety
• Dizziness	
• Tinnitus	
• Hypersensitivity to light or noise	

Adapted from Ghajar and Ivry.[76]

toms (Table 2). Primary symptoms are suggested to arise directly from the physical brain injury, which is suspected to occur in the white matter tracts that connect the prefrontal–cerebellar network. The result of this disruption is considered to be impairment in predictive timing, which causes increased distractibility (attention deficits), working memory deficits, and problems with balance and coordination: symptoms commonly displayed by mTBI patients. An inability to correctly time or anticipate sensory events would result in a temporal mismatch of sensory expectation to actual sensory input, potentially leading to dizziness, tinnitus, and sensory hypersensitivity. Secondary symptoms could arise from increased activation of the prefrontal cortex (PFC), which might occur because of an increase in error signals and performance variability. Serving as a compensatory mechanism, the PFC could be recruited to help bridge the moment-to-moment temporal discrepancies. This increased effort might underlie fatigue, headache, irritability, anxiety, and when prolonged, depression.

Behavior: eye tracking

Frequent lapses in attention are a characteristic symptom of TBI.[77] Traditional measures that use discrete responses are unable to detect momentary lapses in attention. This limitation may contribute to the relative insensitivity of neuropsychological tests in detecting mTBI.[1,2,50,51] Anti-saccades tasks, a type of eye-movement paradigm sensitive to frontal lobe dysfunction,[78] rely on discrete stimulus-response sets. Anti-saccades tasks may be useful once subjects have perceived PCS symptoms[79]; however, this paradigm may not be sensitive to acute mTBI.[80] Because attention varies over time, a relatively continuous measure of performance is needed to detect moment-to-moment fluctuations in attention within individuals.[76]

The examination of performance of visual tracking of a moving target may provide a supplement to conventional behavioral assessments of mTBI patients.[79,81] Using video-oculography, eye movement can be monitored easily, precisely, and continuously. In contrast to the anti-saccade paradigm, visual tracking does not rely on discrete stimulus-response sets during the maintenance phase. Visual tracking of a moving target requires the integration of multiple sensory inputs and one's own motor efforts.[82] Visual tracking also requires cognitive processes including target selection, sustenance of attention, spatio-temporal memory, and expectation.[83–85]

Quantification of visual tracking performance using a circular target trajectory[86,87] provides a continuous behavioral assessment metric. The motion of a target traveling at a constant velocity with a fixed radius from the center is highly predictable. This movement can continue indefinitely within the orbital range of the eye, which makes the stimulus particularly suitable for studying the processes required to maintain predictive visual tracking. Predictive visual tracking requires both attention and working memory,[85] processes for which the PFC is considered to be an important substrate.[88] These cognitive functions are often compromised in mTBI patients.[17,89]

Visual tracking performance can be objectively quantified using parameters, such as smooth pursuit velocity gain, phase error, and root-mean-square error. Because TBI is known to increase intra-individual performance variability on visuomotor tasks,[77,90] we measured the variability of visual tracking performance in terms of gaze positional error relative to the target to grade the level of performance.[81] Good visual tracking was characterized by overall tight clustering of the gaze positions around the target (Fig. 1A). In contrast, poor visual tracking in mTBI subjects was generally characterized by a wide distribution of the gaze along

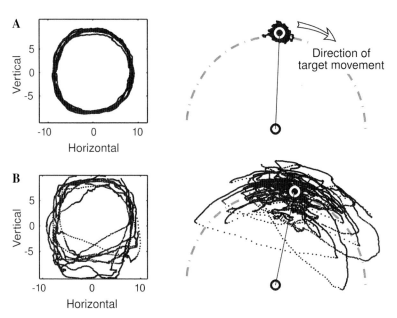

Figure 1. Visual tracking of a target moving in a circular trajectory of 8.5° radius at 0.4 Hz. (A) Example of a good performance by a normal subject. (B) Example of a poor performance by a subject with chronic postconcussive symptoms. Right panel: Two-dimensional trajectory of the gaze superimposed over nine cycles. Left panel: Scattergram of gaze positions relative to the target fixed at the 12 o'clock position. The white circle indicates the average gaze position. The dot–dashed curve indicates the circular path.

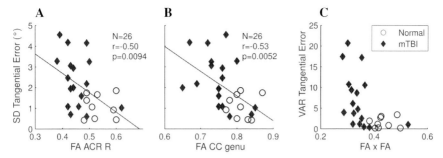

Figure 2. Relationships between FA values and visual tracking performance variability in the tangential direction of the target trajectory. (A) Right ACR. (B) Genu of the corpus callosum (CC). The regression lines were determined from the combined subject population. (C) Cross-factorization of A and B (multiplication of respective abscissa and ordinates). Circles, normal subjects; Diamonds, subjects with chronic postconcussive symptoms; SD, standard deviation; VAR, variance.

the circular path, which indicates spatio-temporal dyssynchrony with the stimulus (Fig. 1B). The spread of visual-tracking gaze errors (variability) can be used as an attention metric and can be correlated with an individual's degree of white matter integrity.

Eye-tracking and DTI

We quantified visual-tracking gaze error variability by the standard deviation of the error distribution and compared this parameter to DTI FA values.[81] Large gaze error variability was associated with low mean FA values in the right anterior corona radiata (ACR; Fig. 2A), the left superior cerebellar peduncle (not shown) and the genu of the corpus callosum (Fig. 2B). The right ACR and left superior cerebellar peduncle are tracts known to support the sustenance of attention and spatial processing.[88,91–93] Both the ACR and genu include fibers connecting to the dorsolateral PFC (DLPFC).[94] Clustering of the normal and mTBI subject populations is observed along both the DTI FA and gaze variability axes (Fig. 2A and B). Because the ACR and the genu are among the most frequently damaged white matter tracts in mTBI,[53] the correlations imply that gaze error variability during visual tracking may provide a useful screening tool for mTBI. When the FA values of the right ACR and the genu are cross-factored, the graph tends to further dissociate the normal and mTBI subject populations (Fig. 2C).

The right DLPFC may be particularly significant to mTBI symptomatology. It is a central site in the synthesis of diverse information needed to carry out complex behaviors[88] and also serves as a node in the attention network.[95] We postulate that increased visual tracking variability is a consequence

of the dyssynchrony between moment-to-moment expectations and incoming sensory input, caused by deficits in the right prefrontal–left cerebellar loop. Given the vulnerability of the frontal white matter to mTBI, the degree to which the connection to the right DLPFC is damaged by the injury may be estimated by visual tracking variability. The function of the DLPFC is also considered to be a convergent factor between posttraumatic stress disorder and persistent PCS.[39] As such, the presence and extent of damage in the right prefrontal cortical connection could potentially serve during the acute stages of mTBI as a predictor of which mTBI patients will develop chronic symptoms.[81]

Individual differences in the outcome of mTBI may be predicted by identifiable risk factors,[39] and therefore it would be useful to measure performance on a predictive visual tracking task acutely after mTBI to compare with longitudinal results. Also, as structural connectivity may be improved by behavioral training,[96] a biofeedback paradigm to improve visual tracking performance could potentially be used therapeutically.

Conclusion

Predictive visual tracking shows promise as an attention metric to assess severity of mTBI. Deficits seen during predictive visual tracking correlate with DTI findings and with observed damage to neural pathways known to carry out cognitive and affective functions that are vulnerable to mTBI. The paradigm we have developed for testing subjects is currently under 5 min in duration for the entire test, which is markedly shorter compared to most neuropsychological tests.

In summary, the approach presented in this paper unifies the anatomical and behavioral deficits characteristic of mTBI, and allows for the design and deployment of preventative, diagnostic, and therapeutic interventions that will improve the outcome of mTBI patients.

Acknowledgments

The work is supported by the Department of Defense Grants W81XWH-08-1-0646, and W81XWH-08-2-0177; James S. McDonnell Foundation grants for the Cognitive Neurobiological Research Consortium in Traumatic Brain Injury and the Attention Dynamics Consortium in Traumatic Brain Injury. Ownership Interest: Sync-Think, Inc. (J.G.).
Patents: United States Patent 7,384,399. Cognition and motor timing diagnosis and training system and method (J.G.).

References

1. Dikmen, S.S., J.E. Machamer, H.R. Winn & N.R. Temkin. 1995. Neuropsychological outcome at 1-year post head injury. *Neuropsychology* **9:** 80–90.

2. Dikmen, S.S., J.D. Corrigan, H.S. Levin, *et al.* 2009. Cognitive outcome following traumatic brain injury. *J. Head Trauma Rehabil.* **24:** 430–438.

3. Borg, J., L. Holm, J.D. Cassidy, *et al.*; WHO Collaborating Centre Task Force on Mild Traumatic Brain Injury. 2004. Diagnostic procedures in mild traumatic brain injury: results of the WHO Collaborating Centre Task Force on Mild Traumatic Brain Injury. *J. Rehabil. Med.* **43**(Suppl.): 61–75.

4. McKeag, D.B. & J.S. Kutcher. 2009. Concussion consensus: raising the bar and filling in the gaps. *Clin. J. Sport Med.* **19:** 343–346.

5. Arfanakis, K., V.M. Haughton, J.D. Carew, *et al.* 2002. Diffusion tensor MR imaging in diffuse axonal injury. *AJNR. Am. J. Neuroradiol.* **23:** 794–802.

6. Ptak, T., R.L. Sheridan, J.T. Rhea, *et al.* 2003. Cerebral fractional anisotropy score in trauma patients: a new indicator of white matter injury after trauma. *AJR. Am. J. Roentgenol.* **181:** 1401–1407.

7. Huisman, T.A., L.H. Schwamm, P.W. Schaefer, *et al.* 2004. Diffusion tensor imaging as potential biomarker of white matter injury in diffuse axonal injury. *AJNR. Am. J. Neuroradiol.* **25:** 370–376.

8. Kraus, M.F., T. Susmaras, B.P. Caughlin, *et al.* 2007. White matter integrity and cognition in chronic traumatic brain injury: a diffusion tensor imaging study. *Brain* **130:** 2508–2519.

9. Okie, S. 2005. Traumatic brain injury in the war zone. *N. Engl. J. Med.* **352:** 2043–2047.

10. Tanelian T. & L.H. Jaycox. 2008. Invisible wounds: mental health and cognitive care needs of america's returning veterans. Santa Monica, CA: Rand Corporation: http://veterans.rand.org.

11. Warden, D.L., L.M. Ryan, K.M. Helick, *et al.* 2005. War neurotrauma: the DVBI experience at Walter Reed Army Medical Center. *J. Neurotrauma* **22:** 1178.

12. Benzinger, T.L.S., D. Brody, S. Cardin, *et al.* 2009. Blast-related injury: imaging for clinical and research applications: report of the St. Louis Workshop 2008. *J. Neurotrauma* **26:** 2127–2144.

13. The Management of Concussion/mTBI Working Group. 2009. VA/DoD clinical practice guideline for management of concussion/mild traumatic brain injury. *J. Rehabil. Res. Dev.* **46:** CP1–CP68.

14. Bazarian, J.J., J. McClung, M.N. Shah, *et al.* 2005. Mild traumatic brain injury in the United States, 1998–2000. *Brain Inj.* **19:** 85–91.

15. Martin, E.M., W.C. Lu, K. Helmick, *et al.* 2008. Traumatic brain injuries sustained in the Afghanistan and Iraq wars. *Am. J. Nurs.* **108:** 40–47.

16. Smith-Seemiller, L., N.R. Fow, R. Kant & M.D. Franzen. 2003. Presence of post-concussion syndrome symptoms in patients with chronic pain vs mild traumatic brain injury. *Brain Inj.* **17:** 199–206.

17. Kushner, D. 1998. Mild traumatic brain injury: toward understanding manifestations and treatment. *Arch. Intern. Med.* **158:** 1617–1624.

18. Bigler, E.D. 2008. Neuropsychology and clinical neuroscience of persistent post-concussive syndrome. *J. Int. Neuropsychol. Soc.* **14:** 1–22.

19. Strich, S.J. 1956. Diffuse degeneration of the cerebral white matter in severe dementia following head injury. *J. Neurol. Neurosurg. Psychiatry* **19:** 163–185.

20. Oppenheimer, D.R. 1968. Microscopic lesions in the brain following head injury. *J. Neurol. Neurosurg. Psychiatry* **31:** 299–306.

21. Gentry, L.R., J.C. Godersky & B. Thompson. 1988. MR imaging of head trauma: review of the distribution and radiopathologic features of traumatic lesions. *AJR. Am. J. Roentgenol.* **150:** 663–672.

22. Adams, J.H., D. Doyle, I. Ford, *et al.* 1989. Diffuse axonal injury in head injury: definition, diagnosis and grading. *Histopathology* **15:** 49–59.

23. Smith, D.H., D.F. Meaney & W.H. Shull. 2003. Diffuse axonal injury in head trauma. *J. Head Trauma Rehabil.* **18:** 307–316.

24. Le, T.H. & A.D. Gean. 2009. Neuroimaging of traumatic brain injury. *Mt. Sinai J. Med.* **76:** 145–162.

25. Povlishock, J.T., D.P. Becker, C.L.Y. Cheng & G.W. Vaughan. 1983. Axonal change in minor head injury. *J. Neuropathol. Exp. Neurol.* **42:** 225–242.

26. Mittl, R.L., R.I. Grossman, J.F. Hiehle, *et al.* 1994. Prevalence of MR evidence of diffuse axonal injury in patients with mild head injury and normal head CT findings. *AJNR. Am. J. Neuroradiol.* **15:** 1583–1589.

27. Rugg-Gunn, F.J., M.R. Symms, G.J. Barker, *et al.* 2001. Diffusion imaging shows abnormalities after blunt head trauma when conventional magnetic resonance imaging is normal. *J. Neurol. Neurosurg. Psychiatry* **70:** 530–533.

28. Chan, J.H., E.Y. Tsui, W.C. Peh, *et al.* 2003. Diffuse axonal injury: detection of changes in anisotropy of water diffusion by diffusion-weighted imaging. *Neuroradiology* **45:** 34–38.

29. Schrader, H., D. Mickeviciene, R. Gleizniene, *et al.* 2009. Magnetic resonance imaging after most common form of concussion. *BMC. Med. Imaging* **9:** 11.

30. Holbourn, A.H.S. 1943. The mechanics of head injuries. *Lancet* **2:** 438–441.

31. Bayly, P.V., T.S. Cohen, E.P. Leister, *et al.* 2005. Deformation of the human brain induced by mild acceleration. *J. Neurotrauma* **22:** 845–856.

32. DePalma, R.G., D.G. Burris, H.R. Champion & M.J. Hodgson. 2005. Blast injuries. *N. Engl. J. Med.* **352:** 1335–1342.

33. Säljö, A., F. Bao, K.G. Haglid & H.A. Hansson. 2000. Blast exposure causes redistribution of phosphorylated neurofilament subunits in neurons of the adult rat brain. *J. Neurotrauma* **17:** 719–726.

34. Moore, D.F., A. Jérusalem, M. Nyein, *et al.* 2009. Computational biology—modeling of primary blast effects on the central nervous system. *Neuroimage* **47**(Suppl. 2):T10–T20.

35. Warden, D.L., L.M. French, L. Shupenko, *et al.* 2009. Case report of a soldier with primary blast brain injury. *Neuroimage* **47**(Suppl. 2): T152–T153.

36. Trudeau, D.L., J. Anderson, L.M. Hansen, *et al.* 1998. Findings of mild traumatic brain injury in combat veterans with PTSD and a history of blast concussion. *J. Neuropsychia. Clin. Neurosci.* **10:** 308–313.

37. Belanger, H.G., T. Kretzmer, R. Yoash-Gantz, *et al.* 2009. Cognitive sequelae of blast-related versus other mechanisms of brain trauma. *J. Int. Neuropsychol. Soc.* **15:** 1–8.

38. Hoge, C.W., D. McGurk, J.L. Thomas, *et al.* 2008. Mild traumatic brain injury in US soldiers returning from Iraq. *N. Engl. J. Med.* **358:** 453–463.

39. Stein, M.B. & T.W. McAllister. 2009. Exploring the convergence of posttraumatic stress disorder and mild traumatic brain injury. *Am. J. Psychiatry* **166:** 768–776.

40. Snell, F.I. & M.J. Halter. 2010. A signature wound of war: mild traumatic brain injury. *J. Psychosoc. Nurs. Ment. Health Serv.* **48:** 22–28.

41. Prigatano, G.P. 1992. Personality disturbances associated with traumatic brain injury. *J. Consult. Clin. Psychol.* **60:** 360–368.

42. Giacino, J.T. & K.D. Cicerone. 1998. Varieties of deficit unawareness after brain injury. *J. Head Trauma Rehabil.* **13:** 1–15.

43. Defense and Veterans Brain Injury Center Working Group on the Acute Management of Concussion/Mild Traumatic Brain Injury (mTBI) in the Deployed Setting. 2008. *Clinical Practice Guideline.* Washington, DC. October 10.

44. Iverson, G.L., J.A. Langlois, M.A. McCrea & J.P. Kelly. 2009. Challenges associated with post-deployment screening for mild traumatic brain injury in military personnel. *Clin. Neuropsychol.* **23:** 1299–1314.

45. Jaffee, M.S., K.M. Helmick, P.D. Girard, *et al.* 2009. Acute clinical care and care coordination for traumatic brain injury within Department of Defense. *J. Rehabil. Res. Dev.* **46:** 655–666.

46. McCrea, M., J.P. Kelly, C. Randolph, *et al.* 1998. Standardized assessment of concussion (SAC): on site mental status evaluation of the athlete. *J. Head Trauma Rehabil.* **13:** 27–35.

47. Schwab, K.A., B. Ivins, G. Cramer, *et al.* 2007. Screening for traumatic brain injury in troops returning from deployment in Afghanistan and Iraq: initial investigation of the usefulness of a short screening tool for traumatic brain injury. *J. Head Trauma Rehabil.* **22:** 377–389.

48. Terrio, H., L.A. Brenner, B.J. Ivins, *et al.* 2009. Traumatic brain injury screening: preliminary findings in a US Army brigade combat team. *J. Head Trauma Rehabil.* **24:** 14–23.

49. Bleiberg, J., A.N. Cernich, K. Cameron, *et al.* 2004. Duration of cognitive impairment after sports concussion. *Neurosurgery* **54:** 1073–1078.

50. Belanger, H.G., G. Curtiss, J.A. Demery, *et al.* 2005. Factors moderating neuropsychological outcomes following mild traumatic brain injury: a meta-analysis. *J. Int. Neuropsychol. Soc.* **11:** 215–227.

51. Ivins, B.J., R. Kane & K.A. Schwab. 2009. Performance on the Automated Neuropsychological Assessment Metrics in a nonclinical sample of soldiers screened for mild TBI after returning from Iraq and Afghanistan: a descriptive analysis. *J. Head Trauma Rehabil.* **24:** 24–31.

52. Van Boven, R.W., G.S. Harrington, D.B. Hackney, *et al.* 2009. Advances in neuroimaging of traumatic brain injury and posttraumatic stress disorder. *J. Rehabil. Res. Dev.* **46:** 717–757.

53. Niogi, S.N., P. Mukherjee, J. Ghajar, *et al.* 2008. Extent of microstructural white matter injury in postconcussive syndrome correlates with impaired cognitive reaction time: a 3T diffusion tensor imaging study of mild traumatic brain injury. *AJNR. Am. J. Neuroradiol.* **29:** 967–973.

54. Scheid, R., K. Walther, T. Guthke, *et al.* 2006. Cognitive sequelae of diffuse axonal injury. *Arch. Neurol.* **63:** 418–424.

55. Lee, H., M. Wintermark, A.D. Gean, *et al.* 2008. Focal lesions in acute mild traumatic brain injury and neurocognitive outcome: CT versus 3T MRI. *J. Neurotrauma* **25:** 1049–1056.

56. Belanger, H.G., R.D. Vanderploeg, G. Curtiss & D.L. Warden. 2007. Recent neuroimaging techniques in mild traumatic brain injury. *J. Neuropsychiatry Clin. Neurosci.* **19:** 5–20.

57. Ptito, A., J.K. Chen & K.M. Johnston. 2007. Contributions of functional magnetic resonance imaging (fMRI) to sport concussion evaluation. *NeuroRehabilitation* **22:** 217–227.

58. Humayun, M.S., S.K. Presty, N.D. Lafrance, *et al.* 1989. Local cerebral glucose abnormalities in mild closed head injured patients with cognitive impairments. *Nucl. Med. Commun.* **10:** 335–344.

59. Gross, H., A. Kling, G. Henry, *et al.* 1996. Local cerebral glucose metabolism in patients with long-term behavioral and cognitive deficits following mild traumatic brain injury. *J. Neuropsychiatry Clin. Neurosci.* **8:** 324–334.

60. Chen, S.H., D.A. Kareken, P.S. Fastenau, *et al.* 2003. A study of persistent post-concussion symptoms in mild head trauma using positron emission tomography. *J. Neurol. Neurosurg. Psychiatry* **74:** 326–332.

61. Ichise, M., D. Chung, P. Wang, *et al.* 1994. Technetium-99m-HMPAO SPECT, CT and MRI in the evaluation of patients with chronic traumatic brain injury: a correlation with neuropsychological performance. *J. Nucl. Med.* **35:** 217–226.

62. Umile, E.M., R.C. Plotkin & M.E. Sandel. 1998. Functional assessment of mild traumatic brain injury using SPECT and neuropsychological testing. *Brain Inj.* **12:** 577–594.

63. Gaetz, M. & D.M. Bernstein. 2001. The current status of electrophysiologic procedures for the assessment of mild traumatic brain injury. *J. Head Trauma Rehabil.* **16:** 386–405.

64. Huang, M., R.J. Theilmann, A. Robb, *et al.* 2009. Integrated imaging approach with MEG and DTI to detect mild traumatic brain injury in military and civilian patients. *J. Neurotrauma* **26:** 1213–1226.

65. Basser, P.J. & C. Pierpaoli. 1996. Microstructural and physiological features of tissues elucidated by quantitative-diffusion-tensor MRI. *J. Magn. Reson. Series B.* **111:** 209–219.

66. Niogi, S.N. & P. Mukherjee. 2010. Diffusion tensor imaging of mild traumatic brain injury. *J. Head Trauma Rehabil.* In press.

67. Song, S.K., S.W. Sun, M.J. Ramsbottom, *et al.* 2002. Dysmyelination revealed through MRI as increased radial (but unchanged axial) diffusion of water. *Neuroimage* **17:** 1429–1436.

68. Lipton, M.L., E. Gellella, C. Lo, *et al.* 2008. Multifocal white matter ultrastructural abnormalities in mild traumatic brain injury with cognitive disability: a voxel-wise analysis of diffusion tensor imaging. *J. Neurotrauma* **25:** 1335–1342.

69. Rutgers, D.R., F. Toulgoat, J. Cazejust, *et al.* 2008. White matter abnormalities in mild traumatic brain injury: a diffusion tensor imaging study. *AJNR. Am. J. Neuroradiol.* **29:** 514–519.

70. Lipton, M.L., E. Gulko, M.E. Zimmerman, *et al.* Diffusion-tensor imaging implicates prefrontal axonal injury in executive function impairment following very mild traumatic brain injury. *Radiology* **252:** 816–824.

71. Bigler, E.D. & J.J. Bazarian. 2010. Diffusion tensor imaging: a biomarker for mild traumatic brain injury? *Neurology* **74:** 626–627.

72. Mayer, A.R., J. Ling, M.V. Mannell, *et al.* 2010. A prospective diffusion tensor imaging study in mild traumatic brain injury. *Neurology* **74:** 643–650.

73. Miles, L., R.I. Grossman, G. Johnson, *et al.* 2008. Short-term DTI predictors of cognitive dysfunction in mild traumatic brain injury. *Brain Inj.* **22:** 115–122.

74. Stuss, D.T. & C.A. Gow. 1992. Frontal dysfunction after traumatic brain injury. *Neuropsychia. Neuropsychol. Behav. Neurol.* **5:** 272–282.

75. Fork, M., C. Bartels, A.D. Ebert, *et al.* 2005. Neuropsychological sequelae of diffuse traumatic brain injury. *Brain Inj.* **19:** 101–108.

76. Ghajar, J. & R.B. Ivry. 2008. The predictive brain state: timing deficiency in traumatic brain injury? *Neurorehabil. Neural Repair* **22:** 217–227.

77. Stuss, D.T., L.L. Stethem, H. Hugenholtz, *et al.* 1989. Reaction time after head injury: fatigue, divided and focused attention, and consistency of performance. *J. Neurol. Neurosurg. Psychiatry* **52:** 742–748.

78. Munoz, D.P. & S. Everling. 2004. Look away: the anti-saccade task and the voluntary control of eye movement. *Nat. Rev.* **5:** 218–228.

79. Heitger, M.H., R.D. Jones, A.D. Macleod, *et al.* 2009. Impaired eye movements in post-concussion syndrome indicate suboptimal brain function beyond the influence of depression, malingering or intellectual ability. *Brain* **132:** 2850–2870.

80. Crevits, L., M.C. Hanse, P. Tummers & G.V. Maele. 2000. Anti-saccades and remembered saccades in mild traumatic brain injury. *J. Neurol.* **247:** 179–182.

81. Maruta, J., M. Suh, S.N. Niogi, *et al.* 2010. Visual tracking synchronization as a metric for concussion screening. *J. Head Trauma Rehabil.* In press.

82. Lisberger, S.G., E.J. Morris & L. Tychsen. 1987. Visual motion processing and sensory-motor integration for smooth pursuit eye movements. *Annu. Rev. Neurosci.* **10:** 97–129.

83. Chen, Y., P.S. Holzman & K. Nakayama. 2002. Visual and cognitive control of attention in smooth pursuit. *Prog. Brain Res.* **140:** 255–265.

84. Krauzlis, R.J. 2005. The control of voluntary eye movements: new perspectives. *Neuroscientist* **11:** 124–137.

85. Barnes, G.R. 2008. Cognitive processes involved in smooth pursuit eye movements. *Brain Cogn.* **68:** 309–326.

86. Umeda, Y. & E. Sakata. 1975. The circular eye-tracking test. I. Simultaneous recording of the horizontal and vertical component of eye movement in the eye-tracking test. *ORL. J. Otorhinolaryngol. Relat. Spec.* **37:** 290–298.

87. Van Der Steen, J., E.P. Tamminga & H. Collewijn. 1983. A comparison of oculomotor pursuit of a target in circular real, beta or sigma motion. *Vis. Res.* **23:** 1655–1661.

88. Miller, E.K. & J.D. Cohen. 2001. An integrative theory of prefrontal cortex function. *Annu. Rev. Neurosci.* **24:** 167–202.

89. McAllister, T.W., M.B. Sparling, L.A. Flashman, *et al.* 2001. Differential working memory load effects after mild traumatic brain injury. *Neuroimage* **14:** 1004–1012.

90. Robertson, I.H., T. Manly, J. Andrade, *et al.* 1997. 'Oops!': performance correlates of everyday attentional failures in traumatic brain injured and normal subjects. *Neuropsychologia* **35:** 747–758.

91. Pardo, J.V., P.T. Fox & M.E. Raichle. 1991. Localization of a human system for sustained attention by positron emission tomography. *Nature* **349:** 61–64.

92. Jonides, J., E.E. Smith, R.A. Koeppe, *et al.* 1993. Spatial working memory in humans as revealed by PET. *Nature* **363:** 623–625.

93. Stoodley, C.J. & J.D. Schmahmann. 2009. Functional topography in the human cerebellum: a meta-analysis of neuroimaging studies. *Neuroimage* **44:** 489–501.

94. Barbas, H. & D.N. Pandya. 1984. Topography of commissural fibers of the prefrontal cortex in the rhesus monkey. *Exp. Brain Res.* **55:** 187–191.

95. Fox, M.D., M. Corbetta, A.Z. Snyder, *et al.* 2006. Spontaneous neuronal activity distinguishes human dorsal and ventral attention systems. *Proc. Natl. Acad. Sci. USA* **103:** 10046–10051.

96. Takeuchi, H., A. Sekiguchi, Y. Taki, *et al.* 2010. Training of working memory impacts structural connectivity. *J. Neurosci.* **30:** 3297–3303.

Ann. N.Y. Acad. Sci. ISSN 0077-8923

ANNALS OF THE NEW YORK ACADEMY OF SCIENCES

Issue: *Psychiatric and Neurologic Aspects of War*

Posttraumatic stress disorder: a history and a critique

Nancy C. Andreasen

Psychiatric Iowa Neuroimaging Consortium, Iowa City, Iowa

Address for correspondence: Nancy C. Andreasen, M.D., Ph.D., Andrew H. Woods Chair of Psychiatry Psychiatric Iowa Neuroimaging Consortium, 200 Hawkins Drive, Room W278 GH, Iowa City, Iowa 52242. nancy-andreasen@uiowa.edu

Although posttraumatic stress disorder (PTSD) is sometimes considered to be a relatively new diagnosis, as the name first appeared in 1980, the concept of the disorder has a very long history. That history has often been linked to the history of war, but the disorder has also been frequently described in civilian settings involving natural disasters, mass catastrophes, and serious accidental injuries. The diagnosis first appeared in the official nomenclature when *Diagnostic and Statistical Manual of Mental Disorders* (DSM)-I was published in 1952 under the name gross stress reaction. It was omitted, however, in the next edition in 1968, after a long period of relative peace. When DSM-III was developed in the mid-1980s the recent occurrence of the Vietnam War provoked a more thorough examination of the disorder. PTSD was defined as a stress disorder that is a final common pathway occurring as a consequence of many different types of stressors, including both combat and civilian stress. The definition of PTSD has filled an important niche in clinical psychiatry. Its definition continues to raise important questions about the relationship between a stressor, the individual experiencing it, and the characteristic symptoms.

Keywords: PTSD; history; DSM-III; DSM-IV

Introduction

Although posttraumatic stress disorder (PTSD) is sometimes considered to be a relatively new diagnostic concept, given that it was first described using that name in the third edition of the *Diagnostic and Statistical Manual of Mental Disorders* (DSM-III),[1] the concept of the disorder is considerably older. In order to understand where we are now, it is helpful to consider where we have been in the past. The disorder that we now know as PTSD has had a long and interesting history.

Historical antecedents to diagnostic manuals

Early descriptive accounts of stress-related disorders are often linked to the history of warfare. Stephen Crane's introspective accounts of a youth's reaction to the stress of a battle during the Civil War provides an early example. The Youth (Henry Fleming), the main character in *The Red Badge of Courage,* describes a range of anxiety symptoms that he experiences during combat.[2] The horrors of trench warfare during World War I, and their resultant psychological consequences, led to formulation of the concept of "shell shock," initially thought to be a consequence of exposure to intense artillery. Subsequently clinicians realized that the symptoms were due to the stress of the combat experience.

Interest in shellshock waned as memories of World War I receded, but it was reawakened by the advent of World War II. As had happened previously, soldiers who were chronically exposed to combat experienced a syndrome characterized anxiety, intense autonomic arousal, reliving, and sensitivity to stimuli that are reminiscent of the original trauma.[3] This syndrome was given a variety of different names: traumatic war neurosis, combat fatigue, battle stress, and gross stress reaction. When the war drew to its end, another type of stress was discovered: the experience of death camp survivors.[4]

In the pre-DSM era a literature also accumulated on psychiatric disorders that occurred as a consequence of exposure to noncombat injuries. Alexandra Adler wrote seminal papers on the psychological effects of stress in civilian settings, beginning with

doi: 10.1111/j.1749-6632.2010.05699.x

her work on the Cocoanut Grove fire, and described both the clinical picture and the epidemiology.[5] She also compared the effects of stress reactions occurring as a consequence of head injuries with those that occurred because of psychological stress, thereby anticipating current discussions of the relationship between PTSD and traumatic brain injury (TBI) in the context of the conflicts in Iraq and Afghanistan.[6,7] Nemiah[8] wrote about the effects of industrial accidents, and Hamburg *et al.*[9] wrote about the effects of burn injuries. The descriptions of the syndromes occurring as a consequence of these diverse stressors were surprisingly similar.

During this time conceptual frameworks for understanding the effects of stress as a predisposing factor for mental illness also developed and matured. Two main positions were articulated. The first position (the "biological school"), represented by thinkers such as Selye, emphasized the role of physical mechanisms.[10] Selye coined the term "stress" and hypothesized that it was mediated by the hypothalamic–pituitary–adrenal (HPA) axis. He described the general adaptation syndrome as a healthy response to stress, and he considered the traumatic neuroses to be a consequence of chronic or severe stress. The second position (the "psychological school") had its roots in the psychodynamic tradition.[11] It emphasized the role of the unconscious, and of repressed memories and early childhood traumata. It led eventually to descriptions of mechanisms of defense and of their role in producing or preventing disease. These two conceptual frameworks set the stage for the history that was to follow.

Defining gross stress reaction

Because World War II brought together psychiatrists from all over the world and from all over the United States, it became clear that they could differ in training, conceptual framework, and in approaches to diagnosis and treatment. A consensus developed that some standardization was needed, and this challenge led to the creation of the first diagnostic manual, developed by the Veterans' Administration. This provided an incentive to the American Psychiatric Association (APA) to develop its own manual: the first Diagnostic and Statistical Manual of the APA, or DSM-I, which appeared in 1952.[12] This manual included a category called gross stress reaction. It was defined as a stress syndrome that is a response

to an exceptional physical or mental stress, such as a natural catastrophe or battle; it occurs in people who are otherwise normal; and it must subside in days to weeks; if it persists, another diagnosis should be made.

The first revision of this manual, DSM-II, was published in 1968.[13] Without any explanation, the diagnosis of gross stress reaction was omitted. The most plausible explanation for the omission is that the concept was closely linked to warfare and combat, and DSM-II was written in a peaceful era. Consequently, between 1968 and 1980 no official diagnosis for stress disorders was available.

This change in the official APA nosology and classification occurred just as the Vietnam War was beginning its escalation. The publication of DSM-II and the Tet Offensive occurred in the same year. The war refocused attention on postcombat stress disorders. As the war became more unpopular, returning veterans were often greeted with contempt. No accepted diagnosis was available for those who had psychiatric symptoms, and treatment facilities were minimal. Activists began to note the inequity created by sending men to war without recognizing the psychiatric consequences and the need to provide adequate treatment for them. When the DSM-III Task Force was assembled in the mid-1980s, the status of gross stress reaction was one of the issues that it faced. Should this diagnosis be included again? And if so, should the old DSM-I definition be modified in any way?

Because I had studied stress disorders in burn patients,[14–17] I was assigned the task of determining whether the diagnosis should be reintroduced and, if so, how it should be defined. The task required addressing three major issues.

The stressor

How severe should it be? Does the type of stressor matter? For example, if the stressor involves a cruelty inflicted by human beings, does that create more psychological stress than one occurring by accident? Does being in a death camp create more distress than experiencing a natural disaster such as a hurricane? Does the duration of the stressor matter? What is the relationship between the time of occurrence of the stressor and the onset of symptoms? Must the onset be immediate, or can it be delayed, as often occurs in postcombat situations? Should there be a specific diagnosis for each of the many different kinds of stressors? Should there be a specific diagnosis of "Post-Vietnam Syndrome," as the pro-Vietnam veteran activists were advocating?

The stressed

DSM-I specified that gross stress reaction should only be diagnosed in individuals who were normal prior to experiencing the stress. If they had another psychiatric disorder, such as depression, the stress reaction would be treated as secondary to that and would not be given an independent diagnosis. Implicitly, this approach suggested that gross stress reaction was a diagnosis that should not confer any stigma; it implied that people who developed it were normal healthy individuals who had simply been temporarily overcome by a stress that was overwhelming. If this approach were to be adopted in DSM-III, it would ignore the accumulating evidence that protective and predisposing factors could play a role in response to stress. Might it not be the case that people with preexisting disorders, such as depression, are more vulnerable to stress and therefore more prone to develop an independent pathological response to it that should also be recognized and treated?

The symptoms

In the context of the biological versus psychodynamic interpretations of the stress response, how should the characteristic symptoms be described and defined? Should these emphasize the physical symptoms of the stress response, such as the intense autonomic arousal? Or should they emphasize the more psychological symptoms, such as dissociation, reliving, and psychic numbing? How should they be described in terms of time of onset? Should acute reactions be the only ones emphasized? Or should a delayed onset also be recognized? How long might the symptoms persist? DSM-I had specified that the disorder should subside in days to weeks, and that another diagnosis should be given if the symptoms did not remit. Should this also be the model for DSM-III?

DSM-III and the definition of PTSD

The decision to include a diagnosis that described a psychiatric syndrome occurring as a consequence of an exposure to a significant stressor was very easy to make. By the mid-1970s there was an extensive research literature describing both the epidemiology

and symptomatology of syndromes occurring as a consequence of stress.[3–9,14–17] Although the absence of a diagnosis for stress disorders was a problem for government systems such as the Department of Veterans Affairs (VA), during the 1970s most of psychiatry in fact took little note of the DSM-II classification system. The absence of an "official" diagnosis for stress disorders did not preclude their study by researchers. Consequently, there was a great deal of evidence indicating that stress disorders were common, that they had characteristic symptoms, and that they were a final common pathway reached by experiencing a variety of different types of stressors: combat, death camps, industrial accidents, natural disasters, mass catastrophes, and violent acts against individuals. The issue was simply how to incorporate all this evidence into the definition and description of the disorder.

The stressor was defined relatively narrowly: as so severe that it would produce significant symptoms in almost anyone, as outside the range of normal human experience. It could be physical or psychological or both. In recognition that a stress syndrome is a final common pathway with many entry points reflecting the variety of stressors that can produce it, there was no specific "post-Vietnam syndrome." Instead the new diagnosis was given the very general name of "post-traumatic stress disorder." For the stressed, there was no requirement of preexisting normality; this decision was based on the recognition that individuals vary in vulnerability and resilience. The symptoms were divided into three general categories: reexperiencing (including dissociative-like states), numbing of responsiveness, and cognitive or autonomic symptoms. The onset could be either acute or delayed.

The reemergence of a diagnostic category for stress syndromes after 22 years of absence clearly filled a niche. The diagnosis soon became widely used clinically, and it also became the object of many research studies.[18] The rapid and widespread acceptance also led to some unintended consequences. Despite the narrow definition of the stressor specified in the diagnostic criteria, the concept of was steadily broadened by clinicians (and also researchers) to include milder stressors that were not intended for inclusion (e.g., auto accidents, childhood abuse). The concept of dissociation was increasingly emphasized, which introduced a psychodynamic coloring that was not intended, given that DSM-III attempted to avoid alliances with any of the various competing models of disease mechanisms that were available. The temporal juxtaposition between the stressor and the symptoms was allowed to become longer and longer, so that a delayed onset became the norm. As a consequence, dissociative syndromes after "childhood abuse" (broadly defined and sometimes poorly documented) were reported with increasing frequency. The diagnosis, assumed to be relatively rare in peacetime, became much more common.

When DSM-III-R appeared just 7 years later, in 1987, many of these unintended modifications were reified in new diagnostic criteria.[19] It was now 42 years after the conclusion of World War II and 24 years after the end of the Vietnam War, both of which had shaped the conceptualization of PTSD in DSM-III. Clinicians were more interested in the problems of here-and-now, and so the diagnosis of PTSD was steadily changing in that direction. DSM-III-R broadened the definition of the stressor; it was no longer defined as so severe that it would produce symptoms in almost anyone. It emphasized the psychological nature of the stressor and minimized physical components. It expanded the range of symptoms to include a stronger emphasis on dissociation, and it eliminated the acute form of the disorder. These revisions raised several concerns about the degree and rapidity of the change in conceptualization. The plight of Nazi death camp victims and the combat stress of Normandy or Iwo Jima had been the prototype for the DSM-III definition of PTSD. Had the diagnosis become too broad? Had the diagnosis become too psychodynamic at the expense of its biological underpinnings? Does using the same diagnosis for death camp survivors and victims of auto accidents trivialize the diagnosis?

The process of change continued when DSM-IV was completed in 1994.[20] It too was written in a time of relative peace, and this was reflected in the modifications made to the definition of PTSD. The definition of the stressor was further modified, but still open to a broad interpretation; for example, it was expanded so that the stress was no longer limited to one experienced by the patient himself; it could be "a threat to the physical integrity of self or others" (p. 427).[20] Acute stress disorder was added, but with an emphasis on dissociative symptoms.

Consequently, these changes raised concerns similar to those created by DSM-III-R.

PTSD at present

The occurrence of 9/11 and other acts of international terrorism have changed the context for conceptualizing stressors. The United States is now at war again in both Iraq and Afghanistan, and consequently combat-induced PTSD is now very much on the public and psychiatric radar screen. The biological aspects of the disorder have also reemerged in importance. For example, the relationship between TBI and PTSD requires exploration.[7] Furthermore, advances in neuroscience have facilitated the identification of stress circuitry in the brain through neuroimaging and animal studies.[21] The rising rates of PTSD in military personnel have set off alarm bells, and they have also caused some to question the validity of the diagnosis. Others point to valid reasons for the rise, such as prolonged deployments, the frustrations inherent in counterterrorist warfare, and the recruitment of reservists and National Guard members who did not expect to engage in combat when they joined. The burden on VA Hospitals has become so heavy that an Institute of Medicine study was requested and completed. This study, in three volumes, supports the validity of the diagnosis and the increased need for services.[22–24]

At present the existence of a valid syndrome occurring as a consequence of severe stress can not be questioned. The diagnosis of PTSD fills an important niche in psychiatric nosology. But there are also still many ambiguities that must be resolved and gray areas that must be clarified. These include the interplay between physical and psychological components, the perils of over diagnosing versus under diagnosing, and the complex interaction between the severity and duration of the stressor and the ego strength and coping mechanisms of the individual who is stressed.

Conflicts of interest

The author declares no conflicts of interest.

References

1. American Psychiatric Association Committee on Nomenclature and Statistics. 1980. *Diagnostic and Statistical Manual of Mental Disorders*, 3rd ed. American Psychiatric Association. Washington, DC.

2. Crane, S. 1977. The red badge of courage. In *The Portable Stephen Crane*. Penguin Books. New York.

3. Grinker, R.R. & J.P. Spiegel. 1944. Brief psychotherapy in war neuroses. *Psychsom. Med.* **6:** 123–131.

4. Kral, V.A. 1951. Psychiatric observations under severe chronic stress. *Am. J. Psychiatry* **108:** 185–192.

5. Adler, A. 1943. Neuropsychiatric complications in victims of Boston's Cocoanut Grove disaster. *JAMA* **123:** 1098–1101.

6. Adler, A. 1945. Two different types of post-traumatic neuroses. *Am. J. Psychiatry* **102:** 237–240.

7. Bhattacharjee, Y. 2008. Shell shock revisited: solving the puzzle of blast trauma. *Science* **319:** 406–408.

8. Nemiah, J.C. 1963. Psychological complications in industrial injuries. *Arch. Environ. Health* **7:** 481–487.

9. Hamburg, D.A., C.P. Artz, E. Reiss, *et al.* 1953. Clinical importance of emotional problems in the care of patients with burns. *N. Engl. J. Med.* **248:** 355–359.

10. Selye, H. 1956. Stress and psychiatry. *Am. J. Psychiatry* **113:** 423–427.

11. Fenichel, O. 1996. *The Psychoanalytic Theory of Neurosis*, 2nd ed. Routledge. London.

12. American Psychiatric Association Committee on Nomenclature and Statistics. 1952. *Diagnostic and Statistical Manual of Mental Disorders*. American Psychiatric Association. Washington, DC.

13. American Psychiatric Association Committee on Nomenclature and Statistics. 1968. *Diagnostic and Statistical Manual of Mental Disorders*, 2nd ed. American Psychiatric Association. Washington, DC.

14. Andreasen, N.J.C., R. Noyes, C.E. Hartford, *et al.* 1972. Management of emotional reactions in seriously burned adults. *N. Engl. J. Med.* **286:** 65–69.

15. Andreasen, N.J.C. 1974. Neuropsychiatric complications in burn patients. *Int. J. Psychiatry Med.* **5:** 161–171.

16. Andreasen, N.J.C., R. Noyes & C.E. Hartford. 1972. Factors influencing adjustment of burn patients during hospitalization. *Psychosom. Med.* **34:** 517–525.

17. Andreasen, N.J.C., A.S. Norris & C.E. Hartford. 1971. Incidence of long-term psychiatric complications in severely burned adults. *Ann. Surg.* **174:** 785–793.

18. Andreasen, N.C. 1985. Posttraumatic stress disorder. In *Comprehensive Textbook of Psychiatry*, 3rd ed. H.I. Kaplan & B.J. Sadock, Eds.: 918–924. Williams and Wilkins. New York.

19. American Psychiatric Association Committee on Nomenclature and Statistics. 1987. *Diagnostic and Statistical Manual of Mental Disorders*, 3rd ed. revised. American Psychiatric Association. Washington, DC.

20. American Psychiatric Association Committee on Nomenclature and Statistics. 1994. *Diagnostic and Statistical Manual of Mental Disorders*, 4rd ed. American Psychiatric Association. Washington, DC.

21. Etkin, A & T.D. Wager. 2007. Functional neuroimaging of anxiety: a meta-analysis of emotional processing in PTSD, social anxiety disorder, and specific phobia. *Am. J. Psychiatry* **164:** 1476–1488.

22. Institute of Medicine. 2006. Posttraumatic stress disorder: diagnosis and assessment. Washington, DC.

23. Institute of Medicine. 2007. Treatment of PTSD: an assessment of the evidence. Washington, DC.

24. Institute of Medicine. 2007. PTSD compensation and military service. Washington, DC.

Ann. N.Y. Acad. Sci. ISSN 0077-8923

ANNALS OF THE NEW YORK ACADEMY OF SCIENCES

Issue: *Psychiatric and Neurologic Aspects of War*

Posttraumatic stress disorder and traumatic stress: from bench to bedside, from war to disaster

Robert J. Ursano, Matthew Goldenberg, Lei Zhang, Janis Carlton, Carol S. Fullerton, He Li, Luke Johnson, and David Benedek

Center for the Study of Traumatic Stress, Department of Psychiatry, Uniformed Services University School of Medicine, Bethesda, Maryland

Address for correspondence: Robert J. Ursano, M.D., Center for the Study of Traumatic Stress and Chairman, Department of Psychiatry, Uniformed Services University School of Medicine, 4301 Jones Bridge Rd, Bethesda, Maryland 20814. rursano@usuhs.mil

War is a tragic event and its mental health consequences can be profound. Recent studies indicate substantial rates of posttraumatic stress disorder and other behavioral alterations because of war exposure. Understanding the psychological, behavioral, and neurobiological mechanism of mental health and behavioral changes related to war exposure is critical to helping those in need of care. Substantial work to encourage bench to bedside to community knowledge and communication is a core component of addressing this world health need.

Keywords: posttraumatic stress disorder; disaster; treatment; neurobiology

The ongoing war in Iraq and Afghanistan has led to high rates of posttraumatic stress, posttraumatic stress disorder (PTSD), depression, suicide, comorbid concussions, traumatic brain injuries (TBIs), and other combat-related mental and behavioral health needs. Stigma associated with these problems and other barriers to care heighten the complexity of addressing these mental and behavioral health needs. War inflicts a serious toll on society, particularly among the soldiers who must fight and their families. The physical effects of war—battle injuries and fatalities—have long been known and counted, but the psychological and behavioral effects of conflict—always known and often scorned—have only, more recently, been the focus of societal medical attention.

The behavioral and psychological outcomes of exposure to traumatic events are complex and multifactorial. The effects range from presumed epigenetic alterations to the impact of exposure to life threat and altered interpersonal and social support systems. In addition, a significant body of research indicates that the psychological effects of repeated traumatic event exposure are cumulative.[1,2] However, repeated exposure to traumatic events has rarely been studied. In addition, while there are multiple animal models of stress-associated illnesses, such as PTSD, depression, and substance abuse, these models replicate components of the human disorders but do not represent total models of the disease.

While the majority of soldiers and veterans exhibit significant resilience in the face of trauma and growth as a result of their military service, many develop significant psychological and behavioral problems related to their war experience. These problems include mental disorders, such as PTSD, depression and substance abuse, as well as risk behaviors, and increased rates of suicide. War veterans also show increased risk of physical health problems and early death. Understanding how and why such problems occur can help to identify those service members at highest risk and lead to the development of interventions to prevent and mitigate adverse outcomes.

Disorders, illness, and distress

In the last few decades we have gained a great deal of knowledge about the effects of war, although the observation of war syndromes span hundreds of

doi: 10.1111/j.1749-6632.2010.05721.x

 Ann. N.Y. Acad. Sci. 1208 (2010) 72–81 © 2010 Association for Research in Nervous and Mental Disease.

years and include the "thousand yard stare," "soldier's heart," "shell shock," and "combat fatigue."[3] Perhaps the most studied of these modern descriptions of war and trauma-related disorders is PTSD. PTSD, formally defined in the early 1980s, is a mental condition that develops following a traumatic event and is characterized by intrusive recollections of the event, avoidance of event-related stimuli, and hyperarousal including irritability, startle response, and sleep disturbance. PTSD may come in mild and severe forms and may be one of the "common colds" of psychiatric illness. That is, many may get it in a lifetime, most will recover, but for some, this common cold can become pneumonia with serious morbidity and impairment.

One of the most vexing questions surrounding the return of our nation's warriors to the home front is the detection and management of emerging PTSD and other posttraumatic distress symptoms, which persist and disrupt social, occupational, or interpersonal function. The process by which we reintegrate returning soldiers and screen for potential long-term adjustment problems has undergone considerable scrutiny and reform during our prolonged military operations in Iraq and Afghanistan. Studies suggest that between 10 and 20% of combat veterans in the current conflicts in Iraq and Afghanistan develop PTSD.[4] There is increasing evidence that there is a relationship between PTSD and other adverse psychosocial outcomes of war including substance abuse, aggression, and suicide. Many soldiers who do not meet criteria for a diagnosis of PTSD also experience significant psychological difficulties related to their war experiences, including depression, anxiety, and adjustment problems. Using data on predeployment mental health utilization the Mental Health Advisory Team (MHAT)-VI demonstrated that population-level mental health after a 1-year deployment begins to return to predeployment levels after approximately 2 years at home station and essentially resets after 3 years at home station.[5] Thus, the Army has identified a "Boots-on-the-Ground to Home Station Dwell Time" or "BOG: Dwell" ratio of 1 : 2 or 1 : 3 as critical to reestablishing the mental health of the fighting force.

Suicide

In the present wars of Iraq and Afghanistan, suicide behaviors have been of increasing concern, particularly in the U.S. Army and U.S. Marine Corps.

Since 2005, the suicide rates in the U.S. Army have climbed steadily in the face of ongoing wars in Iraq and Afghanistan and now (20 per 100,000 per year) are about double the prewar rate. Suicide prevention is a major priority of the military leadership and several prevention programs have been implemented in recent years.[6] The Army has also devoted unprecedented resources (including a recent $50 million grant) to studying suicide in hopes of better understanding the phenomenon and preventing future tragedy.[7] The new 5-year study funded by the National Institutes of Mental Health, the Army STARRS (Study to Assess Risk and Resilience in Service Members) is the largest study ever to address suicide in the Army and perhaps suicide in general as a national problem. The study is a "Framingham" type study, meant to identify risk and resilience factors—psychological, interpersonal, community, and neurobiological—for suicidal behaviors and also for PTSD, depression, and substance abuse.

Suicide is a multidetermined outcome that usually occurs as a result of a number of factors including individual vulnerabilities (e.g., distress intolerance or the presence of a mental disorder, such as depression or PTSD) and stressful life experiences (e.g., relationship problems or financial difficulties). For decades, service members committed suicide more infrequently than their civilian counterparts, but in 2008 the suicide rate in the U.S. Army reached a 28-year high and exceeded the rate in the age-matched general population. That the military had lower rates of suicide than the civilian population suggests that (1) the military may have comprised fewer vulnerable persons, (2) the benefits of service in the military in terms of steady work and social support/cohesion outweighed the inherent stress of military life, or most likely, (3) some combination of the two. What, then, has changed to account for the significant rise in the suicide rate? Numerous possible contributors are present: the stressors associated with prolonged war—multiple deployments, longer separation from family supports, increased combat exposure, more available fatal means in combat theaters and elevated rates of mental disorders, such as PTSD, as well as potentially altered recruitment standards. Veterans who screen positive for PTSD have been found to be four times more likely to experience suicidal ideation as those without PTSD.[8]

One factor that has often been implicated in suicides is the distress caused by problems in soldiers" intimate relationships, especially infidelity or breakups. This risk factor is also prominent in civilian suicides. Service members whose relationships are characterized by excessive enmeshment (i.e., they are particularly reliant on their intimate relationships for their identity) may be particularly vulnerable to a change in relationship status.[9] War can strain even strong, previously healthy relationships as well. The long-term physical separation necessitated by deployment is often quite difficult, especially for young couples and those with young children. Soldiers who are informed of family stressors, such as illness or financial problems while in theater, may not be able to assist their families from afar, resulting in feelings of inadequacy, helplessness, and depression.

Upon return from deployment, some soldiers have a difficult time readjusting to their noncombat life and some spouses/partners have trouble relating to their soldiers" experiences of war including any psychological difficulties that have arisen. The divorce rate among service members has been reported to be slowly increasing throughout the course of the current wars,[10] although this is often a difficult index to track as it may drop to below average postwar. The fact that the war effort is being executed by such a small portion of society and that much of American society is largely unengaged may also contribute to feelings of isolation among soldiers and veterans. Although this is much less prominent than post Vietnam, it may still be a risk factor in some groups. This may be especially true for reservists and members of the National Guard who after deployment return to their homes, jobs, and communities often without their military colleagues.

Another factor that may lead to adverse outcomes for returning soldiers is physical injury. One of the great triumphs of modern military medicine has been the increasing survival rates of soldiers who sustain physical injuries on the battlefield. But while many service members are surviving wounds that would have previously been fatal, they are often left with prolonged physical disability. The psychological consequences of these injuries including loss of limb(s), paralysis, burns, or other disfigurement are beginning to be appreciated. Veterans with significant limitations in physical activity have higher rates of suicide than those without such limitations,[11] and

almost certainly suffer increased rates of psychiatric illness and adjustment difficulties. Another common physical injury in the recent conflicts is TBI and the psychological and behavioral consequences of TBI have been a focus of increasing study.[12]

Aggression and violence

As with suicide, violence toward others by service members and recent veterans has also been attracting increased attention, especially in the wake of the killing of several service members at a mental health clinic in Iraq by an Army sergeant in 2009. There is some, but not sufficient, evidence that war experience may contribute to an increased propensity toward aggression and violence. Some argue that a key task of effective warrior training is to overcome a natural disinclination for harming others. Soldiers therefore can have a difficult time "turning off" their aggressive ways upon returning from deployment.[13] Increased aggression may also be a result of PTSD, substance abuse, or other mental problems. Veterans of recent conflicts in Iraq and Afghanistan who screened positive for PTSD or subthreshold PTSD were more likely to report significantly greater anger, hostility, and aggression.[14] PTSD also substantially increases risk for suicide attempts even after adjusting for depression and also completed suicides reported as high as 9.8 times greater risk.[15–18]

Domestic or intimate partner violence (IPV) has been an issue of interest in the military for some time and has also been brought to attention by several high profile cases including the murder of several military spouses by their soldier husbands in 2004. Estimates of IPV among service members vary widely (13–58%), but most point to somewhat higher rates among service members than among demographically matched civilian controls.[19] More dramatic, though, are rates of IPV among veterans, especially those with PTSD. A survey as part of the National Vietnam Veterans Readjustment Study showed that about one-third of veterans with PTSD perpetrated IPV in the previous year, nearly three times the rate of both veterans without PTSD and the civilian general public.[20] Rates were even higher among the subset of veterans who were hospitalized for psychiatric illness or substance abuse. Another related issue that will require more study is that of war's effect on parent–child relationships. How does war exposure affect a soldier's ability to parent? Is child abuse and/or neglect more frequent among war-exposed soldiers?

Other adverse outcomes

Soldiers exposed to certain war experiences including violent combat, killing another person, or witnessing human trauma demonstrated more risk-taking behaviors upon returning home than those who were less exposed.[21] It is not clear why this is the case, but the disinhibition seems to be not merely the result of the increased substance use in this population.

Accidents are just one cause of increased morbidity and mortality among veterans, especially those with PTSD. Vietnam veterans with PTSD have been found to have a more than twofold risk of all-cause mortality including significantly elevated risks of cardiovascular death, cancer death, and death from "external causes" including homicides, suicides, and accidents.[22] TBI has also been called a "signature injury" of the present conflict and in its mild form is presently hotly debated as to its contributions to PTSD and to the morbidity of returning veterans.[12]

From bench to bedside: new areas for mechanisms, biomarkers, and treatment

Stress-related disorders are associated with changes in brain structure and function in key areas associated with stress responses, fear learning, and extinction: the hippocampus, amygdala, prefrontal cortex (PFC), hypothalamus, and cerebellum.

Substance abuse: cannabinoids

The comorbidity of stress-induced disorders and substance abuse is of particular importance in service members and is well documented but poorly understood. Cannabis use in particular has often been noted in soldiers after return from Iraq and Afghanistan. The endocannabinoid system is involved in complex modulation of stress responses, emotion, learning and memory, and reward/addiction pathways through the cannabinoid receptor type 1 (CBR-1). Abundant expression of CB1 has been reported in all key brain regions known to govern anxiety and stress response including the amygdala, hippocampus, interior cingulated cortex, PFC, periacqueductal gray matter, basal ganglia, and cerebellum.

The endocannabinoids are involved in a wide variety of physiological functions including pain, appetitive behaviors, reward, addictions, motor control, emotion, and learning and memory through the presynaptic CB1 receptor (e.g., Iversen[23]). The brain produces at least five endocannabinoids with submicromolar affinity for cannabinoid receptors. Anandamide is the best-studied endocannabinoid and has a high affinity for the CB1 receptor. The endocannabinoids may also be involved in cue-induced fear conditioning[24] and extinction of fear memories.[25–27]

CB1 knockout mice lack the CB1 receptor and shows vulnerability to stress and behavioral preservation after chronic stress associated with downregulation of CB1 receptors and 2-AG levels suggesting that CB1 activation is necessary for adaptation to stress.[28] Furthermore CB1 knockout mice show impaired extinction of aversive learning and their response to stress increases over time rather than developing adaptation and also show marked inability to extinguish fear conditioning.[29] Further evidence supports the role of endocannabinoids in anxiolytic-like effects in adult rats and in rat pups with isolation-induced stress.

Our group has initiated studies of the cerebellar cannabinoid systems and their relation to stress. There is evidence that the cerebellum may exert a significant influence on emotional memory and cognitive processing as well as mediate the altered time perception that is frequently associated with severe stress and is the most commonly reported symptom of peritraumatic dissociation. We carried out a series of experiments utilizing an animal model of repeated stress focusing on sex-related differences in brain regional CBR-1 expression and function particularly in the cerebellum. We found sex-related differences in CBR-1 mRNA in brain regions involved in mediation of stress responses and addiction including the cerebellum. We found basal rates of protein kinase C (PKC) phosphorylation of CBR-1 were higher in the cerebella of females and there were sex-related differences in PKC subtype activity associated with exposure to stress. CBR-1 signaling may have a role in stress-induced alterations in neurotransmission and behavior changes further implicating endocannabinoids in mediating aspects of the stress response including substance abuse, peritraumatic events, and development of PTSD.

Role of p11: a potential molecular mechanism and biomarker in PTSD

There is no objective laboratory biomarker test for PTSD. Strategies for systematic development of biomarkers are needed.[30] Currently, clinicians rely upon symptom checklists, clinical histories, mental status, patient self-reports, and symptom duration to make a diagnosis. Development of a blood-based biomarker test is a potential tool to aid in PTSD diagnosis. Previous studies have shown downregulation of p11, an S-100 calcium-binding protein, in depression,[31] a common comorbid disorder of PTSD.

Over the last decade many studies have reported abnormal hypothalamic–pituitary–adrenal axis activity in PTSD, but these studies do not always report changes in the same direction. A recent study demonstrated that dexamethasone (Dex), a synthetic glucocorticoid, can upregulate p11.[32] These observations led to our hypothesis that in PTSD patients there may be an altered expression of p11 that is mediated by glucocorticoid receptors (GRs). To test this idea, we determined levels of p11 mRNA expression in the postmortem PFC of PTSD patients. In our previous study,[33] we demonstrated that stress, induced by 3 days of inescapable shock, increases both p11 mRNA levels in the PFC of rats and corticosterone levels in their blood. Importantly, p11 expression was also upregulated in the postmortem cortex of patients with a history of PTSD. Dex upregulated p11 expression in SH-SY5Y cells through glucocorticoid response elements (GREs) within the p11 promoter, which could be attenuated by either a GR antagonist, RU486, or by mutating two of the three glucocorticoid response elements (GRE2 and GRE3) in the p11 promoter.[33] This work demonstrated that PTSD is associated with increased p11 expression that is regulated by glucocorticoids through GREs within the p11 promoter. Therefore, our basic scientific observation of p11's molecular mechanism in PTSD has led to further translational research and may lead to larger clinical studies.

Some of the symptoms of PTSD are similar to symptoms in a number of disorders, particularly in respect to emotional dysregulation. Therefore, we examined expression of p11 in the peripheral blood mononuclear cells (PBMCs) of PTSD, bipolar disorder (BP), major depressive disorder (MDD), and schizophrenia (SCZ) patients.[34] Those with PTSD had lower levels of p11 mRNA in PBMCs than control subjects, while those with BP, MDD, and SCZ had significantly higher p11 levels than the controls. In addition, p11 expression was positively correlated with the score of the Hamilton Depression Rating Scale, the Chinese Davison Trauma Scale-Frequency, and the Chinese Davison Trauma Scale-Severity. GR mRNA expression levels in PBMCs of PTSD were significantly downregulated compared to control subjects. These findings suggest that PBMC p11 mRNA levels may serve as a potential biomarker to distinguish PTSD from BP, MDD, and SCZ.

5-HT$_{2A}$ receptor: pharmacological target for the treatment of exaggerated fear in PTSD

Most of the research in stress-related psychiatric disorders such as PTSD, thus far has focused on the effectiveness of a few classes of compounds in alleviating the symptoms instead of preventing the pathogenesis of stress-induced disorders. However, prevention of the disorder is theoretically very possible because of knowing the onset timing (e.g., exposure to the traumatic event).

Dysregulation of the serotonergic system has long been recognized in the occurrence of stress-related psychiatric syndromes including depressive disorders and PTSD.[35] Among various 5-HT receptor subtypes, alterations in central 5-HT$_{2A}$ receptor signaling are particularly relevant to the pathophysiology of stress-related psychiatric syndromes. There is a general consensus among many positron emission tomography scan studies that there is decreased brain 5-HT$_{2A}$ receptor density in drug-naïve depressed patients.[36,37] Animal studies further suggest that diminished 5-HT$_{2A}$ receptor signaling is closely associated with the occurrence of stress-induced psychiatric symptoms. For example, inescapable stress induces a decrease in 5-HT$_{2A}$ receptor expression in the hippocampus and the decrease of 5-HT$_{2A}$ receptors in the hypothalamus and hippocampus appears to be specifically associated with behavioral depression after exposure to stress.[38]

Recently, utilization of a restraint/tail shock–stress protocol in young adult male rats together with 5-HT$_{2A}$ receptor blockade with MDL 11,939 prior to exposure to stress could prevent subsequent behavioral and physiological abnormalities.[39] In addition, it was subsequently shown that the development of behavioral and physiological abnormalities, such as enhanced startle response and reduced body weight after exposure to a 3-day restraint/tail shock protocol, could be averted by administration of the 5-HT$_{2A}$ receptor antagonist, MDL 11,939, thus indicating a critical role of 5-HT$_{2A}$ receptor activation in the pathophysiological response to traumatic stress.[39] Thus, administration of 5-HT$_{2A}$ receptor antagonists, such as MDL 11,939, to block/protect these receptors from excessive 5-HT$_{2A}$ receptor activation, appears to be a promising prophylactic and/or therapeutic agent for stress-associated psychiatric disorders, such as PTSD.

Localizing fear memory and stress to microcircuits of the amygdala

A wealth of data from both rodent and human studies have described the key role that the amygdala plays in the emotion of fear.[40] Fearful faces and threatening words activate the amygdala in humans. Moreover the presentation of subliminal fearful stimuli is also detectable by the amygdala, suggesting rapid and perhaps unique neural circuits that activate the amygdala to rapidly warn the body of unconditioned and conditioned threats.[41] The lateral nucleus (LA) of the amygdala is at an apex for sensory input and motor output for fear behavior and is thus a strong candidate for the storage of key aspects of associative memories linking the unconditioned stimuli and conditioned stimuli in classically conditioned fear. Recent data have also begun to reveal the circuits and networks interconnected with the amygdala that are responsible for fear-conditioning associated behaviors including contextual fear learning and fear extinction.[42]

Much less is known about intraamygdala microanatomy and circuitry. Of all the amygdala nuclei the microcircuits of the LA have been the most extensively studied. The LA is divided into three subnuclei, dorsal (LAd), ventromedial (LAvm), and ventrolateral (LAvl) on the basis of histologic appearance. The LAd is further subdivided into superior and inferior on the basis of network behavior and functional properties.[42–45] The most progress has been made in the LA in part because this nucleus has been a focus for its role in conditioned fear memory. The LA most likely contains a network of interconnected neurons. These networks likely form the networks upon which both normal and pathological fear memories are formed. While the identification of these potential amygdala networks is an important step in understanding the microcircuitry of fear; more work is needed to fully understand these networks and their role in fear pathology.

How stress interacts with these amygdala networks to influence the fear memories is an important question for understanding normal and pathological fear responses. The interaction between stress and the amygdala is mediated in part by the adrenal hormone cortisol and its receptors. Both genomic and membrane-acting mineralocorticoid (gMR and mMR) and glucocorticoid (gGR and mGR) receptors have been identified as part of the cellular signal transduction mechanism in the stress response.[46] Extensive evidence from animal models indicates that adrenal hormones modulate memory consolidation. Memory consolidation is enhanced when corticosterone and GR antagonists are administered during memory acquisition, but is impaired when the same drugs are administered during stored memory retrieval and tasks that include activation of the amygdala. Both mMR and gMR as well as mGR and gGR have been identified in the amygdala including at amygdala synapses. How these receptors interact with the micronetworks of the LA during fear memory and behavior is an important area for future research.

Prevention and treatment of PTSD

Recent guidelines summarize present knowledge of the treatment of PTSD and Acute Stress Disorder, two primary concerns for war-exposed soldiers.[47,48]

Early intervention and prevention

No medication has been shown to prevent the development of PTSD. A potential role for propranolol in preventing PTSD was suggested by a pilot study,[49] in which 32 emergency department patients received a 10-day course of propranolol or placebo, beginning within 6 h of a trauma. Propranolol treatment did not change CAPS (Clinician Administered PTSD Scale) scores at 1 month but did decrease physiological response to script-driven imagery 3 months after the trauma. Similarly, a 14-day randomized-controlled trial[50] of propranolol compared with gabapentin compared with placebo failed to demonstrate the superiority of either medication over placebo.

There has been recent interest in a specific preventive approach for disaster survivors called Psychological First Aid (PFA). The principles from which PFA has been derived—the fostering of safety, calmness, self- and community-efficacy, social connectedness, and optimism in the aftermath of disaster—are supported by considerable empirical evidence comprehensively summarized by Hobfoll *et al.*[51] However, questions surrounding optimal delivery format and which type of responder (clinician versus emergency responder versus community leader) might be best suited to deliver the various elements of a public health intervention targeting the adverse psychological consequences of trauma exposure must also be addressed.[52] Thus, PFA must at present be considered an evidence-informed, rather than evidence-based intervention.

Recent data from Bryant *et al.*[53] indicate that cognitive-behavioral therapy (CBT) administered about 3 weeks after traumatic event exposure is effective in preventing PTSD. However, no systematic studies have addressed this in war-exposed populations. It is a clinically applied strategy based on the evidence of these studies.

Pharmacological treatments

Various PTSD treatment practice guidelines published in the last decade support the use of CBT and of pharmacological treatment (usually with selective serotonin reuptake inhibitors (SSRIs)) as effective treatments for PTSD. The most recent meta-analyses and randomized-controlled trials augment prior support for the efficacy of CBT and of SSRIs, and add support for the efficacy of serotonin–norepinephrine reuptake inhibitors (SNRIs) over placebo for noncombat-related PTSD.

An Institute of Medicine review has questioned whether medications are as effective as in combat-related PTSD.[54] In contrast, a randomized-controlled trial[55] of 144 combat veterans of the Balkan Wars recruited at eight sites in Bosnia-Herzegovina and Croatia and randomized to fluoxetine or placebo. Two recent studies have also found efficacy for venlafaxine.[56,57]

Recently, a series of placebo-controlled augmentation trials have demonstrated the efficacy of the α-adrenergic antagonist prazosin for the treatment of trauma-related nightmares and sleep disruption[58–60] in PTSD. Beyond sleep, total PTSD symptoms improved significantly with augmentation.

Additional studies (references available) comparing nefazodone and sertraline, venlafaxine and sertraline, the SNRI reboxetine and fluvoxamine, fluoxetine, moclobemide, and tianeptine have generally demonstrated some evidence for superiority of antidepressants to placebo but have done little to clarify the relative utility of these different antidepressants. Trials with anticonvulsants and second-generation antipsychotics are limited and have not established a primary role for these agents in the treatment of PTSD.

Psychotherapy

Psychotherapy, perhaps one of the most elegant methods for brain change, has been studied extensively for treatment of PTSD. Most of the well-designed randomized-controlled trials of psychotherapy published have examined variations of CBT. Therapeutic approaches and techniques overlap across psychotherapies and there is no consensus on how these psychotherapies should be categorized. Cognitive Processing Therapy is considered by some[54] to be one form of exposure-based CBT and prolonged exposure another. Both approaches are supported by considerable evidence established through multiple randomized-controlled trials.[47,48] The multiple positive trials of exposure-based CBTs have included components of psychoeducation, breathing, and relaxation training. By definition, these therapies also incorporate some form of reexposure to past traumatic experience (e.g., imaginal, *in vivo*, written, verbal, or taped narrative recounting) into sessions. In addition, homework is often included.

Eye-movement desensitization and reprocessing (EMDR) has also been examined as a treatment for PTSD. It has been shown to be effective; however, a dismantling study has shown the eye movements are not a part of the effectiveness.[47,48] Therefore, EMDR is best seen as a form of CBT. Some evidence also exists that traditional CBT with exposure leads to more sustained symptom remission than does EMDR (Rothbaum *et al.*[61]).

Applied treatment for a special population: mortuary affairs soldiers

Mortuary affairs (MA) soldiers are small in number compared to the extent of their responsibilities. The current conflicts in Iraq and Afghanistan have required MA soldiers to have repeated deployments to the war zone. In fact, since the beginning of the terrorist attacks in 2001, many MA soldiers have been deployed to not only Iraq and Afghanistan but also the site of the Pentagon attack and the attacks on the World Trade Centers in New York City on September 11, 2001 and the Katrina hurricane. Their exposure to the toxic effects of death combined with the war zone stressors, exceeds all conflicts since the Vietnam era.

During the past two decades a number of studies have examined the effects of handling remains on military personnel and disaster workers.[62–65] Overall, findings suggest that regardless of profession, training, or past experience, duties involving recovery and identification of human remains are associated with acute and long-term psychological distress and psychiatric disorders.[66]

Our group has conducted the only study to date that examined pre- and postresponses of noncombat exposed mortuary workers handling bodies during the Persian Gulf War.[67,68] Posttraumatic symptoms, including intrusion and avoidance increased significantly for the exposed mortuary workers even when age, gender, volunteer status, and prior experience working with the dead were controlled. Importantly, even after controlling for stress prior to exposure to the dead, exposure itself was associated with increased posttraumatic symptoms.

No empirically informed interventions have been developed to address the specific needs of this well-identified high-risk group, MA soldiers returning from deployment. Our group has initiated a study of a unique intervention, TEAM (Troop Education for Army Morale: Units and Individuals Working Together) designed to meet the specific needs of MA soldiers returning from deployment. This intervention, designed to speed recovery, return to work, and limit barriers to care, is unique in that it is based on evidence-informed interventions that not only involve working with the soldier on an individual level, but also it integrates building resources within the unit (enhanced buddy care) and within the home (spouse support).

TEAM draws theory from evidence-based and evidence-informed clinical trials that have shown that in order to modify individual behavioral risk factors, such as drug, alcohol and tobacco use, diet, and physical activity, the most successful approaches have been those which incorporated elements of social organizational interventions and changes. For example, people who are socially isolated are more likely to engage in health risk behaviors and less likely to engage in behaviors that promote health.[69] Therefore, in order to alter or affect behavioral change in individuals, it is important to consider the social context or environment. TEAM, builds resources within the unit (buddy care) and family (spouse) environments as well as the individual. TEAM may have applicability to other high-stress-exposed first responders and disaster workers working with or exposed to the dead including firefighters, law enforcement, professional mortuary teams, and disaster workers.

Conclusion: need systems of care across stages of illness and recovery

Knowledge of the psychological, behavioral, and neurobiological mechanisms of brain change and treatment are needed for the medical care of those exposed to war and other disasters and traumatic events. "Trauma informed care" integrated into our health care systems must span from primary care to mental health. Comprehensive health care for trauma-related disorders, such as PTSD, must address all elements that affect health and behavior: the disorder, symptoms, comorbid conditions, impairment, disability, and the various trajectories of symptoms and disorders. By developing treatment plans for each of these domains we will better care for those affected by traumatic events. This will require much more scientific knowledge, organizational sophistication, continuities of services, and expanded models of care to best help those with PTSD and traumatic stress.

Conflicts of interest

The authors declare no conflicts of interest.

References

1. Milliken, C.S., J.L. Auchterlonie & C.W. Hoge. 2007. Longitudinal assessment of mental health problems among active and reserve component soldiers returning from the Iraq War. *JAMA* **298:** 2141–2190.
2. Williams, S.L., D.R. Williams, D.J. Stein, *et al.* 2007. Multiple traumatic events and psychological distress: the South Africa stress and health study. *J. Trauma. Stress* **20:** 845–855.
3. Shephard, B. 2001. *A War of Nerves: Soldiers and Psychiatrists in the Twentieth Century.* Harvard University Press. Cambridge, MA.
4. Hoge, C.W., C.A. Castro, S.C. Messer, *et al.* 2004. Combat duty in Iraq and Afghanistan, mental health problems, and barriers to care. *N. Engl. J. Med.* **351:** 13–22.

5. Mental Health Advisory Team VI. 2009. Mental health advisory team report (MHAT) VI, Operation Iraqi Freedom 07-09, Report. Army Medicine Reports http://www.armymedicine.army.mil/reports/mhat/mhat_vi/MHAT_VI-OIF_Redacted.pdf (accessed August 20, 2010).

6. Carden, M. J. 2009. *Army Continues Focus on Suicide Prevention.* American Forces Press Service. Washington.

7. Kuehn, B.M. 2009. Soldier suicide rates continue to rise. *JAMA* **301:** 1111–1113.

8. Jakupcak, M., J. Cook, Z. Imel, *et al.* 2009. Posttraumatic stress disorder as a risk factor for suicidal ideation in Iraq and Afghanistan War veterans. *J. Trauma. Stress* **22:** 303–306.

9. Ledgerwood, D.M. 1999. Suicide and attachment: fear of abandonment and isolation from a developmental perspective. *J. Contemp. Psychother.* **29:** 65–73.

10. Jelinek, P. 2009. *Military Divorce Rate Edges Higher.* Associated Press. Washington.

11. Sher, L. 2009. Suicide in war veterans: the role of comorbidity of PTSD and depression. *Expert Rev. Neurother.* **9:** 921–923.

12. Tanielian, T., L.H. Jaycox, T.L. Schell, *et al.* 2008. *Invisible Wounds of War: Psychological and Cognitive Injuries, their Consequences, and Services to Assist Recovery.* RAND. Santa Monica.

13. Grossman, D. 1995. *On Killing: The Psychological Cost of Learning to Kill in War and Society.* Back Bay Books. New York.

14. Jakupcak, M., D. Conybeare, L. Phelps, *et al.* 2007. Anger, hostility, and aggression among Iraq and Afghanistan War veterans reporting PTSD and subthreshold PTSD. *J. Trauma. Stress* **20:** 945–954.

15. Gradus, J.L., P. Qin, A.K. Lincoln, *et al.* 2010. Posttraumatic stress disorder and completed suicide. *Am. J. Epidemiol.* **171:** 721–727.

16. Nock, M.K., K. Hwang, N.A. Sampson, *et al.* 2009. Cross-national analysis of the associations among mental disorders and suicideal behavior: findings from the WHO world mental health surveys. *PLoS Med.* **6:** 1–17.

17. Nock, M.K., K. Hwang, N.A. Sampson & R.C. Kessler. 2010. Mental disorders, comorbidity and suicidal behavior: results from the National Comorbidity Survey Replication. *Mol. Psychiatry.* **15:** 868–876.

18. Wilcox, H.C., C.L. Storr & N. Breslau. 2009. Posttraumatic stress disorder and suicide attempts in a community sample of urban young adults. *Arch. Gen. Psychiatry* **66:** 305–311.

19. Marshall, A.D., J. Panuzio & C.T. Taft. 2005. Intimate partner violence among military veterans and active duty servicemen. *Clin. Psychol. Rev.* **25:** 862–876.

20. Jordan, B.K., C.R. Marmar, J.A. Fairbank, *et al.* 1992. Problems in families of male Vietnam veterans with posttraumatic stress disorder. *J. Consult. Clin. Psychol.* **60:** 916–926.

21. Killgore, W.D., D.I. Cotting, J.L. Thomas, *et al.* 2008. Post-combat invincibility: violent combat experiences are associated with increased risk-taking propensity following deployment. *J. Psychiatr. Res.* **42:** 1112–1121.

22. Boscarino, J.A. 2006. Posttraumatic stress disorder and mortality among U.S. Army veterans 30 years after military service. *Ann. Epidemiol.* **16:** 248–256.

23. Iversen, L. 2003. Cannabis and the brain. *Brain* **126:** 1252–1270.

24. Phillips, R.G. & J.E. LeDoux. 1992. Differential contribution of amygdala and hippocampus to cued and contextual fear conditioning. *Behav. Neurosci.* **106:** 274–285.

25. Davis, M., D.L. Walker & K.M. Myers. 2003. Role of the amygdala in fear extinction measured with potentiated startle. *Ann. N.Y. Acad. Sci.* **985:** 218–232.

26. Chhatwal, J.P., M. Davis, K.A. Maguschak & K.J. Ressler. 2005. Enhancing the cannabinoid neurotransmission augments the extinction of conditioned fear. *Neuropsychopharmacology* **30:** 516–524.

27. Mikics, E., T. Dombi, B. Barsvari, *et al.* 2006. The effects of cannabinoids on contextual conditioned fear in CB1 knock-out and CD1 mice. *Behav. Pharmacol.* **17:** 223–230.

28. Fride, E., R. Suris, J. Weidenfeld & R. Mechoulam. 2005. Differential response to acute and repeated stress in cannabinoid CB1 receptor knockout newborn and adult mice. *Behav. Pharmacol.* **16:** 431–440.

29. Marsciano, G., C.T. Wotjak, S.C. Azad, *et al.* 2002. The endogenous cannabinoid system controls extinction of aversive memories. *Nature* **418:** 530–534.

30. Zhang, L., H. Li, D. Benedek, *et al.* 2009. A strategy for the development of biomarker tests for PTSD. *Med. Hypotheses* **73:** 404–409.

31. Svenningsson, P., K. Chergui, I. Rachleff, *et al.* 2006. Alterations in 5-HT1B receptor function by p11 in depression-like states. *Science* **311:** 77–80.

32. Yao, X.L., M.J. Cowan, M.T. Gladwin, *et al.* 1999. Dexamethasone alters arachidonate release from human epithelial cells by induction of p11 protein synthesis and inhibition of phospholipase A2 activity. *J. Biol. Chem.* **274:** 17202–17208.

33. Zhang, L., H. Li, T.P. Su, *et al.* 2008. p11 is up-regulated in the forebrain of stressed rats by glucocorticoid acting via two specific glucocorticoid response elements in the p11 promoter. *Neuroscience* **153:** 1126–1134.

34. Su, T.P., L. Zhang, M.Y. Chung, *et al.* 2009. Levels of the potential biomarker p11 in peripheral blood cells distinguish patients with PTSD from those with other major psychiatric disorders. *J. Psychiatr. Res.* **43:** 1078–1085.

35. Southwick, S.M., S. Paige, C.A. Morgan III, et al. 1999. Neurotransmitter alterations in PTSD: catecholamines and serotonin. *Semin. Clin. Neuropsychiatry* **4:** 242–248.

36. Malone, K.M., S.P. Ellis, D. Currier & J.J. Mann. 2006. Platelet 5-HT2A receptor subresponsivity and lethality of attempted suicide in depressed in-patients. *Int. J. Neuropsychopharmacol.* **10:** 335–343.

37. Messa, C., C. Colombo, R.M. Moresco, *et al.* 2003. 5-HT(2A) receptor binding is reduced in drug-naive and unchanged in SSRI-responder depressed patients compared to healthy controls: a PET study. *Psychopharmacology* **167:** 72–78.

38. Dwivedi, Y., A.C. Mondal, G.V. Payappagoudar & H.S. Rizavi. 2005. Differential regulation of serotonin (5HT)2A receptor mRNA and protein levels after single and repeated stress in rat brain: role in learned helplessness behavior. *Neuropharmacology* **48:** 204–214.

39. Jiang, X., Z.J. Zhang, S. Zhang, *et al.* 2009. 5-HT2A receptor antagonism by MDL 11,939 during inescapable stress prevents subsequent exaggeration of acoustic startle response and reduced body weight in rats. *J. Psychopharmacol.* **0:** 1–9 [E-pub ahead of print].

40. Fanselow, M.S. & J.E. LeDoux. 1999. Why we think plasticity underlying Pavlovian fear conditioning occurs in the basolateral amygdala. *Neuron* **23:** 229–232.

41. LeDoux, J. 2007. The amygdala. *Curr. Biol.* **17:** R868–R874.

42. Johnson, L.R. 2009. The micro anatomy of fear: circuits underlying fear acquisition and extinction. *Cell Sci. Rev.* **5:** 1742–1748.

43. Repa, J.C., J. Muller, J. Apergis, *et al.* 2001. Two different lateral amygdala cell populations contribute to the initiation and storage of memory. *Nat. Neurosci.* **4:** 724–731.

44. Johnson, L.R. & J.E. LeDoux. 2004. *Fear and Anxiety: The Benefits of Translational Research.* J.M., Gorman, *et al.*, Eds.: 227–250. APA Press. Washington.

45. Johnson, L.R., J.E. Ledoux & V. Doyere. 2009. Hebbian reverberations in emotional memory micro circuits. *Front. Neurosci.* **3:** 198–205.

46. Prager, E.M. & L.R. Johnson. 2009. Stress at the synapse: signal transduction mechanisms of adrenal steroids at neuronal membranes. *Sci. Signal.* **2:** re5.

47. American Psychiatric Association. 2002. *Diagnostic and Statistical Manual of Mental Disorders, Fourth Edition, Text Revision.* American Psychiatric Association. Washington.

48. Benedek, D.M., M.J. Friedman, D. Zatzick & R.J. Ursano. 2009. Guideline watch: practice guideline for the treatment of patients with acute stress disorder and posttraumatic stress disorder. *Am. Psychiatr. Assoc. FOCUS* **7:** 1–9.

49. Pitman, R.K., K.M. Sanders, R.M. Zusman, *et al.* 2002. Pilot study of secondary prevention of posttraumatic stress disorder with propranol. *Biol. Psychiatry* **51:** 189–192.

50. Stein, M.B., C. Kerridge, J.E. Dimsdale & D.B. Hoyt. 2007. Pharmacotherapy to prevent PTSD: results from a randomized controlled proof-of-concept trial in physically injured patients. *J. Trauma. Stress* **20:** 923–932.

51. Hobfoll, S.E., P. Watson, C.C. Bell, *et al.* 2007. Five essential elements of immediate and mid-term mass trauma intervention: empirical evidence. *Psychiatry* **70:** 283–315.

52. Benedek, D.M. & C.S. Fullerton. 2007. Translating five essential elements into programs and practice: commentary on "Five essential elements of immediate and mid-term mass trauma intervention: empirical evidence" by Hobfoll et al. *Psychiatry* **70:** 345–349.

53. Bryant, R.A., J. Mastrodomenico, K.L. Felmingham, *et al.* 2008. Treatment of acute stress disorder: a randomized controlled trial. *Arch. Gen. Psychiatry* **65:** 659–667.

54. Institute of Medicine. 2007. *Treatment of PTSD: An Assessment of the Evidence.* National Academies Press. Washington.

55. Martenyi, F. & V. Soldatenkova. 2006. Fluoxetine in the acute treatment and relapse prevention of combat-related posttraumatic stress disorder: analysis of the veteran group of a placebo-controlled, randomized clinical trial. *Eur. Neuropsychopharmacol.* **16:** 340–349.

56. Davidson, J., D. Baldwin, D.J. Stein, *et al.* 2006. Treatment of posttraumatic stress disorder with venlafaxine extended release: a 6-month randomized controlled trial. *Arch. Gen. Psychiatry* **63:** 1158–1165.

57. Pavcovich, L.A. & R.J. Valentino. 1997. Regulation of a putative neurotransmitter effect of corticotropin-releasing factor: effects of adrenalectomy. *J. Neurosci.* **17:** 401–408.

58. Raskind, M.A., E.R. Peskind, E.D. Kanter, *et al.* 2003. Reduction of nightmares and other PTSD symptoms in combat veterans by prazosin: a placebo-controlled study. *Am. J. Psychiatry* **160:** 371–373.

59. Raskind, M.A., E.R. Peskind, D.J. Hoff, *et al.* 2007. A parallel group placebo controlled study of prazosin for trauma nightmares and sleep disturbance in combat veterans with post-traumatic stress disorder. *Biol. Psychiatry* **61:** 928–934.

60. Taylor, F.B., P. Martin, C. Thompson, *et al.* 2008. Prazosin effects on objective sleep measures and clinical symptoms in civilian trauma posttraumatic stress disorder: a placebo-controlled study. *Biol. Psychiatry* **63:** 629–632.

61. Rothbaum, B.O., M.C. Astin & F. Marsteller. 2005. Prolonged exposure versus eye movement desensitization and reprocessing (EMDR) for PTSD rape victims. *J. Trauma. Stress* **18:** 607–616.

62. Bryant, R.A. & A.G. Harvey. 1996. Posttraumatic stress reactions in volunteer firefighters. *J. Trauma. Stress* **9:** 51–62.

63. Fullerton, C.S., J.E. McCarroll, R.J. Ursano & K.M. Wright. 1992. Psychological responses of rescue workers: fire fighters and trauma. *Am. J. Orthopsychiatry* **62:** 371–378.

64. Marmar, C.R., D.S. Weiss, T.J. Metzler, *et al.* 1996. Stress responses of emergency service personnel to the Loma Prieta earthquake Interstate 880 freeway collapse and control traumatic incidents. *J. Trauma. Stress* **9:** 63–85.

65. McCarroll, J.E., R.J. Ursano & C.S. Fullerton. 1995. Symptoms of PTSD following recovery of war dead: 13–15 month follow-up. *Am. J. Psychiatry* **152:** 939–941.

66. Ursano, R.J., J.E. McCarroll & C.S. Fullerton. 2007. *Textbook of Disaster Psychiatry.* R.J. Ursano, *et al.*, Eds.: 227–246. Cambridge University Press. New York.

67. McCarroll, J.E., R.J. Ursano, C.S. Fullerton, *et al.* 2001. Effects of exposure to death in a war mortuary on posttraumatic stress disorder symptoms of intrusion and avoidance. *J. Nerv. Ment. Dis.* **189:** 44–48.

68. McCarroll, J.E., R.J. Ursano, C.S. Fullerton, *et al.* 2002. Somatic symptoms in Gulf War mortuary workers. *Psychosom. Med.* **64:** 29–33.

69. Adler, N., T. Boyce, M.A. Chesney, *et al.* 1994. Socioeconomic status and health: the challenge of the gradient. *Am. Psychol.* **49:** 15–24.

Ann. N.Y. Acad. Sci. ISSN 0077-8923

Evidence-based treatments for PTSD, new directions, and special challenges

Judith Cukor, Megan Olden, Francis Lee, and JoAnn Difede

Department of Psychiatry, Weill Cornell Medical College of Cornell University, New York, New York

Address for correspondence: Judith Cukor, Ph.D., Weill Cornell Medical College, 525 East 68th Street, Box 200, New York, New York 10065. juc2010@med.cornell.edu

This paper provides a current review of existing evidence-based treatments for posttraumatic stress disorder (PTSD), with a description of psychopharmacologic options, prolonged exposure therapy, cognitive processing therapy, and eye movement desensitization and reprocessing, especially as they pertain to military populations. It further offers a brief summary of promising treatments with a developing evidence base, encompassing both psychotherapy and pharmacotherapy. Finally, challenges to the treatment of PTSD are summarized and future directions suggested.

Keywords: posttraumatic stress disorder; evidence-based treatment; PE; novel treatments

Introduction

Posttraumatic stress disorder (PTSD) is estimated to affect 8–9% of individuals in the population at some point in their lives.[1,2] It is characterized by a pattern of symptoms arising in the aftermath of a trauma that causes significant functional impairment and distress to the individual.[3] PTSD is associated with high rates of comorbidity and increased risk for suicide[4] and is often chronic in nature, with more than one-third of cases continuing to meet diagnostic criteria after many years.[5]

In the 30 years since its diagnostic criteria was first outlined in the Diagnostic and Statistical Manual of Mental Disorders, Third Edition (DSM-III), a body of research has emerged, identifying rates of PTSD in various populations, isolating risk factors for its development, and developing effective methods for its treatment. These three decades of research have revealed that psychotherapy, and specifically exposure-based therapies have the most compelling evidence base and should be used as the first line treatment for PTSD[6,7] with limited evidence for the efficacy of any of the U.S. Food and Drug Administration (FDA) approved pharmacologic agents.[8] Yet, despite the unparalleled success of these interventions, treatment failures persist. A meta-analysis of 26 studies with 44 treatment conditions found that overall, 56% of those enrolled in treatment

and 67% of those who completed treatment no longer met criteria for PTSD after treatment and 44% of enrollees and 54% of completers had clinically meaningful improvement by standards defined by the authors.[9] At best, then, one-third of patients who complete these evidence-based therapies retain a diagnosis of PTSD at completion of treatment, offering compelling reason to continue to pursue alternative treatments or augmentations to current interventions.

With recent events in the nation and world history, and the high rates of PTSD in returning military from Operation Iraqi Freedom/Operation Enduring Freedom (OIF/OEF), the urgency of identifying effective treatment options for PTSD is imperative.

Evidence-based treatments for PTSD

Treatment recommendation guidelines indicate that psychotherapy is the most effective treatment for PTSD.[7] Among the various modalities of psychotherapy, cognitive behavioral therapy (CBT) has the strongest evidence base, as highlighted by a recent meta-analysis encompassing 26 treatment outcome studies.[9] Similarly, a report by the Institute of Medicine[6] concluded that exposure therapy is the only treatment with sufficient evidence to recommend for the treatment of PTSD.

doi: 10.1111/j.1749-6632.2010.05793.x

Bisson *et al.*,[10] in a meta-analysis of 38 studies, reported that CBT for trauma was significantly more effective than waitlist or usual care groups in improving symptoms of PTSD. Eye movement desensitization and reprocessing (EMDR) was also significantly effective, though the evidence base for EMDR was not as strong as that for CBT. Stress management/relaxation and group CBTs showed success on some measures but to a lesser degree, while other therapies, including supportive therapy/nondirective counseling, psychodynamic therapies, and hypnotherapy, did not show clinically significant effects on PTSD symptoms.

CBTs for PTSD place varying emphases on the exposure or behavioral components versus the cognitive elements, and have garnered different amounts of support. Prolonged exposure (PE), a treatment protocol developed by Foa *et al.*,[11] was one of the first techniques to amass an evidence base and is widely accepted as the gold standard for CBT treatment. The theoretical basis for PE relies upon the learning model, and views PTSD as a disorder of extinction, whereby the individual's response to crisis does not diminish sufficiently, and the association between the memory of the event and a message of danger has not been extinguished even when the danger has passed. The main components of PE, imaginal exposure and *in vivo* exposure, entail the revisiting of trauma memories and triggers to extinguish this response, by facilitating habituation to the memory, decreasing avoidance, and eliminating associations with danger by providing corrective information about safety. During imaginal exposure, patients are instructed to relate their trauma experience in detail with their eyes closed, while trying to engage emotionally in the memory. The patient retells his/her trauma experience repeatedly over the course of a number of sessions, thereby allowing the processing of the trauma experience. *In vivo* exposure entails approaching activities, people, and/or places the patient may have been avoiding to allow habituation to the environment, and the assimilation of the corrective information regarding safety.

Within cognitive behavioral treatments for PTSD, an impressive evidence base supports the use of prolonged imaginal exposure as a specific therapeutic technique in various populations including sexual assault and motor vehicle accidents.[12] In one of the few randomized controlled trials of CBT in mili-

tary populations,[13] female veterans and active duty service personnel receiving 10 sessions of PE were more likely to no longer meet PTSD diagnostic criteria and to achieve total PTSD remission than those in the supportive arm.

A recent meta-analysis of PE[14] found large effect sizes for PE as compared to control conditions with patients receiving PE treatment improving at a rate of 86% greater than those in the control condition. There was no evidence of the superiority of PE over other treatments (i.e., cognitive processing therapy (CPT), cognitive therapy, stress inoculation training, and EMDR) though a very small number of studies were available for comparison, so further research is necessary to provide conclusive answers regarding comparability of treatments. Based on the overall positive findings related to PE, the Veterans' Administration Office of Mental Health Services has introduced a program to disseminate PE treatment to its providers so it can be delivered as a treatment of choice in Veterans Affairs establishments.[15]

CPT is another exposure-based protocol with a strong emphasis on increasing the cognitive components and decreasing the amount of exposure necessary for treatment, which some believe will be more palatable to individuals with PTSD. CPT consists of a 12-session protocol that was originally developed as a treatment for PTSD related to sexual assault,[16] but has more recently been applied to military trauma and motor vehicle accidents. It comprises two integrated elements. The cognitive therapy component focuses on deconstructing assimilated distorted beliefs, such as guilt, and more global beliefs about the world and self, and generating more balanced statements. The exposure component entails having the patient write the trauma memory and read it to their therapist and to themselves and then examine the writing for "stuck points."[17]

Initial case studies and clinical trials were promising and led to a randomized controlled trial comparing CPT to PE and a minimal attention waitlist control for the treatment of PTSD in a sample of chronically distressed rape victims.[17] Results found that both PE and CPT were highly successful in treating PTSD and comorbid depressive symptomatology. Applications to a military population with chronic PTSD have been encouraging. In one randomized trial of CPT versus waitlist control, 40% of patients receiving CPT no longer met criteria for

PTSD at the study's end and 50% demonstrated a reliable drop in PTSD symptoms at posttreatment assessment 1 month later, with further significant improvements in comorbid depression, anxiety, guilt, and social adjustment.[18] Similarly to PE, dissemination efforts are providing training in CPT for veteran providers nationwide.

EMDR has been at the center of considerable controversy since its inception. EMDR is an eight-stage information processing treatment proposed by Shapiro[19] that entails focusing on a vivid image of the memory while the therapist leads the patient through a series of eye movements, tones, tapping, or other tactile stimulation. The treatment is said to work by enhancing processing of the trauma memory when new connections are made with more positive information and the associations with the memory no longer hold emotional or physiological arousal.[20]

The evidence base for EMDR seems to support its effectiveness for the treatment of PTSD, with some studies finding it comparable to exposure-based CBT,[21] and others finding it less effective.[10] The central question at the heart of the debate surrounding EMDR is whether the effectiveness of the treatment is due solely to the exposure to the trauma memory during the exercise, thereby rendering the treatment merely a disguised exposure therapy, or whether there is in fact added benefit to the dual stimulation.[22] Due to the nature of the treatment, it would be difficult to separate the elements to evaluate their independent contributions.

Psychopharmacology

Only two pharmacologic agents are FDA approved for the treatment of PTSD: sertraline and paroxetine. These selective serotonin reuptake inhibitors (SSRIs) primarily act upon the serotonin neurotransmitter system and have the strongest empirical support in the treatment literature. Indeed, response rates are low and rarely reach above 60% with less than 30% achieving full remission.[23] Overall, less than 50% of PTSD patients improve on SSRIs.[8] In addition, maintenance of effects is only achieved through continued medication treatment,[24] which one might attribute to the medication addressing symptoms rather than the source of the problem, which is the trauma experience.

Surprisingly little consensus has been reached on second line treatments for PTSD. An encompass-

ing systematic review of open and controlled trials found some support for the use of risperidone, which was effective in four of six reviewed trials.[23] Short-term trials of antipsychotic medications revealed some effects but Berger and colleagues[23] suggest this may reflect treatment of nonspecific symptoms, such as insomnia, and not those specifically related to PTSD. In addition, severe side effects with longer trials could be problematic. The authors indicate that anticonvulsants seem helpful when used as an augmentation to other therapeutic regimens, but studies using it as a monotherapy were largely insignificant. They also caution against the use of benzodiazepenes because of its potentially addictive nature and the question of whether it may contribute to the development of PTSD.[23] In practice, medication is frequently used to target more isolated symptoms (i.e., sleep difficulty), rather than the overall disorder.

Barriers to implementation of evidence-based treatments

Dissemination and acceptance of evidence-based treatments pose a significant obstacle to implementation of best practices. van Minnen *et al.*[25] presented 255 trauma experts with case examples, and found that despite the evidence noted above, exposure was underutilized, there was a lack of training in the technique, and providers were more likely to offer medication than exposure when the PTSD presented with a comorbid depression. Becker *et al.*[26] surveyed 217 psychologists and found only 17% used exposure therapy for the treatment of PTSD, and even among those who had received training in exposure, 38–46% did not implement its use. Reasons cited among the trained psychologists included hesitancy to use manualized treatments and the concern that patients would decompensate, despite the existence of evidence to the contrary. In training a large cohort of psychologists to use PE therapy in the aftermath of 9/11, Cahill *et al.*[27] found that discomfort in using exposure and cognitive restructuring techniques, concerns about decompensation, and a disinclination to use manualized treatments served as significant barriers to the implementation of treatment.

Promising directions

A recent proliferation in studies of novel and innovative treatments for PTSD suggests an awareness of the need for alternatives to supplement the current evidence-based treatments. Some emerging treatments will be summarized here, selected because of their growing evidence base and persuasive scientific rationale, though they represent only a small number of interventions that are currently being proposed. Due to the preliminary nature of these studies, there is insufficient evidence to draw conclusions about the efficacy of these treatments, but there is reason to be optimistic about the possibility for new treatment options.

While treatment outcome studies seek to identify novel, effective interventions, exciting translational research has directed its attention to identifying neurocircuitry involved in fear conditioning that may shed light on propensity to develop PTSD or failure to improve with treatment. In light of the conceptualization of PTSD as a disorder of fear extinction or inhibition, findings on genetic and neurobiological factors related to fear inhibition may provide more information that may be used to address risk factors or treatment failures.[28]

Emerging pharmacotherapies

Prazosin. Prazosin, an alpha-1 adrenergic receptor blocker, has recently been investigated as a tool in targeting insomnia and nightmares following a traumatic event. Originally marketed to treat hypertension and benign prostate hyperplasia,[29] prazosin's role in inhibiting adrenergic activity suggests it may also prove efficacious in treating sleep-related PTSD symptoms. These symptoms are believed to be moderated by increased central nervous system adrenergic activity, resulting in greater release of norepinephrine and increased sensitivity to norepinephrine at receptor sites.[30] Prazosin's effectiveness for the treatment of nightmares has been reported in case studies, retrospective chart reviews, and open label trials.[31] Preliminary evidence exists for its effectiveness in military populations[32,33] with reports of 50% decrease in nightmares after 8 weeks of treatment.[34] Prazosin demonstrates a promising adjunct to target insomnia and trauma-related nightmares in patients with PTSD. Further studies are needed to determine optimal dosing regimens as well as the applicability of this treatment across a wide variety of traumas.

D-cycloserine. The cognitive enhancer D-cycloserine (DCS; trade name Seromycin) shows promise among pharmacologic agents for PTSD for its potential to facilitate extinction learning. Originally developed as an antituberculosis antibiotic, DCS is a partial agonist for the N-methyl-D-aspartate (NMDA) glutamate receptor, which has a crucial role in learning and memory functions. DCS has been shown to facilitate extinction learning in animal models of conditioned fear and in some human trials of other types of learning.[35–41]

In the first double-blind randomized controlled trial,[42] patients with acrophobia in the DCS condition reported significantly lower anxiety and demonstrated reduced galvanic skin response when in the virtual environment than those receiving a placebo, and reported increased real-life exposure to heights at 3 months. Positive results were also demonstrated in a double-blind randomized controlled trial of 27 patients with social phobia ($N = 27$)[43] and a randomized controlled trial of 56 patients with social anxiety.[44]

Existing research highlights the potential role of DCS in facilitating fear extinction and reducing posttreatment relapse.[36] Studies are under way to investigate the use of DCS in PTSD patients to augment PE and virtual reality therapy, with the hope that its use may improve or accelerate treatment effects through enhancement of extinction learning on a biological level.

Emerging psychotherapies

Couples and family therapy. PTSD frequently negatively impacts marital and family relationships, sometimes resulting in isolating behaviors and increased anger and irritability.[45] In fact, upwards of 75% of OIF/OEF veterans report relationship difficulties.[46] Family interventions for PTSD sufferers may focus treatment on reducing stress to the family system, or they may target the individual with PTSD, building support for this person within the family.[47]

Several couples-based treatments have been developed, including cognitive behavioral conjoint therapy (CBCT) for PTSD.[45] This 15-session protocol treats couples with behavioral and communication techniques, and cognitive interventions addressing maladaptive thoughts about the trauma and their impact on the relationship and symptoms of PTSD. CBCT has obtained preliminary support, with one pilot study of married Vietnam veterans and their spouses ($N = 7$)[48] finding significant improvement in PTSD scores by clinician and spouse ratings. Adaptations are under way to apply this therapy to OIF/OEF veterans and assess its efficacy.[45]

Despite a lack of systematic investigations, the use of family- and couples-based treatments for PTSD has a strong theoretical base, particularly for use with military service members struggling to communicate wartime experiences to family members.

Interpersonal psychotherapy. As individuals with PTSD frequently experience disrupted relationships with family, friends, and colleagues, interpersonal psychotherapy (IPT), with its focus on social functioning, has been a focus of empirical inquiry. One pilot study of a 14-week IPT treatment for patients suffering from a variety of traumas,[49] found that 69% of patients demonstrated a 50% reduction in PTSD symptoms. Group applications of IPT have been more mixed, with one study reporting greater reductions in PTSD and depression symptoms for a group IPT intervention than a waitlist control group[50] and another finding that IPT was only moderately effective in reducing PTSD symptoms.[51]

Future work will be needed to determine whether an interpersonal focus is effective in reducing the full range of PTSD symptoms, or whether IPT is best used as a supplementary treatment tool to address relational deficits in patients following a traumatic experience.

Virtual reality. Virtual reality exposure therapy (VRET) uses technological advances to augment traditional imaginal exposure treatment. In imaginal exposure, the patient relies upon his/her imaginal capacities to retell the trauma experience in a manner that evokes emotional engagement. Virtual reality enhanced exposure facilitates this emotional engagement by adding visual, auditory, olfactory, and even haptic computer-generated simulation experiences as the patient relates the trauma memory, thereby increasing presence in the memory. Evidence for the efficacy of VRET has been shown for Vietnam veterans,[52,53] survivors of the World Trade Center attacks,[54] and OIF/OEF veterans.[55]

VRET has garnered interest especially in the military population for the treatment of returning OIF/OEF veterans. It is hypothesized that virtual reality technology may increase engagement in the exposure exercises, an advantage to a subset of individuals who are trained to keep emotions at bay to think clearly in life-threatening situations.[56] It is fur-

ther hypothesized that virtual reality may represent a palatable alternative treatment for a generation of active duty personnel who are concerned about stigma of mental health treatment, and have grown up with gaming technology.[57] Current efforts are targeting dissemination of VRET to military bases nationwide. Ongoing randomized controlled trials will shed light on the potential independent contribution of this treatment above that of imaginal exposure. Virtual reality is discussed in detail elsewhere in this volume.

Special considerations

Specific issues related to special populations may necessitate further research on the applicability of current treatments. The challenge of treating PTSD is further amplified by the presence of comorbid disorders, which frequently occur with a diagnosis of PTSD. Rates of lifetime Major Depression are cited by the National Comorbidity Survey[5] as 48% in men and 49% in women with PTSD, making it the most common comorbidity. More than 51% of men and 27% of women with PTSD met criteria for alcohol abuse or dependence and over 34% of men and 26% of women met criteria for drug abuse or dependence.

Despite the high rates of comorbid PTSD and depression, there is little to no examination of the use of therapies in populations with this comorbidity.[58] With little exception,[59] most studies focus on a PTSD population and examine depressive symptomatology as a secondary outcome. A recent meta-analysis of PTSD outcome studies suggests that these treatments may also improve symptoms of depression,[10] but this is far from a certainty.

Debate has centered over the best method of addressing comorbid PTSD and substance use. General practice has been to use sequential treatment, requiring the patient to first complete substance-use treatment, and then refer them to a PTSD treatment program. Yet, clinical wisdom and recent evidence[60] suggest that gains made in substance-use treatment are at great risk for relapse at cues related to the trauma memory that may serve as triggers for substance use and self-medication.[61] A recent study of a trauma-focused treatment found that as PTSD symptoms improved, substance use showed significant improvement; however, the reciprocal relationship was not found.[62]

Evidence suggests that treating the problems concurrently is the best strategy. Integrated treatment trials of PTSD and substance use have been largely positive, but are still in preliminary stages. Positive effects on both PTSD and substance use have been reported using the Seeking Safety treatment,[61,62] PE,[63–65] and a CBT protocol[66] and further trials are under way using COPE (concurrent treatment with PE),[60] behavioral couples therapy,[67] and PE.[68]

Physical impairment in the aftermath of a trauma with physical injuries may also complicate the course of mental health treatment as the patient copes with scarring or disfigurement, pain, and functional impairment that prohibits functioning in premorbid roles.[69] Research has indicated that the physical injury itself impacts treatment for PTSD as more severely injured patients, while more likely to develop PTSD, are also less likely to benefit from traditional CBT treatment.[70] Yet, despite the effect physical injury may have upon PTSD, there exists no guide for treatment of PTSD in the context of a physical injury.

With the recent increase in its occurrence due to military related injuries, more attention is being given to the comorbid presentation of PTSD and traumatic brain injury (TBI). To date, little work has focused on effective treatment strategies for both, and due to the common exclusion of individuals with TBI from PTSD treatment studies, little is known of the efficacy of PTSD treatment in this population.[71] Future research must address whether treatments are effective in their current form, or must be modified to some extent or changed completely to be effective for individuals with mild TBI with or without lasting cognitive deficits.[72]

Conclusions

The evidence base for the treatment of PTSD offers effective options in the form of exposure therapies. Novel treatments, including couples and interpersonal therapies, virtual reality therapy, and the use of prazosin and DCS, are being developed and evaluated through outcome trials. Yet, the task before us remains great. Chronic PTSD exists in large numbers throughout the world and especially among those sent to battle to protect our national interests. Our responsibility lies in the further development of alternative treatments and the dissemination of current evidence-based practices. Failure of providers to use established treatments is a barrier to effective care that as a community must be addressed. Controlled trials of new therapies need to be conducted before they can be added to the list of tools at the disposal of a clinician. Close examination of applications of current protocols to special populations may yield the development of modified treatments that can increase efficacy. While translational research stands to provide exciting contributions to our knowledge base, it must then be applied clinically to the implementation of differential therapeutics. In conclusion, exposure therapy is a powerful tool in the treatment of PTSD, and novel treatments are filling in the gap left by treatment failures. It remains incumbent upon the scientific community to put evidence-based treatments in the hands of the clinicians and to develop and evaluate broader treatment options.

Conflicts of interest

The authors declare no conflicts of interest.

References

1. Hidalgo, R.B. & J.R. Davidson. 2000. Posttraumatic stress disorder: epidemiology and health-related considerations. *J. Clin. Psychiatry* **61**(Suppl. 7): 5–13.
2. Yule, W. 2001. Posttraumatic stress disorder in the general population and in children. *J. Clin. Psychiatry* **62**(Suppl. 17): 23–28.
3. American Psychological Association. 1994. *Diagnostic and Statistical Manual of Mental Disorders* (4th ed.). American Psychiatric Association. Washington, DC.
4. Kessler, R.C. 2000. Posttraumatic stress disorder: the burden to the individual and to society. *J. Clin. Psychiatry* **61**(Suppl. 5): 4–12; discussion 13–14.
5. Kessler, R.C., A. Sonnega, E. Bromet, *et al.* 1995. Posttraumatic stress disorder in the National Comorbidity Survey. *Arch. Gen. Psychiatry* **52**: 1048–1060.
6. Institute of Medicine (IOM). 2008. *Treatment of Posttraumatic Stress Disorder: An Assessment of the Evidence.* The National Academies Press. Washington, DC.
7. National Collaborating Centre for Mental Health. 2005. *Post-Traumatic Stress Disorder: The Management of PTSD in Adults and Children in Primary and Secondary Care.* 167 National Institute for Clinical Excellence (NICE). London (UK).
8. Foa, E.B., M.E. Franklin & J. Moser. 2002. Context in the clinic: how well do cognitive-behavioral therapies and medications work in combination? *Biol. Psychiatry* **52**: 987–997.
9. Bradley, R., J. Greene, E. Russ, *et al.* 2005. A multidimensional meta-analysis of psychotherapy for PTSD. [erratum appears in *Am. J. Psychiatry.* 2005;**162**:832] *Am. J. Psychiatry* **162**: 214–227.
10. Bisson, J.I. *et al.* 2007. Psychological treatments for chronic post-traumatic stress disorder. Systematic review and meta-analysis. *Br. J. Psychiatry* **190**: 97–104.

11. Foa, E., E. Hembree & B. Rothbaum. 2007. *Prolonged Exposure Therapy for PTSD: Emotional Processing of Traumatic Experiences, Therapist Guide*. Oxford University Press. New York.

12. Difede, J. & J. Cukor. 2009. Evidence-based long-term treatment of mental health consequences of disasters among adults. In *Mental Health and Disasters*. Y. Neria, S. Galea & F. Norris, Eds.: 336–349. Cambridge University Press. New York.

13. Schnurr, P.P. *et al.* 2007. Cognitive behavioral therapy for posttraumatic stress disorder in women: a randomized controlled trial. *JAMA* **297:** 820–830.

14. Powers, M., J.M. Halpern, M.P. Ferenschak, *et al.* 2010. A meta-analytic review of prolonged exposure for posttraumatic stress disorder. *Clin. Psychol. Rev.* **30:** 635–641.

15. Nemeroff, C.B. *et al.* 2006. Posttraumatic stress disorder: a state-of-the-science review. *J. Psychiatr. Res.* **40:** 1–21.

16. Resick, P.A. & M.K. Schnicke. 1993. *Cognitive Processing Therapy for Rape Victims: A Treatment Manual*. Sage. Thousand Oaks, CA.

17. Resick, P.A., P. Nishith, T.L. Weaver, *et al.* 2002. A comparison of cognitive-processing therapy with prolonged exposure and a waiting condition for the treatment of chronic posttraumatic stress disorder in female rape victims. *J. Consult. Clin. Psychol.* **70:** 867–879.

18. Monson, C.M. *et al.* 2006. Cognitive processing therapy for veterans with military-related posttraumatic stress disorder. *J. Consult. Clin. Psychol.* **74:** 898–907.

19. Shapiro, F. 2001. *EMDR: Eye Movement Desensitization of Reprocessing: Basic Principles, Protocols and Procedures*. 2nd ed. Guilford Press. New York.

20. Maxfield, L. 2003. Clinical implications and recommendations arising from EMDR research findings. *J. Trauma. Pract.* **2:** 61–81.

21. Seidler, G.H. & F.E. Wagner. 2006. Comparing the efficacy of EMDR and trauma-focused cognitive-behavioral therapy in the treatment of PTSD: a meta-analytic study. *Psychol. Med.: J. Res. Psychiatry Allied Sci.* **36:** 1515–1522.

22. Nowill, J. 2010. A critical review of the controversy surrounding eye movement desensitization and reprocessing. *Couns. Psychol. Rev.* **25:** 63–70.

23. Berger, W. *et al.* 2009. Pharmacologic alternatives to antidepressants in posttraumatic stress disorder: a systematic review. *Prog. Neuropsychopharmacol. Biol. Psychiatry* **33:** 169–180.

24. Davidson, J. *et al.* 2001. Efficacy of sertraline in preventing relapse of posttraumatic stress disorder: results of a 28-week double-blind, placebo-controlled study. *Am. J. Psychiatry* **158:** 1974–1981.

25. van Minnen, A., L. Hendriks & M. Olff. 2010. When do trauma experts choose exposure therapy for PTSD patients? A controlled study of therapist and patient factors. *Behav. Res. Ther.* **48:** 312–320.

26. Becker, C.B., C. Zayfert & E. Anderson. 2004. A survey of psychologists' attitudes towards and utilization of exposure therapy for PTSD. *Behav. Res. Ther.* **42:** 277–292.

27. Cahill, S.P. *et al.* 2006. Dissemination of exposure therapy in the treatment of posttraumatic stress disorder. *J. Trauma. Stress* **19:** 597–610.

28. Jovanovic, T. & K.J. Ressler. 2010. How the neurocircuitry and genetics of fear inhibition may inform our understanding of PTSD. *J. Psychiatry* **167:** 648–662.

29. Miller, L. 2008. Prazosin for the treatment of posttraumatic stress disorder sleep disturbances. *Pharmacology* **28:** 656–666.

30. Taylor, H., M. Freeman & M. Cates. 2008. Prazosin for treatment of nightmares related to posttraumatic stress disorder. *Am. J. Health Syst. Pharmacy* **65:** 716–722.

31. Taylor, F. *et al.* 2008. Prazosin effects on objective sleep measures and clinical symptoms in civilian trauma posttraumatic stress disorder: a placebo-controlled study. *Biol. Psychiatry* **63:** 629–632.

32. Raskind, M.A. *et al.* 2003. Reduction of nightmares and other PTSD symptoms in combat veterans by prazosin: a placebo-controlled study. *Am. J. Psychiatry* **160:** 371–373.

33. Thompson, C.E., F.B. Taylor, M.E. McFall, *et al.* 2008. Nonnightmare distressed awakenings in veterans with posttraumatic stress disorder: response to prazosin. *J. Trauma. Stress* **21:** 417–420.

34. Raskind, M.A. *et al.* 2007. A parallel group placebo controlled study of prazosin for trauma nightmares and sleep disturbance in combat veterans with post-traumatic stress disorder. *Biol. Psychiatry* **61:** 928–934.

35. Davis, M., M. Barad, M. Otto & S. Southwick. 2006. Combining pharmacotherapy with cognitive behavioral therapy: traditional and new approaches. *J. Trauma. Stress* **19:** 571–581.

36. Davis, M., K. Ressler, B.O. Rothbaum & R. Richardson. 2006. Effects of D-cycloserine on extinction: translation from preclinical to clinical work. *Biol. Psychiatry* **60:** 369–375.

37. Ledgerwood, L., R. Richardson & J. Cranney. 2005. D-cycloserine facilitates extinction of learned fear: effects on reacquisition and generalized extinction. *Biol. Psychiatry* **57:** 841–847.

38. Flood, J.F., J.E. Morley & T.H. Lanthorn. 1992. Effect on memory processing by D-cycloserine, an agonist of the NMDA/glycine receptor. *Eur. J. Pharmacol.* **221:** 249–254.

39. Lelong, V., F. Dauphin & M. Boulouard. 2001. RS 67333 and D-cycloserine accelerate learning acquisition in the rat. *Neuropharmacology* **41:** 517–522.

40. Monahan, J.B., G.E. Handelmann, W.F. Hood & A.A. Cordi. 1989. D-cycloserine, a positive modulator of the N-methyl-D-aspartate receptor, enhances performance of learning tasks in rats. *Pharmacol. Biochem. Behav.* **34:** 649–653.

41. Walker, D.L., K.J. Ressler, K.-T. Lu & M. Davis. 2002. Facilitation of conditioned fear extinction by systemic administration or intra-amygdala infusions of D-cycloserine as assessed with fear-potentiated startle in rats. *J. Neurosci.* **22:** 2343–2351.

42. Ressler, K.J. *et al.* 2004. Cognitive enhancers as adjuncts to psychotherapy: use of D-cycloserine in phobic individuals to facilitate extinction of fear. *Arch. Gen. Psychiatry* **61:** 1136–1144.

43. Hofmann, S.G. *et al.* 2006. Augmentation of exposure therapy with D-cycloserine for social anxiety disorder. *Arch. Gen. Psychiatry* **63:** 298–304.

44. Guastella, A.J. *et al.* 2008. A randomized controlled trial of D-cycloserine enhancement of exposure therapy for social anxiety disorder. *Biol. Psychiatry* **63:** 544–549.

45. Monson, C., S. Fredman & K. Adair. 2008. Cognitive-behavioral conjoint therapy for PTSD: application to operation enduring and Iraqi Freedom service members and Veterans. *J. Clin. Psychol.* **64:** 958–971.

46. Sayers, S., V. Farrow, J. Ross & D. Oslin. 2009. Family problems among recently returned military veterans referred for a mental health evaluation. *J. Clin. Psychiatry* **70:** 163–170.

47. Riggs, D. 2000. Marital and family therapy. In *Effective Treatments for PTSD.* E. Foa, T. Keane & M. Friedman Eds.: 280–301. Guilford Press. New York.

48. Monson, C.M., P.P. Schnurr, S.P. Stevens & K.A. Guthrie. 2004. Cognitive-behavioral couple's treatment for posttraumatic stress disorder: initial findings. *J. Trauma. Stress* **17:** 341–344.

49. Bleiberg, K. & J. Markowitz. 2005. A pilot study of interpersonal psychotherapy for posttraumatic stress disorder. *Am. J. Psychiatry* **162:** 181–183.

50. Krupnick, J.L. *et al.* 2008. Group interpersonal psychotherapy for low-income women with posttraumatic stress disorder. *Psychother. Res.* **18:** 497–507.

51. Robertson, M., P. Rushton, D. Batrim, *et al.* 2007. Open trial of interpersonal psychotherapy for chronic post traumatic stress disorder. *Aust. Psychiatry* **15:** 375–379.

52. Rothbaum, B.O. *et al.* 1999. Virtual reality exposure therapy for PTSD Vietnam veterans: a case study. *J. Trauma. Stress* **12:** 263–271.

53. Rothbaum, B.O., L.F. Hodges, D. Ready, et al. 2001. Virtual reality exposure therapy for Vietnam veterans with posttraumatic stress disorder. *J. Clin. Psychiatry* **62:** 617–622.

54. Difede, J. *et al.* 2007. Virtual reality exposure therapy for the treatment of posttraumatic stress disorder following September 11, 2001. *J. Clin. Psychiatry* **68:** 1639–1647.

55. Gerardi, M., B.O. Rothbaum, K. Ressler, *et al.* 2008. Virtual reality exposure therapy using a virtual Iraq: case report. *J. Trauma. Stress* **21:** 209–213.

56. Cukor, J., J. Spitalnick, J. Difede, *et al.* 2009. Emerging treatments for PTSD. *Clin. Psychol. Rev.* **29:** 715–726.

57. Rizzo, A. 2009. CyberSightings. *Cyberpsychol. Behav.* **12:** 113–118.

58. Brady, K.T., T.K. Killeen, T. Brewerton & S. Lucerini. 2000. Comorbidity of psychiatric disorders and posttraumatic stress disorder. *J. Clin. Psychiatry* **61**(Suppl. 7): 22–32.

59. Dunn, N.J. *et al.* 2007. A randomized trial of self-management and psychoeducational group therapies for co-morbid chronic posttraumatic stress disorder and depressive disorder. *J. Trauma. Stress* **20:** 221–237.

60. Back, S.E. 2010. Toward an improved model of treating co-occurring PTSD and substance use disorders. *Am. J. Psychiatry* **167:** 11–13.

61. Najavits, L.M. 2002. *Seeking Safety: A Treatment Manual for PTSD and Substance Abuse.* The Guilford Press. New York, NY.

62. Hien, D. *et al.* 2010. Do treatment improvements in PTSD severity affect substance use outcomes? A secondary analysis from a randomized clinical trial in NIDA's Clinical Trials Network. *Am. J. Psychiatry* **167:** 95–101.

63. Triffleman, E., K. Carroll & S. Kellogg. 1999. Substance dependence posttraumatic stress disorder therapy: an integrated cognitive-behavioral approach. *J. Subst. Abuse Treat.* **17:** 3–14.

64. Brady, K.T., B. Dansky, S. Back, *et al.* 2001. Exposure therapy in the treatment of PTSD among cocaine-dependent individuals: preliminary findings. *J. Subst. Abuse Treat.* **21:** 47–54.

65. Najavits, L., M. Schmitz, S. Gotthardt & R. Weiss. 2005. Seeking Safety plus exposure therapy: an outcome study on dual diagnosis men. *J. Psychoactive Drugs* **37:** 425–435.

66. McGovern, M.P. *et al.* 2009. A cognitive behavioral therapy for co-occurring substance use and posttraumatic stress disorders. *Addict. Behav.* **34:** 892–897.

67. Rotunda, R.J., T.J. O'Farrell, M. Murphy & S.H. Babey. 2008. Behavioral couples therapy for comorbid substance use disorders and combat-related posttraumatic stress disorder among male veterans: an initial evaluation. *Addict. Behav.* **33:** 180–187.

68. Foa, E.B. & M.T. Williams. 2010. Methodology of a random ized double-blind clinical trial for comorbid posttraumatic stress disorder and alcohol dependence. *Ment. Health Subst. Use: Dual Diagn.* **3:** 131–147.

69. Difede, J., J. Cukor, F. Lee & R. Yurt. 2009. Treatments for common psychiatric conditions among adults during acute, rehabilitation, and reintegration phases. *Int. Rev. Psychiatry* **21:** 559–569.

70. Wagner, A., D.F. Zatzick, A. Ghesquiere & G.J. Jurkovich. 2007. Behavioral activation as an early intervention for posttraumatic stress disorder and depression among physically injured trauma survivors. *Cogn. Behav. Pract.* **14:** 341–349.

71. McAllister, T. 2009. Psychopharmacological issues in the treatment of TBI and PTSD. *Clin. Neuropsychol.* **23:** 1338–1367.

72. Vasterling, J.J., M. Verfaellie & K.D. Sullivan. 2009. Mild traumatic brain injury and posttraumatic stress disorder in returning veterans: perspectives from cognitive neuroscience. *Clin. Psychol. Rev.* **29:** 674–684.

Ann. N.Y. Acad. Sci. ISSN 0077-8923

ANNALS OF THE NEW YORK ACADEMY OF SCIENCES

Issue: *Psychiatric and Neurologic Aspects of War*

Buddy-to-Buddy, a citizen soldier peer support program to counteract stigma, PTSD, depression, and suicide

John F. Greden,[1,3] Marcia Valenstein,[1,2] Jane Spinner,[1] Adrian Blow,[4] Lisa A. Gorman,[4] Gregory W. Dalack,[1] Sheila Marcus,[1] and Michelle Kees[1]

[1]University of Michigan Department of Psychiatry and Comprehensive Depression Center, University of Michigan, Ann Arbor, Michigan. [2]Ann Arbor Veterans Administration Hospital, University of Michigan, Ann Arbor, Michigan. [3]Molecular and Behavioral Neurosciences Institute, University of Michigan, Ann Arbor, Michigan. [4]Michigan State University, Lansing, Michigan

Address for correspondence: John F. Greden, M.D., University of Michigan Health System, 4250 Plymouth Road, Ann Arbor, Michigan 48109. gredenj@umich.edu

Citizen soldiers (National Guard and Reserves) represent approximately 40% of the two million armed forces deployed to Afghanistan and Iraq. Twenty-five to forty percent of them develop PTSD, clinical depression, sleep disturbances, or suicidal thoughts. Upon returning home, many encounter additional stresses and hurdles to obtaining care: specifically, many civilian communities lack military medical/psychiatric facilities; financial, job, home, and relationship stresses have evolved or have been exacerbated during deployment; uncertainty has increased related to future deployment; there is loss of contact with military peers; and there is reluctance to recognize and acknowledge mental health needs that interfere with treatment entry and adherence. Approximately half of those needing help are not receiving it. To address this constellation of issues, a private–public partnership was formed under the auspices of the Welcome Back Veterans Initiative. In Michigan, the Army National Guard teamed with the University of Michigan and Michigan State University to develop innovative peer-to-peer programs for soldiers (Buddy-to-Buddy) and augmented programs for military families. Goals are to improve treatment entry, adherence, clinical outcomes, and to reduce suicides. This manuscript describes training approaches, preliminary results, and explores future national dissemination.

Keywords: citizen soldiers; peer-to-peer; PTSD; depression; suicide

Introduction

Forty percent or more of the approximate two million troops that have been deployed to military conflicts in Afghanistan and Iraq have been members of America's National Guard or military Reserve units.[1] These "citizen soldiers" experience traumas and stresses comparable to those encountered by active duty soldiers, such as battlefield conflicts and injuries; improvised explosive device explosions; deaths among fellow soldiers in their units; "downrange funerals" (a colloquial term used by some deployed military soldiers); and prolonged separation from loved ones.

The clinical and social consequences of these experiences include posttraumatic stress disorder (PTSD) symptoms, clinical depression, sleep dysregulation and nightmares, self-medication, sub-stance use and abuse, and suicide thoughts, acts, and occasional tragic deaths by suicide. For some, co-occurring traumatic brain injuries confound the clinical presentation.[2–5]

Military personnel experience major psychiatric disorders at rates comparable to the general population, but these rates increase following deployment.[6,7] In one study, combat experience during Operation Enduring Freedom (OEF) and Operation Iraqi Freedom (OIF) was significantly associated with use of mental health services and military attrition following deployment.[6] Forty-two percent of citizen soldiers from Reserve and National Guard units report mental health issues suggesting the need for evaluation and possible treatment; yet, many do not initiate treatment.[5,8] Only 54% of soldiers referred through the Post Deployment Health Assessment screening process subsequently followed

doi: 10.1111/j.1749-6632.2010.05719.x

Ann. N.Y. Acad. Sci. 1208 (2010) 90–97 © 2010 Association for Research in Nervous and Mental Disease.

through with a mental health visit,[6] and only 30% with identified need reported receiving minimally adequate treatment (adequate medication trial or at least eight psychotherapy sessions).[5]

Although research is needed to improve effectiveness of available treatments, innovative programs to overcome stigma and associated barriers to treatment entry and adherence are arguably as crucial.

Unique stresses and barriers to treatment entry and adherence among citizen soldiers

Citizen soldiers commonly encounter additional stressors or barriers that are different from active duty soldiers and interfere with entry and adherence into treatment. Perhaps most important is the inexorable stigma associated with seeking care. Although a common barrier to active duty soldiers as well, stigma may be even more difficult to overcome in community settings. Other postdeployment stresses include financial pressures and for some, income reductions; concerns about job availability or job security upon returning from deployment; home foreclosures; future prospects of being deployed; and absence of the readily available medical and psychiatric facilities that would have been available had they returned to an active duty military post. For those in rural areas, clinical services sometimes are available only at great distances, generating long travel times that make appointments difficult to keep. Finally, the dispersal and separation across large state regions and loss of everyday contact with military buddies mean that citizen soldiers do not have colleagues and comrades readily available for valuable sharing of experiences and support. A key consequence is that many of those needing professional treatment are reluctant, and far less likely to receive it unless these barriers are overcome; without treatment, clinical and functional deterioration is more likely.

This report does not focus upon specific treatment interventions for PTSD, depression, suicide, or their co-occurrence. Available treatments are described in detail elsewhere and extensive Department of Defense projects are under way to improve available treatments.[9] Instead, we aim to describe refinements and innovations in peer-to-peer strategies to help counter the unique barriers faced by citizen soldiers to aid them in overcoming stigma and

promote essential entry into and adherence with appropriate treatments.

Michigan Army National Guard: a prototype of citizen soldier in America

The Michigan Army National Guard's (MI ARNG) experiences illustrate the growing importance of citizen soldiers in ongoing military conflicts. Since 2001, around 90% of the approximate 9,000 members of the MI ARNG have deployed to Afghanistan and/or Iraq, many on multiple occasions. Citizen soldiers, as already summarized, manifest symptoms compatible with PTSD, depression, substance use, and interpersonal conflicts to a greater degree as active duty soldiers. Such symptoms are sometimes not evident until after significant time delays. Some returning soldiers also have manifestations of traumatic brain injury, sometimes referred to as a new signature injury in the OEF/OIF conflict.[2,5] To help respond to these concerns and proactively address these "silent injuries," MI ARNG leaders forged collaborations with faculty and staff members of Michigan State University and the University of Michigan; steps involved in forging such collaborations are described in a separate report.[9]

A survey tool was used to understand the scope of veterans' problems and mental health needs. This survey was completed by 926 returning MI ARNG soldiers and spouses. Approximately, 40% of this sample screened positive for a mental health problem of some kind translating to approximately 3,500 of the 9,000 MI ARNG soldier force. Approximately, 8% of those assessed for a mental health problem reported suicidal thoughts (Table 1).

A crucial issue was identified: only 47% of returned citizen soldiers with reported clinical problems had sought any help. The most common reported reasons for not seeking help were linked to

Table 1. Reported reasons for not seeking help

- Do not want it in military records (27%)
- Unit leadership might treat me differently (20%)
- Too embarrassing (17%)
- Harm career (17%)
- Costs (15%)
- Do not know where to go to get help (6%)
- No providers in my community (6%)
- Transportation (5%)

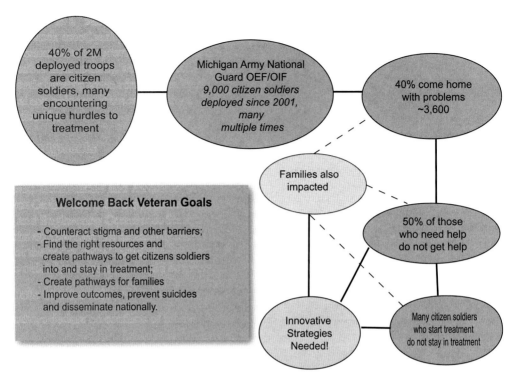

Figure 1. Scope of problems among citizen soldiers and families: need for innovative peer-to-peer programs and national dissemination strategies. (In color in Annals online.)

stigma, fear of being seen as weak, concerns about confidentiality of military records, fears about damaging their future careers, and for a much smaller percentage, uncertainty about where to go for treatment or practical barriers in getting there.

Efforts to counteract these stigma barriers appear fundamental if we are to successfully identify and treat PTSD, depression, suicide, and related problems among returning veterans. Treatments can not work unless they are delivered; innovative strategies are required. A summary of the issues is portrayed in Figure 1.

Welcome Back Veterans: a private–academic–military partnership to address mental health problems of returning veterans

Responding to the well-reported problems of returning military veterans nationally, start-up philanthropic funding was provided in a national initiative known as "Welcome Back Veterans" (WBV) (www.welcomebackveterans.org). WBV leadership worked in partnership with Major League Baseball, the McCormick Foundation, and initially the Ad Council to generate funding. The University of Michigan, Weill-Cornell, and Stanford University were selected as three "WBV core centers" to help mobilize clinical outreach and national dissemination efforts to address some of the unmet needs of returning veterans. The aims were to integrate and disseminate gains and specialty knowledge from each university, coordinate with advances occurring elsewhere, and augment the veterans administration programs available to returning veterans. A University of Michigan team and a Michigan State University team collaborated with the leadership of the MI ARNG to design and implement an innovative peer-to-peer program for returning soldiers. Although not the focus of this report, the University of Michigan team also forged accompanying strategies to reach out to families and children of MI ARNG citizen soldiers.

Buddy-to-Buddy: a peer-to-peer program for returning citizen soldiers

The collaborative team hypothesized that the crucial steps of counteracting stigma and improving treatment entry and adherence might best be enhanced by "using culture to change culture." When discussing their OEF/OIF deployments, many soldiers conveyed, that "if you haven't been there, you don't get it," "we believe in taking care of our own," and "other veterans can be trusted." For many, the nation's established system of medical and psychiatric programs and traditional clinical teams of medical, psychology, or social work leaders are not necessarily starting points. Correlative comments occasionally conveyed optimism, such as "another veteran who has been there may make it easier to get help." A logical extension of these observations led to the realization that when cultural barriers impeded treatment entry or adherence, peer-to-peer influences may be a crucial cultural starting point in overcoming them.[10]

For these reasons, university partners worked with the MI ARNG leaders and staff to develop what became known as "Buddy-to-Buddy." More detailed descriptions of Buddy-to-Buddy will be described in forthcoming publications. This manuscript aims to summarize Buddy-to-Buddy concepts, goals, acceptance, and dissemination to date; future steps required to confirm the clinical effectiveness of peer-to-peer strategies; and future recommendations as to how this and other related programs may play crucial roles for returning veteran populations. We also hypothesize that these initiatives may be a valuable adjunct and foundation in efforts to reduce veteran suicides.

Buddy-to-Buddy components, goals, principles, and philosophies: a brief summary

Buddy-to-Buddy ensures contact with every returning MI ARNG soldier by using soldier peers. Trained peers regularly contact their assigned panel of soldiers to "check in," help identify those with clinical needs, encourage registration and entry into Veterans Administration Hospital (VAH) or military programs, and develop strategies to enhance enrollment in community treatment programs that are perceived as safe and acceptable should other alternatives be unworkable or unacceptable. In addition, soldier peers support adherence after starting treatment.

The program also seeks to identify and train selected community clinicians, orienting them to military culture and combat issues. This serves to enhance the resource pool and optimizes the like-

lihood for readily available interventions. These efforts build on earlier efforts initiated by Michigan State University and MI ARNG to emphasize collaboration with an array of quality providers, because community resources and a geographically dispersed network of clinical providers are essential to address the approximately 50% of citizen soldiers that need and would benefit from clinical intervention but are not currently receiving it. More such efforts are planned.

Consistent with military traditions, "buddies, families, and resiliency" became constant messages, accompanied by the messages of "you are not alone, treatment works, it has helped many of your buddies, and pursuing help is a sign of strength." Another major thrust sought to link veterans with other concrete resources they need to reduce stressors, such as employment benefits, housing, and financial guidance.

Creating and training the pool of Buddy Ones and Buddy Twos

A starting principle of the Buddy-to-Buddy outreach program was to ensure that all soldiers were contacted, not just the ones who were exhibiting clear and unmistakable signs of needing help. A two-tier program was created. The first tier of peer-to-peer, called Buddy Ones, consists of soldiers within each National Guard unit. The recruitment, operation, and oversight are provided by the MI ARNG. A second, smaller tier, called Buddy Twos or Volunteer Veterans, is operated by veterans outside of the Guard, and is overseen by University of Michigan staff.

"Buddy-One" individuals were identified for further training by their Chain of Command. They were chosen either by their position in the chain of command or because they were informal leaders of their units, depending on the preferences of the Command of each specific Battalion. Care was taken that peers supporters and their soldiers did not have great disparity in rank.

Training for Buddy Ones approximates 3 h and conveys the program rationale and philosophy, roles, communications skills, including what to do in case of emergencies, and an overview of resources of all types. A manual and quick reference cards were prepared and are distributed to Buddy One personnel. These are available online or upon request. Support and retraining are provided during drill weekends and ongoing consultation continues to be integral to refinements.

"Check-in" calls are incorporated into the design. A strong message for Buddy One personnel is that "your job is not to give help, it's to get help." Special strategies emphasize earlier identification of worrisome behavior, believing that those who know the soldier can assess whether something is wrong; legitimize seeking help; communicate knowledge of referral sources; and follow-up to aid adherence. Buddy Twos are veterans from outside the Guard who serve as back up for the Buddy Ones. They receive more intensive training in communication skills, including motivational interviewing, and become well-versed in both military and community resources that they can use as needed. The Buddy Twos staff the National Guard Armories statewide during drill weekends and serve as on-site resources to address concerns. Buddy Twos often help individuals navigate systems, such as the Veterans Administration in order to facilitate access. To date, approximately 350 Buddy Ones and 32 Buddy Twos have been trained.

Importantly, MI ARNG command leaders have been invested in identifying and supporting citizen soldiers with these "invisible injuries." Their leadership and partnership have been essential. Individual soldiers identified as potential Buddy Ones or Buddy Twos have been similarly invested, helpful, and committed to helping their returning veteran colleagues; their participation and suggestions were instrumental in planning, shaping, and implementing the program as well as suggesting modifications.

Buddy-to-Buddy: preliminary observations and evaluations

Among the Buddy-to-Buddy participants surveyed, 9 of 10 understand the intent of the program; approximately two-thirds are receiving regular calls from their Buddy and feel comfortable talking with their Buddy. More than half reported using resources or services suggested by their Buddy. In many cases, these were referrals for concrete resources, such as assistance with benefits, job-placement services, financial assistance, or legal help. Of primary relevance to this report, more than 20% have been referred to formal treatment by their Buddy, reflecting previously unmet clinical needs. These referrals have been made to VAHs and Vet Centers, community-based mental health

providers, military-sponsored agencies, such as Military One Source, and to community clinical resources. These referrals are in the process of being evaluated in greater detail and longer-term outcome evaluations are being proposed.

MI ARNG leaders and participants have endorsed these initiatives, conveying that they merge favorably with the fundamentals of National Guard culture. Predictably, not all returning citizen soldiers are likely to be responsive to peer-to-peer initiatives, but clearly more of those in need of treatment are being reached by this use of buddy culture. Even more would be reached with extensions of the program. Synergy with adjunct innovative strategies may be required to reach those not yet receptive to the Buddy-to-Buddy approach. Examples include family outreach programs, incorporation of respected speakers to help counteract stigma, and others.

Potential role of peer-to-peer programs in reduction of suicides among citizen soldiers

Rates of suicide in active military personnel have been increasing since 2003 and now surpass age- and gender-matched nonveterans. These increases have led to a fervent search for new interventions.[11–14] In a recent Department of Defense and Veterans Administration Conference on Suicide Prevention among Veterans, Shinsheki conveyed that of the approximate 85 deaths a day by suicide in America, about 18 are by veterans and most are not currently receiving treatment in the VAH.[15]

It is our hypothesis that the Buddy-to-Buddy program has strong potential to augment suicide prevention programs by applying the previously described, that is, the "use of culture to change the culture of treatment avoidance." Strategies would emphasize earlier identification of worrisome, threatening or self-injurious behaviors, knowing about referral sources, "helping show the way," and longer-term support of adherence to treatment once started.[16]

Determining whether suicide prevention efforts among returning soldiers are effective requires close attention to co-occurring diagnoses or comorbidities. PTSD and clinical depression commonly coexist among returning soldiers.[17,18] Stresses during and after deployment play a role in both, and may precipitate both PTSD and/or major depressive disorder (MDD). MDD is the diagnosis most closely associated with suicide and its primary ages of onset (15–24 years of age) overlap closely with the age range for most soldiers and returning veterans.[19–21] In the general population, 80% or more of those who die by suicide are struggling with MDD[19]; yet, depression often remains undiagnosed in all populations.[22] Reasons are multiple: depressive symptoms may be mild and sporadic in early stages so they may be overlooked or attributed exclusively to external stresses. In some cases, symptoms may be clouded or "hidden" by co-occurring diagnoses. PTSD, for example, may have greater cultural acceptance in military populations than a diagnosis of depression, although this has not been adequately studied. Unfortunately, co-occurring clinical depression, when untreated, routinely evolves over subsequent years into an episodic, recurrent, worsening chronic illness that becomes more difficult to treat.[22]

Because co-occurrence is the norm, concomitant treatment of all prevailing clinical syndromes should be the norm. Treatment of the individual citizen soldiers should be as comprehensive as possible, addressing all existing contributors. This includes PTSD, depression, sleep dysregulation, and substance misuse.

Another potential rationale for developing Buddy-to-Buddy type programs to aid suicide prevention is that the goals, culture, and strategies are parallel to those emphasized by suicide prevention programs encountered by veterans during their military deployments. Examples are ACE (Ask, Care, Escort),[23] ACT (Ask, Care, Treat),[24] and R.A.C.E. (Recognize, Ask, Care, Escort)[25].[10]

In essence, we hypothesize that coupling Buddy-to-Buddy or comparable documented peer support programs with evidence-based treatment interventions would help address many untreated individuals; improve entry and adherence into treatment; accelerate clinical improvements by enabling exposure to effective treatments for PTSD, depression and other risk variables; and hopefully reduce suicides for returning veterans. Lessons learned to date are summarized in Table 2.

Augmenting strategies: family outreach and use of spokespersons

Survey data indicate high levels of parenting and marital stress at the time of reintegration. In addition, spouses uniformly report a desire to have increased support during deployment, suggesting

Table 2. Buddy-to-Buddy program summary highlights

- *Similar risks:* Citizen soldiers struggle with PTSD, clinical depression, sleep dysregulation, substance use disturbances, and increased risk of suicide upon returning from deployment at rates comparable or greater than active duty soldiers. Comorbidity (co-occurrence of one or more diagnostic syndromes) is the norm, not the exception.
- *Unique barriers and stresses:* Citizen soldiers encounter additional stresses and unique hurdles to receiving treatment upon returning to their community, including financial and family stresses, stigma, unavailability of treatment resources, and separation from military support systems. Stigma remains formidable.
- *Inadequate treatment entry and adherence:* Only about half of those in need enter treatment. Overcoming stigma-related barriers is an essential first step for these returning citizen soldiers if clinical help is to be provided and suicides and other problems prevented.
- *Prevailing culture is a barrier:* Advice to seek treatment often ignored. The prevailing culture remains "If you haven't been there you don't get it."
- *"Buddy-to-Buddy:" using culture to change culture:* Buddy-to-Buddy uses military culture to change the stigma culture; peer-to-peer appears to be a powerful approach to addressing stigma and associated barriers.
- Goals of Buddy-to-Buddy are to get help, not to give help.
- *Private–Public–Academic–Military partnerships are fundamental:* When dealing with citizen soldiers in the National Guard and Reserves, collaborations, mutual respect, and understanding are essential. Involvement of military leadership is fundamental at all stages.
- *Buddy-to-Buddy may aid suicide prevention:* studies are required but treatment entry is essential if treatments are to work.
- *Dissemination strategies are needed:* Because of national scope, dissemination strategies must be developed. Multiple voices must be recruited to help counteract stigma. Emerging clinical networks are positioned to aid and would greatly accelerate dissemination strategies.

that early interventions both preceding and during deployment may reduce symptom severity in spouses. Such interventions also could target risk factors for parenting and marital strain. These prevention strategies might reduce marital dyadic and parenting stress upon reintegration, in turn reducing stresses impacting the soldier. Moreover, providing spouses with resources needed for their own symptoms often serves as a motivation for spouses to encourage their soldier partners toward intervention.

Other trusted spokespersons similarly can be recruited and educated in mental health literacy to help destigmatize these silent brain injuries, and to emphasize the importance of early treatment and maintenance of wellness, support systems, and suicide prevention strategies. They often are equally valuable in helping community members understand the problems being faced by returning veterans. These may be celebrities, athletes, politicians, or local citizens willing to lend their voices to help educate the public while simultaneously decreasing stigma.

Future recommendations

Citizen soldiers live in coexisting cultures. They are military personnel who spend most of their lives in civilian settings. They have played crucial roles in ongoing military conflicts. During deployment and postdeployment, they experience similar clinical problems to active duty soldiers, but upon returning home often lack the available support systems of military posts. Although Veterans Administration and community resources are available for most, among many there is prevailing reluctance to use them. A major national initiative is needed to enable a far greater percent of returning citizen soldiers with mental health problems to break through their internal resistance, enter, and hopefully benefit from available treatments.

We strongly recommend that Buddy-to-Buddy be thoroughly evaluated for efficacy and that if it is effective in improving soldier outcomes, that it be disseminated nationally, national training programs be launched, efforts be linked with evaluation outcome assessments, and proxy serial evaluation measures be used when seeking to evaluate possible suicide risk.[11,21] Suicide has a low base rate so truly large samples must be studied, accompanied by serial assessments of suicide ideation, acts, prior history of suicide attempts, and identification of well-documented risk variables, such as depression, PTSD, substance abuse, and sleep dysregulation. Dissemination predictably can be acceler-

ated if already existing national networks are incorporated into these academic-military-community partnerships.

We also recommend that flexibility and individual preference be recognized as important variables when seeking to get reluctant individuals into treatment. Stigma promotes strong recalcitrance to treatment, so it may be essential to match referral resources to the veterans' and family members' preferences. Motivational interviewing can be used effectively as an approach to encourage treatment entry.[26] Finally, to maintain follow-up when geographic barriers exist, telemedicine interventions may be essential.[27,28]

The strategy we are emphasizing uses trusted fellow veterans (buddies) and augmenting supporting personnel as allies to improve treatment entry and adherence. Evidence to date indicates that this approach may help many overcome prevailing stigma. Consistent with both military culture and centuries-old clinical values, the goals are that no citizen soldiers will be left behind and that those struggling with invisible wounds of war will be welcomed back to a healthier future.

Acknowledgments

The authors acknowledge indispensable contributions from academic colleagues at Michigan State University, the Ann Arbor Veterans Administration Hospital, University of Michigan, in addition to Weill-Cornell and Stanford, the other core centers in the Welcome Back Veterans collaboration. We also acknowledge support from Health Services Research and Development Service, Department of Veterans Affairs. RRP 09-420, Families and Communities Together Coalition, Michigan State University, Department of Human Development and Family Studies and Biomedical Research Informatics Center at Michigan State University. Major League Baseball, the McCormick Foundation, the Meader Research Fund, and the Entertainment Industry Foundation (EIF) provided critical financial support. Finally, and most importantly, the participation of returning citizen soldiers and leaders of the Michigan Army National Guard (MI ARNG) made it possible to develop and steadily refine the Buddy-go-Buddy and family programs.

Conflicts of interest

The authors declare no conflicts of interest.

References

1. Waterhouse, M. & J. O'Bryant. 2008. National Guard personnel and deployments: fact sheet. Congressional Research Service, The Library of Congress. Order Code RS22451. January.

2. Hoge, C.W., D. McGurk, J.L. Thomas, *et al.* 2008. Mild traumatic brain injury in U.S. soldiers returning from Iraq. *N. Engl. J. Med.* **358:** 453–463.

3. Jacobson, I.G., M.A. Ryan, T.I. Hooper, *et al.* 2008. Alcohol use and alcohol-related problems before and after military combat deployment. *JAMA* **300:** 663–675.

4. Schneiderman, A., E. Braver & H. Kang. 2008. Understanding sequelae of injury mechanisms and mild traumatic brain injury incurred during the conflicts in Iraq and Afghanistan: persistent postconcussive symptoms and posttraumatic stress disorder. *Am. J. Epidemiol.* **167:** 1446–1452.

5. Tanielian, T. & L.H. Jaycox. eds. 2008. *Invisible Wounds of War: Psychological and Cognitive Injuries, Their Consequences, and Services to Assist Recovery.* RAND. Santa Monica, CA. iii–iv; 3–7; 123–134.

6. Hoge, C.W., J.L. Auchterlonie & C.S. Milliken. 2006. Mental health problems, use of mental health services, and attrition from military service after returning from deployment to Iraq or Afghanistan. *JAMA* **295:** 1023–1032.

7. Riddle, J.R., T.C. Smith, B. Smith, *et al.* for the Millenium Cohort Study Team. 2007. Millenium cohort: the 2001–2003 baseline prevalence of mental disorders in the U.S. military. *J. Clin. Epidemiol.* **60:** 192–201.

8. Milliken, C.S., J.L. Auchterlonie & C.W. Hoge. 2007. Longitudinal assessment of mental health problems among active and reserve component soldiers returning from the Iraq war. *JAMA* **298:** 2141–2148.

9. Dalack, G.W., A. Blow, M. Valenstein, *et al.* 2010. Working together to meet the needs of Army National Guard soldiers: an academic-military partnership. *Psychiatric Services* Accepted.

10. Emmanuel, L.O. 2009. *VA hires vets to go find comrades who need help.* Mar 24 2009. Associated Press. http://www.armytimes.com/news/2009/03/ap_va_veterans_outreach_032509/(accessed August 26, 2010).

11. Army Suicide Prevention Program (ASPP). 2009. Shoulder to Shoulder: no soldier stands alone. http://www.armyg1.army.mil/hr/suicide/(accessed April 6, 2009).

12. Basu, S. 2009. Suicide rate among soldiers at all-time high. *U.S. Medicine.* March. http://www.usmedicine.com/articles/suicide-rate-among-soldiers-at-all-time-high.html (accessed August 17, 2010).

13. Kuehn, B.M. 2009. Soldier suicide rates continue to rise: military, scientists work to stem the tide. *JAMA* **301:** 1111–1113.

14. US Army(b), Wright, LT COL G., Media Relations Division, OCPA. 2009. Army releases March suicide data. News release.

http://www.army.mil/newsreleases/2009/04/10/19537-army-releases-march-suicide-data/(accessed April 30, 2009).

15. Shinsheki, E. 2010. Department of Defense/VA Suicide Prevention Conference: Building Strong and Resilient Communities. January 11. Washington, DC. http://www1.va.gov/opa/speeches/2010/10_0111hold.asp (accessed August 17, 2010).

16. Valenstein, M., D. Eisenberg, J.F. McCarthy, *et al.* 2009. Service implications of providing intensive monitoring during high-risk periods for suicide among VA patients with depression. *Psychiatr. Serv.* **60:** 439–444.

17. Keane, T.M., A.D. Marshall & C.T. Taft. 2006. Posttraumatic stress disorder: etiology, epidemiology, and treatment outcome. *Annu. Rev. Clin. Psychol.* **2:** 161–197.

18. Kilpatrick, D.G., K.C. Koenen, K.J. Ruggiero, *et al.* 2007. The serotonin transporter genotype and social support and moderation of posttraumatic stress disorder and depression in hurricane-exposed adults. *Am. J. Psychiatry* **164:** 1693–1699.

19. Joiner, T.E. 2005. *Why People Die by Suicide.* Harvard University Press. Cambridge, MA.

20. Oquendo, M.A., D. Currier & J.J. Mann. 2006. Prospective studies of suicidal behavior in major depressive and bipolar disorders: what is the evidence for predictive risk factors? *Acta Psychiatr. Scand.* **114:** 151–158.

21. Valenstein, M., H.M. Kim, D. Ganoczy, *et al.* 2009. Higher-risk periods for suicide among VA patients receiving depression treatment: prioritizing suicide prevention efforts. *J. Affect Disord.* **112:** 50–58.

22. Greden, J.F. 2001. The burden of disease for treatment-resistant depression. *J. Clin. Psychiatry* **62**(Suppl. 16): 26–31.

23. Department of Veterans Affairs. 2009. ACE, suicide prevention for veterans and their families and friends. http://www.mentalhealth.va.gov/docs/VA_Brochure_08_25_2009.pdf (accessed August 17, 2010).

24. Bureau of Navy Personnel. Life Counts! ACT. http://www.npc.navy.mil/NR/rdonlyres/7A8A1BD2-0E80-4778-8759-779EB66C54E2/0/Suicide_Prevention_Trifold.pdf (accessed August 17, 2010).

25. United States Marine Corps. Never Leave a Marine Behind, R.A.C.E., Suicide Prevention. 2010. http://www.usmc-mccs.org/display_files/R_A_C_E%20BI-Fold%20with%20Explanation%20Page.pdf. May 12, 2010 (accessed August 17, 2010).

26. Hettema, J.E., J.M. Steele & W.R. Miller. 2005. Motivational interviewing. *Annu. Rev. Clin. Psychol.* **1:** 91–111.

27. Ludman, E.J., G.E. Simon, L.C. Grothaus, *et al.* 2007. A pilot study of telephone care management and structured disease self-management groups for chronic depression. *Psychiatr. Serv.* **58:** 1065–1072.

28. Hunkeler, E.M., J.F. Meresman, W.A. Hargreaves, *et al.* 2000. Efficacy of nurse telehealth care and peer support in augmenting treatment of depression in primary care. *Arch. Fam. Med.* **9:** 700–708.

Ann. N.Y. Acad. Sci. ISSN 0077-8923

ANNALS OF THE NEW YORK ACADEMY OF SCIENCES

Issue: *Psychiatric and Neurologic Aspects of War*

Suicide risk and prevention in veteran populations

Martha L. Bruce

Department of Psychiatry, Weill Cornell Medical College, White Plains, New York

Address for correspondence: Martha L. Bruce, Ph.D., M.P.H., Department of Psychiatry, Westchester Division, Weill Cornell Medical College, 21 Bloomingdale Road, White Plains, New York 10605. mbruce@med.cornell.edu

Rates of suicide among veterans of Operation Enduring Freedom (OEF) and Operation Iraqi Freedom (OIF) rose significantly from 2005 to 2007, adding to existing concerns about veteran suicide risk by the Department of Veterans Affairs. This paper summarizes the available data about risk and rates of suicide in veterans, including the choice of appropriate comparison groups and the identification of risk factors. The data suggest that taking into account the selection bias of who enters the military (known as the healthy soldier effect), rates of suicide in veterans are higher than expected, especially among activity duty OEF/OIF veterans and even more so among those who experienced injuries and trauma. Thus, the experiences of war and the downstream sequelae, in particular the individuals' psychological reactions and societal responses, lead to suicide risk. This paper describes the VA's response to these data in developing and implementing suicide prevention interventions.

Keywords: suicide; veterans; military

Introduction

In January 2010, the Department of Veterans Affairs (VA) released new data indicating that the rate of suicide among United States military veterans had increased by 26% between 2005 and 2007. The VA estimated that in 2005, the suicide rate per 100,000 veterans among men ages 18–29 was 44.99, but jumped to 56.77 in 2007. "Of the more than 30,000 suicides in this country each year, fully 20 percent of them are acts by veterans," said VA Secretary Eric Shinseki at a VA-sponsored suicide prevention conference. "That means on average 18 veterans commit suicide each day. Five of those veterans are under our care at VA."[1,2] The new data were consistent with a heightened awareness of the VA of the high risk for suicide in veterans, as evidenced by the then-Secretary of Veterans Affairs, James B. Peak, M.D., convening in 2008 a Blue Ribbon Work Group on Suicide Prevention in the Veteran Population. The Report of the Blue Ribbon Work Group addressed the needs of the full population of veterans, across the age span, and included not only those who use the health and mental health services provided by the Veterans Health Administration (VHA) but also those who do not use or are eligible for using the services.[3]

The purpose of this paper is to consider this issue more closely by examining the evidence based on veteran suicide risk, identifying factors associated with any increased risk, and describing the kinds of suicide prevention interventions that are being implemented in response to this need.

Assessing veterans' increased suicide risk

The veteran population is a large and heterogeneous group. The 5.5 million veterans served annually by the VHA represent only 23% of the total veteran population. The full population of veterans includes men and women who served during World War II, the Korean War, the Vietnam War, the Gulf War, Operation Enduring Freedom, and Operation Iraqi Freedom (OEF/OIF). Thus, the individuals served by the VA encompass a wide age range. Their military experience varies widely, and with only some veterans having seen active combat. Thus, the question "Do veterans have an increased risk of suicide?" then, includes "which veterans?" and "compared to whom?" These comparisons are useful to

doi: 10.1111/j.1749-6632.2010.05697.x

Ann. N.Y. Acad. Sci. 1208 (2010) 98–103 © 2010 Association for Research in Nervous and Mental Disease.

prevention efforts in identifying both highest risk groups and potentially modifiable risk factors for suicide.

This type of comparison faces several methodological challenges. One is known as the "Healthy Soldier Effect": factors that are generally known to increase suicide risk (e.g., poor physical health) are also those that keep individuals out of the military. A true comparison needs to take into account such selection biases and any other characteristics that differentiate the military from others in the general population.[4] Similarly, we need to classify the period of risk (e.g., within a set number of years since military discharge or at any given time) and age. In the general population, the two age groups with highest suicide risk are adults ages 20–24 (12.5 suicides/year/100,000) and 65 and over (14.2 suicides/year/100,000) with the very highest rates among non-Hispanic white men age 85 and older (48 suicides/year/100,000).[5] Another methodological problem is that deaths by suicide are not always classified as such on death certificates, either because of uncertainties that suicide caused the death or because the cause of death is misreported.[6] Finally, published analyses of suicide risk among veterans have varied in their approach (analytic strategies, etc.) and data sources. With these issues in mind, the following paragraphs summarize the data overall as well as by veteran group.

All veterans

Kaplan *et al.* analyzed data from a representative sample (the National Health Interview Survey 1986–1994) matched to the National Death Index through 1997.[7] Veteran status was determined by self-report. Using survival analyses that controlled for sociodemographic variables as well as self-rated health and use of physician services, they estimated that veterans had a statistically significant 2.3 increased risk of dying by suicide compared to the rest of the population. In contrast, veterans had no higher risk than others of dying by natural causes. Among all men who died by suicide, veterans were disproportionally white, >65 years old, and died by firearms.[7]

Veterans of the Vietnam War Era

Kang and Bullman's 2009 review of the literature identified three studies that compared suicide deaths of Vietnam Era veterans to the general population using standardized mortality ratios (SMR).[8] None of the three studies reported an increased risk

of suicide for Vietnam veterans. However, among Vietnam veterans, other studies have identified subgroups with an increased relative risk (RR) of suicide.[9,10] Veterans who were deployed to Vietnam had a 1.76 increased risk of suicide compared to other veterans of the same era. Several aspects of the war experience were associated with an increased risk of suicide, including experiencing a diagnosis of posttraumatic stress disorder (PTSD; SMR = 6.74, 95% confidence 4.40–9.87), having been hospitalized for a combat wound (SMR = 1.22, 1.00–1.46), and experiencing two or more wounds (SMR = 12.58, 1.06–0.146).

Veterans of the Gulf War Era

Kang and Bullman's review identified one study that compared suicide deaths of Gulf War Era veterans to the general population using SMR and again found no increased risk for suicide.[8] A study comparing veterans who were deployed to the Gulf War theater compared to other veterans from the same era also found no increased risk of all-cause mortality (RR = 1.03, 0.92–1.15) but did find a small but significant increased risk of mortality from external causes (RR = 1.19, 1.02–1.39). Much of this risk was accounted for by transportation-related deaths (RR = 1.44, 1.13–1.84), such as car accidents, where suicidality may or may not have contributed to risky or fatal behavior.

Veterans of OEF/OIF

The data are more complete for veterans from this most recent era. Table 1 summarizes an analysis reported by Kang and Bullman using data from the Defense Manpower Data Center matched to the National Death Index for deaths though 2005.[11] These data indicate that OEF/OIF veterans have significantly lower risk of all-cause mortality than the general population adjusted for age, race, sex, and year of death (SMR = 0.56, 0.52–0.60). These findings are consistent with the "Healthy Soldier Effect" in that, on average, individuals who enter the military will be in better physical and mental health than the rest of the population and, therefore, at lower risk of all-cause mortality.

In contrast, the total group of OEF/OIF veterans are at equal risk for suicide compared to the general population (SMR = 1.15, 0.97–1.35) suggesting that the "Healthy Soldier Effect" does not protect OEF/OIF veterans from suicide. These findings varied little by military service branch. The risk of

Table 1. Suicide among OEF/OIF veterans identified by defense manpower data center; deaths by NDI through 2005[11]

Cause of death	Subgroup of veterans	No. at risk	Rate per 100,000 person years	Standardized mortality ratio	(95% CI)
All causes	All	490,346	124.5	0.56	(0.52–0.60)
Suicide	All	490,346	21.9	1.15	(0.97–1.35)
	Active duty	212,664	24.7	1.33	(1.03–1.69)
	VA pts w/mental disorder	35,554	31.0	1.77	(1.01–2.97)

NDI, National Death Index.

suicide is actually 33% greater than the general population for active duty OEF/OIF veterans (SMR = 1.33, 1.03–1.69). And among OEF/OIF veterans who had received a mental disorder diagnosis in the VA in patient or outpatient records, the risk of suicide was even greater (SMR = 1.77, 1.01–2.97).

The conclusion from these data form the question of whether veterans are at greater risk for suicide. The first key finding listed in the Report of the Blue Ribbon Panel Work Group in Suicide Prevention in the Veteran Population was the conflicting and inconsistent reporting of veteran suicide rates across various studies, with the recommendation that the VA work with other federal agencies to establish a consistent approach of collecting, analyzing, and reporting suicide attempts in veterans.[3] The inconsistencies across the different reports reflect, in part, their differing levels of capacity to take into account selection bias, that is, the factors that differentiate individuals who enter the military from those who do not. With that caveat, the data reported above, using different sources of data and analytic strategies, suggest that veterans do have a higher risk for suicide than comparable subgroups of the general population. Because the military screens for healthy individuals, the overall mortality risk is generally lower for veterans than nonveterans. The fact that veterans have equal or higher suicide risk than the general population indicates that aspects of the military or postmilitary experience may be a potent risk factor for death by suicide.

The risk of suicide is not shared equally among all veterans. Among all groups of veterans, rates are highest in the oldest age groups as is consistent with data on suicide risk in the United States generally. But relative to nonveteran counterparts, suicide rates are particularly high for OEF/OIF veterans. The data reported here and elsewhere point to several factors that may contribute to the veteran's

elevated suicide risk and/or define high-risk groups. Some relate to the military experience, such as an increased risk associated with prolonged combat or injury.[1–3,9–11] The likelihood of surviving the military with a traumatic brain injury (TBI) may be greater for OEF/OIF veterans than those of earlier eras; clinical observations of high levels of suicide ideation among veterans with TBI suggest that TBI may elevate the risk of suicide.[12–14]

The high risk of suicide among veterans can also be attributed, in part, to experiences occurring "downstream" from a veteran's time in the military. To the extent that known risk factors for suicide occur more frequently in veterans than nonveterans, rates of suicide will also be higher. In these cases, the experience in the military may be a distal risk factor for suicide because it leads to a more proximal risk factor. The most salient examples are psychiatric conditions, such as depression and PTSD. Both conditions are disproportionally prevalent in veterans and both greatly increase the risk of suicide in veterans and others.[15,16] Another example is the availability and knowledge of fire arms, which is associated with both a history in the military and completed suicides.[15] Evidence also suggests that OEF/OIF veterans may be less likely to have the social and psychological resources that serve as protective factors for individuals who may otherwise be a risk for suicide. The specific examples from recent literature include lacking a sense of purpose and control as well as lacking social supports.[15,16]

Interventions to decrease veterans' suicide risk

The data quantifying rates of suicide in veteran populations have heighted concerns of both the public and the VA. The most visible response has been enhancements to its infrastructure to support suicide research and prevention activities. Examples include adding Suicide Prevention Coordinators at VA facilities, increasing the number of mental health professionals across VA settings, funding a Mental Health Center of Excellence in Canandaigua, NY, focused in suicide intervention development and the VA Research Center in Denver focused on clinical and neurobiological suicide risk factors research.

Suicide prevention interventions designed for veterans span the Institute of Medicine's (IOM) 1994 categories.[17] These include *universal interventions* designed for everyone in a defined population regardless of their risk for suicide, such as a health care system, a county, or a school district; *selective interventions* designed for subgroups at increased risk, due to age, gender, ethnicity, or family history of suicide; and *indicated interventions* designed for individuals who have a risk factor that puts them at very high risk. The National Strategy for Suicide Prevention describes biopsychosocial, environmental, and sociocultural interventions that fit each of these categories.[18]

The data on risks factors for suicide within the veteran population have been useful for developing suicide prevention strategies. From a public health perspective, the ideal target for suicide prevention is a risk factor that is strongly association with suicidal outcome, has a high prevalence, and is changeable. Targeting risk factors that significantly but only weakly associated with suicidal outcomes will, by itself, not substantially reduce suicide risk. Targeting risk factors that are rare or occur infrequently may have a big effect on the subgroup experiencing the risk factor but will not reduce the overall population's risk. Trying to modify inflexible or unchangeable risk factors is unlikely to affect either individual-level or population-level risk. Such unmodifiable risk factors (e.g., past events, such as combat duty, injury) are useful, however, for identifying subpopulations to target for Indicated or Selective Interventions. Often these factors are events that occurred in the past (i.e., distal risk factors, such as traumatic injury) that lead to or increase the likelihood of more proximal and modifiable risk factors (e.g., depression). The following paragraphs described recent and ongoing suicide prevention interventions implemented by the VA for each of the IOM categories.

Under the umbrella of *Universal Prevention* include education and outreach, screening, and gate-keeper programs. The VA has enhanced suicide outreach in for its deployment and reintegration points for OEF/OIF soldiers and at the VA health facilities serving veterans from all eras. The Suicide Prevention page on the United States Department of Veterans Affairs website, provides education about suicide warning signs, internet links resources, downloadable brochures and information sheets, and direct access to suicide hotlines.[19]

Another *Universal Prevention* intervention is screening, both for proximal risk factors (e.g., PTSD and depression) or, more selectively, for individuals identified at high risk because of having experienced a serious injury or another factors. Gatekeepers are individuals who are not clinically trained but have jobs that put them into routine contact with veterans. Gatekeeper programs educate such individuals to notice veterans who are demonstrating signs and signals of suicide risk.[20] The program trains gatekeepers in how to make effective referrals to mental health specialists.

Selective prevention targets veterans with known risk factors for suicide. Individuals with only unmodifiable risk factors may be monitored more closely than other veterans. The modifiable risk factors most commonly targeted are PTSD, depression, and other mental health disorders associated with the risk of suicide. Interventions designed to improve the care and outcomes of mental health disorders apply not only to OEF/OIF veterans but also veterans of all eras including the oldest age veterans who are in the demographic subgroup of the general population whose rate of suicide is the highest. Interventions to reduce the symptoms and outcomes of mental disorders include access to evidence-based psychiatric treatments[21–24] as well as evidence-based services delivery models. For example, the VHA supports several primary care models of mental health care, including co-location of mental health professionals into primary care clinics[25,26] and collaborative care models including the use of depression care managers in primary care.[27]

Indicated prevention interventions target individuals who have expressed suicidal thoughts and behaviors. The interventions are therefore focused specifically on suicide and not just proximal risk factors. At the system level, interventions include training clinicians in high suicide risk management and supporting suicide crisis lines for veterans. At the patient level, interventions include intensive monitoring and safety plans for such high-risk patients and evidenced-based pharmacotherapy and psychotherapy treatments for suicidal risk.[28–30]

As of this writing, many of the suicide prevention interventions are newly implemented by the VA or recently enhanced. It is therefore too early to know if they have been effective. As war and the influx of newly discharged OEF/OIF veterans is expected to persist, the need for suicide prevention interventions will continue for years to come. Most modifiable and proximal risk factors for suicide are themselves serious problems. So whether or not they reduce suicide rates, the interventions designed to reduce suicide risk factors, such as depression and PTSD, have value in-and-of themselves. Although such interventions are relevant to the general population and not only veterans, the VHA is the nation's largest health care provider and its huge infrastructure makes in uniquely equipped to implement system-wide interventions effectively. Nonetheless, the VHA services reach on a fraction of veterans. The Blue Ribbon Work Group was charged with addressing the needs of the full population of veterans, across the age span and including not only those who use the VA's health care services but it is not clear whether and how the suicide prevention interventions introduced by the VA will reach this broader population.[3]

Several barriers challenge effective implementation of these interventions. A major concern is confidentiality and the worry among veterans of being stigmatized or experiencing other negative consequences for future military participation or other activities if identified as being "high risk" for suicide.[31] The Blue Ribbon Panel noted that despite VHA efforts to maintain privacy, many OIF/OEF services members who are treated at VHA facilities have concerns about confidentiality. Their report recommended more educational programs to let potential clients/patients who might use these services know about level of confidentiality, especially those in the Reserve and Guard who would fear that their VHA use might affect future service.[3]

Another potential barrier to effective implementation is common to all screening interventions where follow-through mechanisms need to be in place to ensure that individuals who screen positive for suicide risk receive subsequent care. Although this challenge can be addressed structurally, an additional barrier is that clinicians and staff are often resistant to being trained and held responsible for suicide-risk assessment and management. The VHA has implemented special training interventions to address this concern.[32] Finally, the Blue Ribbon Panel also noted that while the VA has focused on identifying high-risk veterans, a mechanism is needed that will change or drop the label of "high risk" for patients who have been successfully treated or otherwise improves overtime.[3] Otherwise veterans may be stuck with the high-risk label and its unforeseen consequences.

Conclusion

Any suicide is an unnecessary tragedy. The public media's concerns about reported suicides among OIF/OEF soldiers and veterans are therefore warranted whether or not the risk of suicide among veterans is higher than nonveterans. But the data reviewed in this paper suggest that the rates of suicide in veterans are indeed higher than would be expected. The military recruits and trains individuals in good physical and mental health. Consistent with this "selection bias," veterans have, on average, lower all-cause mortality rates when compared to their demographic counterparts. But their good physical and mental health upon entering the military does not provide this same level of protection from suicide mortality. Indeed, some veterans, especially activity duty veterans and even more so those who experience injuries and trauma, have disproportionately high rates of suicide.

Understanding suicide risk among veterans is helped with a life course perspective in which experiences and events are viewed in relationship to each other over time. Thus it is not entering the military or even being in the military that increases the risk of suicide: it is the experiences of war and their downstream sequelae. For example, military service increases the risk of injury, which in turn increases the risk of long-term disability, which serves to increase the risk of depression, joblessness, and social isolation—all of which together increase suicide risk. Exposure to horrific events may lead to PTSD, which also increases suicide risk. Each step in this progression offers opportunities to change an individual's course, either through changing the individual's psychological reactions to war experiences or changing how societal and social systems respond to the needs of veterans.

Conflicts of interest

The author declares no conflicts of interest.

References

1. Hefling, K. 2010. Suicide rate of veterans increases significantly for former soldiers 18–29. *Huffington Post.* 1/11/2010. http://www.huffingtonpost.com/2010/01/11/suicide-rate-of-veterans-_n_418780.html (accessed June 30, 2010).

2. Clifton, E. 2010. Suicide rate surged among veterans. *IPSNEWS.net.* 1/13/2010. http://ipsnews.net/news.asp?idnews=49971 (accessed June 30, 2010).

3. Blue Ribbon Work Group on Suicide Prevention. 2008. Report of the Blue Ribbon Work Group on Suicide Prevention in the Veteran Population. Washington, DC: US Department of Veterans Affairs. http://www.mentalhealth.va.gov/suicide_prevention/Blue_Ribbon_Report-FINAL_June-30-08.pdf (accessed June 30, 2010).

4. McLaughlin, R., L. Nielsen & M. Waller. 2008. An evaluation of the effect of military service on mortality: quantifying the healthy soldier effect. *Ann. Epidemiol.* **18:** 928–936.

5. National Institute of Mental Health. 2006. Suicide in the U.S.: Statistics and Prevention. http://www.nimh.nih.gov/health/publications/suicide-in-the-us-statistics-and-prevention/index.shtml#factors (accessed April 26, 2010).

6. Breiding, M.J. & B. Wiersema. 2006. Variability of undetermined manner of death classification in the US. *Inj. Prev.* **12**(Suppl. 2): ii49–ii54.

7. Kaplan, M.S., N. Huguet, B.H. McFarland & J.T. Newsom. 2007. Suicide among male veterans: a prospective population-based study. *J. Epidemiol. Commun. Health* **61:** 619–624.

8. Kang, H.K. & T.A. Bullman. 2009. Is there an epidemic of suicides among current and former U.S. military personnel? *Ann. Epidemiol.* **19:** 757–760.

9. Boehmer, T.K., W.D. Flanders, M.A. McGeehin, *et al.* 2004. Postservice mortality in Vietnam veterans: 30-year follow-up. *Arch. Intern. Med.* **164:** 1908–1916.

10. Bullman, T.A. & H.K. Kang. 1996. The risk of suicide among wounded Vietnam veterans. *Am. J. Public Health* **86:** 662–667.

11. Kang, H.K. & T.A. Bullman. 2008. Risk of suicide among US veterans after returning from the Iraq or Afghanistan war zones. *JAMA* **300:** 652–653.

12. Brenner, L.A., B.Y. Homaifar, L.E. Adler, *et al.* 2009. Suicidality and veterans with a history of traumatic brain injury: precipitants events, protective factors, and prevention strategies. *Rehabil. Psychol.* **54:** 390–397.

13. Gutierrez, P.M., L.A. Brenner & J.A. Huggins. 2008. A preliminary investigation of suicidality in psychiatrically hospitalized veterans with traumatic brain injury. *Arch. Suicide Res.* **12:** 336–343.

14. Warden, D. 2006. Military TBI during the Iraq and Afghanistan wars. *J. Head Trauma Rehabil.* **21:** 398–402.

15. Desai, R.A., D. Dausey & R.A. Rosenheck. 2008. Suicide among discharged psychiatric inpatients in the Department of Veterans Affairs. *Mil. Med.* **173:** 721–728.

16. Pietrzak, R.H., M.B. Goldstein, J.C. Malley, *et al.* 2010. Risk and protective factors associated with suicidal ideation in veterans of Operations Enduring Freedom and Iraqi Freedom. *J. Affect. Disord.* **123:** 102–107.

17. Institute of Medicine. 1994. *Reducing Risks for Mental Disorders: Frontiers for Preventive Intervention Research.* Washington, DC.

18. U.S. Department of Health and Human Services. 2001. *National Strategy for Suicide Prevention: Goals and Objectives for Action.* Washington, D.C.: Substance Abuse and Mental Health Services Administration, National Mental Health Information Center, Center for Mental Health Services.

19. US Department of Veterans Affairs. 2010. Suicide prevention. http://www.mentalhealth.va.gov/suicide_prevention/ (accessed June 30, 2010).

20. Matthieu, M.M., W. Cross, A.R. Batres, *et al.* 2008. Evaluation of gatekeeper training for suicide prevention in veterans. *Arch. Suicide Res.* **12:** 148–154.

21. McAllister, T.W. 2009. Psychopharmacological issues in the treatment of TBI and PTSD. *Clin. Neuropsychol.* **23:** 1338–1367.

22. Cukor, J., J. Spitalnick, J. Difede, *et al.* 2009. Emerging treatments for PTSD. *Clin. Psychol. Rev.* **29:** 715–726.

23. Difede, J., J. Cukor, F. Lee & R. Yurt. 2009. Treatments for common psychiatric conditions among adults during acute, rehabilitation, and reintegration phases. *Int. Rev. Psychiatry* **21:** 559–569.

24. Gibbons, R.D., C.H. Brown, K. Hur, *et al.* 2007. Relationship between antidepressants and suicide attempts: an analysis of the Veterans Health Administration data sets. *Am. J. Psychiatry* **164:** 1044–1049.

25. Krahn, D.D., S.J. Bartels, E. Coakley, *et al.* 2006. PRISM-E: comparison of integrated care and enhanced specialty referral models in depression outcomes. *Psychiatr. Serv.* **57:** 946–953.

26. Oslin, D.W., S. Grantham, E. Coakley, *et al.* 2006. PRISM-E: comparison of integrated care and enhanced specialty referral in managing at-risk alcohol use. *Psychiatr. Serv.* **57:** 954–958.

27. Bruce, M.L., T.R. Ten Have, C.F. Reynolds III, *et al.* 2004. Reducing suicidal ideation and depressive symptoms in depressed older primary care patients: a randomized controlled trial. *JAMA* **291:** 1081–1091.

28. Valenstein, M., D. Eisenberg, J.F. McCarthy, *et al.* 2009. Service implications of providing intensive monitoring during high-risk periods for suicide among VA patients with depression. *Psychiatr. Serv.* **60:** 439–444.

29. Valenstein, M., H.M. Kim, D. Ganoczy, *et al.* 2009. Higher-risk periods for suicide among VA patients receiving depression treatment: prioritizing suicide prevention efforts. *J. Affect. Disord.* **112:** 50–58.

30. Mills, P.D., J.M. DeRosier, B.A. Ballot, *et al.* 2008. Inpatient suicide and suicide attempts in Veterans Affairs hospitals. *Jt. Comm. J. Qual. Patient Saf.* **34:** 482–488.

31. Pietrzak, R.H., D.C. Johnson, M.B. Goldstein, *et al.* 2009. Perceived stigma and barriers to mental health care utilization among OEF-OIF veterans. *Psychiatr. Serv.* **60:** 1118–1122.

32. Matthieu, M.M., Y. Chen, M. Schohn, *et al.* 2009. Educational preferences and outcomes from suicide prevention training in the Veterans Health Administration: one-year follow-up with healthcare employees in Upstate New York. *Mil. Med.* **174:** 1123–1131.

Ann. N.Y. Acad. Sci. ISSN 0077-8923

ANNALS OF THE NEW YORK ACADEMY OF SCIENCES

Issue: *Psychiatric and Neurologic Aspects of War*

Monitoring mental health treatment acceptance and initial treatment adherence in veterans

Veterans of Operations Enduring Freedom and Iraqi Freedom versus other veterans of other eras

Steven Lindley,[1,2] Holly Cacciapaglia,[2] Delilah Noronha,[2] Eve Carlson,[2,3] and Alan Schatzberg[1]

[1]Department of Psychiatry, Stanford University School of Medicine, Stanford, California. [2]Veterans Affairs Palo Alto Health Care System, Menlo Park, California. [3]National Center for PTSD, Menlo Park, California

Address for correspondence: Steven E. Lindley, M.D., Ph.D., MC 116A/MPD, VA Palo Alto Health Care System, 795 Willow Road, Menlo Park, California 94025. lindleys@stanford.edu

Identifying factors that influence mental health outcomes in veterans can aid in the redesign of programs to maximize the likelihood of early resolution of problems. To that end, we examined demographic and clinical process data from 2,684 veterans who scored positive on a mental health screen. We investigated this data set for patterns and possible predictors of mental health referral acceptance and attendance. The majority of patients had not received mental health treatment within the last two years (76%). Veterans of Operations Enduring Freedom and Iraqi Freedom (OEF/OIF) were more likely to accept a mental health referral for depression but were equally likely to attend a mental health visit as other era veterans. Decreased acceptance was associated with provider type and contact method, clinic location, depression only, and specific age ranges (65–74). Among those who accepted a referral, decreased attendance was associated with clinic location, depression only, and retirement. No variables predicted OEF/OIF acceptance/attendance. In conclusion, our findings illustrate the importance of close, continual monitoring of clinical process data to help reveal targets for improving mental health care for veterans.

Keywords: posttraumatic stress disorder; depression; health care technology; primary health care; veterans

Introduction

The Department of Veterans Affairs (VA) has significantly expanded mental health services in recent years, in part to address the needs of veterans returning from the conflicts in Iraq and Afghanistan.[1] The expansion has included mandated screening for posttraumatic stress disorder (PTSD), depression, and alcohol misuse, mental health providers integrated into primary care clinics, increased access to specialty mental health care, and the increased availability of providers trained in evidence-based psychotherapies.[2] A central aim of these efforts is to identify and treat patients with combat-related mental health difficulties earlier to lower overall burden on patients, their families, and society. Improv-ing outcomes for the greatest number of patients with the most efficient use of resources depends on continual redesign efforts based on accurate data on treatment outcomes and clinical processes in "real world" clinical settings, including treatment acceptance and adherence.

Treatment acceptance and adherence has been examined in veteran populations previously, including those who served in Afghanistan and/or Iraq (Operations Enduring Freedom and Iraqi Freedom, OEF/OIF). For example, a study of Army and Marine Corps OEF/OIF service members found that 38–45% of those screening positive for a mental health disorder indicated an interest in receiving help and 23–40% reported having received professional help in the last year.[3] As a point of

doi: 10.1111/j.1749-6632.2010.05692.x

Ann. N.Y. Acad. Sci. 1208 (2010) 104–113 © 2010 Association for Research in Nervous and Mental Disease.

comparison, Garvey Wilson *et al.* explored outpatient behavioral health care visits in military health care facilities *prior to* OIF. Results revealed that less than 12% of the military population used behavioral health services in 2000.[4]

Treatment adherence of veterans receiving care at VA facilities has also been examined. For example, a comparison of OEF/OIF to Vietnam era veterans in an outpatient PTSD clinic found that OEF/OIF veterans had significantly lower rates of session attendance and higher rates of treatment dropout than Vietnam era veterans.[5] An investigation comparing mental health care utilization during the first year after returning from deployment in 2003–2004 in OEF, OIF, and veterans deployed to other locations found that 35% of OIF veterans accessed mental health services compared to 22% of OEF, and 24% veterans deployed to other locations. Of those OIF veterans who were referred for a mental health reason, 56% were documented to have received a mental health evaluation.[6] Another study examining utilization of mental health services in OEF/OIF veterans at a VA medical center found that only 56% of veterans diagnosed with PTSD reported using mental health services.[7]

There have also been investigations of factors that may be affecting treatment acceptance and adherence. Looking at the impact of the location where a diagnosis was made, a review of 20,284 pre-Vietnam, Vietnam, and post-Vietnam era veterans recently diagnosed with PTSD found that patients who were diagnosed in a mental health or specialty PTSD clinic were more likely to accept treatment (either medication or counseling), receive counseling, attend more PTSD-related appointments, and receive more counseling sessions relative to those who were diagnosed in a general medical clinic.[8] Research in both civilian[9] and military samples[3,6,9] has shown that the individuals with more severe mental health symptoms have the greatest concerns about the stigma of accepting mental health care. Similarly, even when mental health problems are severe, a high level of concern about what others think is associated with a lower likelihood of seeking help.[9–11] It has been suggested that stigma is more pronounced in the military population, relative to a civilian population, on the basis of expectations for soldiers to be resilient, strong, and healthy in both mind and body.[12]

In addition to stigma, other factors identified as affecting treatment acceptance and adherence have included uncertainty about where to go for help, inability to get an appointment, inconvenience, and the time-consuming nature of treatment.[9] A recent evaluation of trends in mental health care within the VA system suggested inadequate appointment frequency may contribute to veterans terminating treatment prematurely.[1] The VA has attempted to address some of these issues by developing mental health provider teams located within the primary care setting. By having mental health providers in primary care, patients can often be seen by a mental health provider on the same day and in the same location as their primary care physician. If veterans with mental health needs can be identified and engaged in treatment without early termination, some mental health issues may be resolved before they become entrenched and require long-term mental health care.

Understanding the factors that influence treatment acceptance and adherence can aid in the redesign of programs to maximize the likelihood of early resolution of mental health problems. Likewise, identifying ways in which the OEF/OIF and other era populations differ in respect to treatment acceptance and adherence will help in the development of programs designed specifically to meet the needs of newly returning veterans. The VA's current electronic record system allows analysis of a variety of patient characteristics, and—with further development—could allow for routine analyses of mental health processes and outcomes. As a first step, we report here on referral patterns of all patients presenting with either PTSD or depression in primary care clinics in a regional VA health care system. We examined patterns of OEF/OIF versus other era veterans of treatment acceptance and adherence and investigated possible predictors. We specifically addressed whether OEF/OIF veterans show different patterns of acceptance of a mental health referral and/or attending a mental health session than other era veterans. Second, using available variables from the electronic medical record, we examined whether there are characteristics that predict acceptance and/or attendance and whether they apply to the OEF/OIF population. We focused the analyses on those referred for PTSD and/or depression because these constitute the majority of the referrals and because acceptance and attendance was expected to differ in those referred for alcohol misuse or other mental/behavioral health issues alone.

Methods

Sample and procedures

Data were collected from patients seen by the integrated primary care/mental health (PC/MH) team in eight different regional primary care clinics of the Palo Alto VA Health Care System from January 1 to June 30, 2009. Data was obtained from the PC/MH integrated care program administrative database and the VA's Decision Support Systems (DSS) database for analyses. The investigation was approved by the institutional review board for Stanford University and VA Palo Alto Health Care System Administration Research and Development Committee.

The PC/MH program consists of psychologist and psychology health technician teams located in primary care clinics of the Palo Alto VA health care system. During the period in which the data was collected, five of the eight geographically diverse clinics had integrated teams located on-site and the other three were covered remotely by telephone care. The Veterans Health Administration (VHA) mandates that all veterans seen in primary care be screened annually for depression, PTSD (first 5 years), and alcohol use. This screening is typically completed by nursing staff. When screens are positive the PC/MH team is consulted electronically and a follow-up assessment is conducted either by the primary care provider or the PC/MH team. The follow-up assessments of patients are conducted in person if the PC/MH provider is available to conduct the assessment in person or by telephone if not. The assessment is conducted by either a clinical psychologist or a Master's level psychology technician.

Measures

Demographic characteristics. Demographic data including era served, gender, age, race, marital status, employment status, religious affiliation, service connection, and body mass index (BMI) were collected via patient report and extraction from the patients' medical records.

Depression. The Patient Health Questionnaire-2 (PHQ-2) was the screening measure for depression, a two-item depression screen.[13] For patients screening positive (score of 3 or more out of 6), depressive

symptoms were assessed when clinically feasible and indicated using the PHQ-9. To complete the PHQ-9, patients rate the degree to which they experienced each of nine symptoms during the previous two weeks on a four-point Likert scale (0 = not at all to 3 = every day/nearly every day).[14]

PTSD. The Primary Care-PTSD Screen (PC-PTSD) is a four-item screen for PTSD.[15] For patients screening positive ("yes" to three or four items), PTSD symptoms were assessed when clinically feasible and indicated using the PTSD Checklist-Civilian (PCL-C). To complete the PCL-C, patients rate on a five-point Likert scale the degree to which each of 17 PTSD symptoms bothered them over the past month.[16]

Analyses

Demographic characteristics and clinical characteristics of those accepting or not accepting referral and those attending or not attending mental health sessions were compared using Chi-square for categorical variables and Student's *t*-test for continuous variables. Variables that were significantly associated with acceptance and/or attendance in dichotomous comparisons were entered into logistic regression analyses to determine the relative contribution of individual variables to accepting a referral and to attending a session. All statistical comparisons were two-tailed.

Results

From January 1 to June 30, 2009, 2,684 unique consults were received by the integrated PC/MH providers at the Palo Alto VA Health Care System. Sixteen percent of the patients ($n = 430$) had served in either Afghanistan or Iraq or both (OEF/OIF). The majority of OEF/OIF (77%) and other era veterans (76%) had not received treatment by a mental health provider within the VA in the last 2 years ("new mental health patients"). The primary reason recorded for the referral of the "new mental health patients" ($n = 2,027$) included PTSD and PTSD/depression (53% of OEF/OIF and 22% of other era veterans), depression only (7% of OEF/OIF and 42% of other era veterans), alcohol overuse (19% of OEF/OIF and 24% of other era veterans), or a variety of mental health/behavioral health concerns (21% of OEF/OIF and 12% of other era veterans).

Analyses of acceptance and attendance were conducted on the 1,289 new mental health patients referred for PTSD and/or depression. The demographic information for this population is summarized in Table 1. The OEF/OIF veterans were on average 31 years younger, differed significantly in their declared racial classification and employment status, and were more likely to have a service-connected disability than other era veterans. The declared religion preferences and the percent females were similar between OIF/OEF and other era veterans. The mean BMI of both groups fell into the obese range and was significantly lower in the OEF/OIF group (Table 1).

Of those referred for PTSD evaluations, the OEF/OIF vets were equally likely to accept treatment (58%) compared to the other era veterans [60%; $\chi^2 = 0.3$ ($df = 1$, ns)]. In contrast, of those referred for evaluation of depression only, the OEF/OIF veterans were more likely to accept a mental health referral (68%) than other era veterans [38%; $\chi^2 = 9.7$ ($df = 1$, $P < 0.05$)]. Once accepting a treatment referral to specialty mental health care, OEF/OIF vets referred for PTSD and/or depression were equally likely overall to attend their first outpatient mental health treatment (74%) as other era veterans (71%; $\chi^2 = 0.44$ [$df = 1$, ns]). Likewise, among veterans who attended a first appointment, OEF/OIF

Table 1. Characteristics of veterans referred for PTSD and/or depression

Demographic	OEF/OIF $n = 198$	Other era $n = 1,091$	
Age	30.8 ± 9.0	61.1 ± 13.0	$t = 31.4^{**}$
Female	6.6%	5.4%	$\chi^2 = 0.4$
Marital status			$\chi^2 = 107.0^{**}$
Single/never married	41%	12%	
Married	36%	45%	
Separate/divorced	23%	37%	
Widowed	0%	6%	
Race			$\chi^2 = 18.6^{**}$
White	64%	70%	
Black	6%	10%	
Asian/Pacific islander	13%	6%	
Unknown/declined	16%	15%	
Employment status			$\chi^2 = 62.0^{**}$
Employed	39%	29%	
Unemployed	61%	46%	
Retired	0%	25%	
Religion			$\chi^2 = 3.3$
Protestant	37%	39%	
Catholic	30%	29%	
Judaism	2%	1%	
Eastern	1%	2%	
Other	30%	30%	
Service connection	53%	36%	$\chi^2 = 20.7^{**}$
BMI (under age 65)	28.8 ± 5.1	29.9 ± 6.3	$t = 2.3^{*}$
Accepted referral			
PTSD or PTSD+Dep	58%	60%	$\chi^2 = 0.3$
Depression only	68%	38%	$\chi^2 = 9.7^{*}$

$^{*} P < 0.5.$
$^{**} P < 0.001.$

Table 2. Association of patient/clinical characteristics with accepting/attending a treatment referral

Demographics	Accepting		Attending	
	Comparison		Comparison	
Era	$\chi^2 = 12.3$	$P < 0.001$	$\chi^2 = 0.3$	$P = 0.54$
Age (decades)	$\chi^2 = 71.5$	$P < 0.001$	$\chi^2 = 19.9$	$P < 0.01$
Gender	$\chi^2 = 4.5$	$P < 0.05$	$\chi^2 = 0.1$	$P = 0.71$
Marital status	$\chi^2 = 1.5$	$P = 0.69$	$\chi^2 = 1.2$	$P = 0.76$
Race	$\chi^2 = 8.2$	$P < 0.05$	$\chi^2 = 6.7$	$P = 0.08$
Employment	$\chi^2 = 40.9$	$P < 0.001$	$\chi^2 = 16.4$	$P < 0.001$
Religion	$\chi^2 = 1.7$	$P = 0.43$	$\chi^2 = 8.4$	$P = 0.08$
Service connection	$\chi^2 = 0.5$	$P = 0.48$	$\chi^2 = 0.01$	$P = 0.93$
Referral diagnosis	$\chi^2 = 54.2$	$P < 0.001$	$\chi^2 = 12.9$	$P < 0.01$
BMI	$t = 1.2$	$P = 0.24$	$t = 1.0$	$P = 0.32$
Clinical procedures				
Clinic location	$\chi^2 = 26.6$	$P < 0.001$	$\chi^2 = 30.4$	$P < 0.001$
PC/MC vs. PCP	$\chi^2 = 64.0$	$P < 0.001$	$\chi^2 = 0.5$	$P = 0.50$
Face-to-face vs. phone	$\chi^2 = 4.0$	$P < 0.05$	$\chi^2 = 0.4$	$P = 0.55$
Same day vs. not same day	$\chi^2 = 2.3$	$P = 0.13$	$\chi^2 = 0.1$	$P = 0.81$

vets were as likely to attend a second appointment (74%) as other era veterans (77%; $\chi^2 = 0.33$ [$df = 1$, ns]).

Table 2 shows results of comparisons of baseline demographics and clinical procedure characteristics between those who accepted a mental health referral and those who did not and comparisons of those who attended one mental health sessions to those who attended none. OEF/OIF status, age, gender, race, employment status, the referral diagnosis, PC/MH versus PCP, the clinic location, and phone versus face-to-face all were significantly associated with accepting mental health treatment. Specifically being non-OEF/OIF, male, 66–74 years, white or undeclared race, retired, or referred for depression only was associated with a lower rate of accepting a mental health referral. How and where the assessment was conducted was also significantly associated. Specifically, conducting the assessment by telephone (which occurred if the integrated mental health provider was unavailable and the assessment was not completed by the primary care provider) was less likely to result in an acceptance of mental health treatment than if the triage was completed face-to-face (40% versus 47%). The vast majority of the assessments were completed on the same day (90%). The acceptance rate was similar whether or not the assessment was completed on the same day (data not shown). Patients who were triaged by the integrated PC/MH providers were twice as likely to accept a mental health referral (54%) than if the triage was completed by the primary care provider (27%). There were also significant differences in acceptance rates among the clinic locations.

For patients who accepted a referral to a specialty mental health clinic, age, employment status, the referral diagnosis, and the clinic location were all significantly associated with attending at least one mental health clinic appointment (Table 2). Specifically, being older, retired, and referred for depression only was associated with not completing at least one mental health clinic appointment. OEF/OIF status was not associated with attending a first appointment. Also, the method of triage had no effect on the likeliness of subsequently making the first mental health appointment but there was a difference across clinic locations.

The relative contributions of the variables that were significantly associated with acceptance and attendance were examined in logistic regression models (Table 3A and B). The significant demographic variables were entered in the first step followed by clinical procedures in the second step. For accepting a mental health referral (Table 3A), assessment by the PC/MH provider had the highest likelihood of mental health treatment acceptance whereas assessment by telephone, certain clinic locations, referral for depression only, retirement, and age 65–74 were less likely to result in treatment acceptance (Table 3A). For attending a mental health clinic appointment, referral for depression only, being retired, and certain clinic locations were significantly associated with lower attendance in the logistic regression (Table 3B). Analyses conducted in the OEF/OIF veterans sample revealed no significant associations between any variable and acceptance or attendance (data not shown).

Finally, PCL-C and PHQ-9 scores were obtained by the PC/MH providers when possible and clinically indicated. PCL-C scores were obtained for 70% of the OEF/OIF and 48% of other era veterans referred for PTSD and PHQ-9 scores were obtained for 70% of OEF/OIF and 47% of other era veterans referred for depression. The PCL-C and PHQ-9 scores were highly correlated ($r = 0.79$, $P < 0.001$) in the 421 individuals who completed both. Interestingly, BMI showed a small correlation with the PCL-C in the OEF/OIF ($r = 0.17$, $P < 0.01$) and other era ($r = 0.20$, $P < 0.001$) veterans and with the PHQ-9 in the OEF/OIF ($r = 0.17$, $P < 0.05$) and other era veterans ($r = 0.14$, $P < 0.001$). As expected PLC-C and PHQ-9 scores were significantly higher in those accepting mental health referrals (data not shown). Of veterans who scored 50 or more on the PCL-C, 16% (50/305) of all veterans and 14% of OEF/OIF veterans refused a mental health referral. Of veterans who scored greater than 10 on the PHQ-9 (probable moderate to severe depression), 24% of all veterans and 26% of OEF/OIF refused a mental health referral. PCL-C and PHQ-9 scores were also significantly higher in those who made at least one mental health clinic appointment (data not shown).

Discussion

Our preliminary analyses of treatment acceptance and initial adherence in 2,684 veterans screening positive for mental health concerns in primary care clinics reveal that the screening efforts for depression and PTSD are detecting a high prevalence of untreated mental health concerns. This was true for both the OEF/OIF veterans (77%) and the other era veterans (76%). The high rate is in contrast to a study of veteran mental health care use before 2000. Specifically, Hankin *et al.* found that

only 32% of veterans who screened positive for mental health disorders reported not having had mental health treatment.[17] The difference with the present findings is likely due, in part, to the fact that this study only recorded treatment within the last 2 years, screened with brief, less specific measures, and used an administrative sample rather than a study population. Recently, it has been reported that among OEF/OIF veterans, 80% of those with a PTSD diagnosis and 50% of those with another mental health diagnosis had one or more mental health visits in the year following diagnosis.[18] Our findings suggest that there are a large proportion of OEF/OIF and other era veterans who are primary care patients may have mental health needs but are not receiving services.

Contrary to expectations, we found that OEF/OIF era veterans were either equally or more likely, depending on the reason for the evaluation, to accept a referral for mental health treatment than other era veterans. Likewise, OEF/OIF veterans were equally likely to complete an initial and follow-up visit than other era veterans. Although problems with stigma and other barriers to treatment have been well-documented in the OEF/OIF population,[19] it appears that barriers to treatment may be having similar impacts on veterans of all eras. Perhaps the next step is to examine whether barriers to treatment differ across veterans of different eras and whether different approaches will be required to address them.

Analyses to identify factors associated with failure to accept or attend treatment revealed a number of possible targets for improvements. Some of the strongest associations were with clinical practice variables. For example, telephone evaluations and evaluations by primary care physicians appeared to be associated with less treatment acceptance. Although telephone care has been demonstrated to be a very effective mental health intervention,[20,21] use of the telephone appears to be less effective to engage a veteran in mental health than a face-to-face evaluation, particularly one with a direct handoff from the primary care physicians. In addition, difficulties with conducting telephone assessments include difficulty contacting patients and incorrect phone numbers. The higher rate of acceptance when the evaluations were completed by the PC/MH providers is consistent with data demonstrating the enhanced efficacy of integrated care

Table 3. Multiple logistic regression analyses

Variable	OR	95% CI	*P*-values
A. Predictor variables for accepting referral			
Step 1: Demographics			
Era			
Other era	1.00		
OEF/OIF	0.79	0.46–1.35	$P = 0.40$
Age (years)			
< 26	1.00		
26–35	0.63	0.33–1.20	$P = 0.16$
36–45	0.93	0.44–1.99	$P = 0.86$
46–55	1.10	0.52–2.34	$P = 0.80$
56–65	0.54	0.26–1.12	$P = 0.10$
66–75	0.40	0.18–0.92	$P < 0.05$
>75	0.46	0.20–1.08	$P = 0.07$
Gender			
Female	1.00		
Male	0.75	0.44–1.28	$P = 0.29$
Race			
White	1.00		
Black	1.25	0.82–1.85	$P = 0.30$
Asian/Pacific islander	1.09	0.63–1.62	$P = 0.74$
Unknown/decline	0.88	0.60–1.16	$P = 0.48$
Employment status			
Employed	1.00		
Unemployed	0.97	0.73–1.28	$P = 0.80$
Retired	0.64	0.41–0.98	$P < 0.05$
Reason for referral			
PTSD	1.00		
Depression	0.59	0.41–0.84	$P < 0.005$
Both	1.38	0.96–2.42	$P = 0.072$
Step 2: Clinical			
Clinic region			
Central	1.00		
Southern	1.51	1.10–2.07	$P < 0.05$
Valley	3.12	2.24–4.35	$P < 0.001$
PC/MH team triage	3.85	2.80–5.30	$P < 0.001$
Telephone triage	0.54	0.40–0.73	$P < 0.001$
B. Predictor variables for attending first appointment after accepting treatment			
Step 1: Demographics			
Age categories (years)			
<26	1.00		
26–35	0.82	0.30–2.23	$P = 0.70$
36–45	0.71	0.26–1.92	$P = 0.50$
46–55	1.60	0.62–4.14	$P = 0.34$
56–65	1.08	0.45–2.61	$P = 0.86$
66–75	0.59	0.19–1.83	$P = 0.36$

Continued.

Table 3. *Continued*

Variable	OR	95% CI	P-values
>75	1.01	0.30–3.33	$P = 0.99$
Employment status			
Employed	1.00		
Unemployed	0.97	0.62–1.54	$P = 0.91$
Retired	0.40	0.19–0.82	$P < 0.05$
Reason for referral			
PTSD	1.00		
Depression	0.53	0.29–0.94	$P < 0.05$
Both	1.01	0.55–1.85	$P = 0.99$
Step 2: Clinical			
Clinic region			
Center	1.00		
Southern	2.81	1.67–4.71	$P < 0.001$
Valley	4.38	2.61–7.37	$P < 0.001$

programs for depression, but it also may reflect primary care providers screening out false positive screens before referral to the PC/MH team. Interestingly, neither type of provider or method of evaluation (i.e., telephone) had any significant impact on attending a mental health appointment.

We also observed an association among the locations of the clinic where the care was provided and both acceptance and attendance. Our study took place in a large VA system, which consisted of eight primary care clinics spread across a geographically diverse area. The data indicate there may be a need to modify services depending on clinic variables. Modifications likely need to be related to population demographics, clinic sizes, and staffing resources. Program evaluation, procedural changes, and allocation of resources/staff may help alleviate problems that may arise owing to differences across clinics. Despite differences across clinics, this study highlights that a PC/MH program can be provided across a large VA system.

Patient characteristics associated with treatment acceptance and adherence were also identified. For example, it appears that special interventions are needed to enhance treatment acceptance and attendance for older, retired, and depressed veterans. Services, such as those used in the IMPACT (Improving Mood-Promoting Access to Collaborative Treatment) and PROSPECT (Prevention of Suicide in Primary Care Elderly: Collaborative Trial) protocols, may be helpful as both have proven to be effective interventions in this population.[22,23]

For those patients for whom PCL-C and/or PHQ-9 scores were available, the data suggests that those with more severe symptoms are more likely to both accept treatment and attend appointments than those with milder screening symptom severity. Increased severity of PTSD is associated with decreased ability to function, in part due to mental health concerns, alcohol consumption, and illicit drug use.[24] Decreased psychosocial functioning and increased suffering may motivate veterans to accept and, at least initially, adhere to treatment.

A small association was found between symptom severity and BMI in both OEF/OIF and other era veterans. Obesity has been previously reported to be associated with the likelihood of having a mood disorder in some studies.[25,26] There may be many reasons for an association between PTSD and depression severity and BMI (e.g., stress-induced cortisol, use of psychotropic medications, lifestyle differences) and further research is warranted.

Although OEF/OIF status was independently associated with higher acceptance of a mental health referral, it was not independently associated when accounting for age and other variables.

Surprisingly, none of the variables were associated with treatment acceptance or attendance in the OEF/OIF population. In particular, despite the strong association with many of the clinical procedure variables in the other era veterans, these seemed to have little impact in the OEF/OIF population. This could reflect more homogeneity in the OEF/OIF population in the variables examined. It could also be accounted for, in part, by the increased efforts that are already made to engage these new veterans in treatment. This era of veterans has more education about mental health issues and services during active duty and during the military discharge process when compared to other era veterans. In terms of VA clinical practice, additional resources are available for OEF/OIF veterans (including postdeployment clinics where multidisciplinary evaluations are performed and specialized case managers who serve as a point of contact for OEF/OIF veterans for referrals and information). Furthermore, one could argue that the younger generation of OEF/OIF era veterans has more social exposure to mental health issues as mental health has made strides toward education and destigmatization in recent years.

This study highlights the need for future efforts in identifying additional variables that may be associated with treatment acceptance. Specifically, it will be important to identify variables associated with OEF/OIF treatment acceptance and adherence. Additional variables, such as patient satisfaction, gender ideologies, and help-seeking behaviors, are possible areas of investigation. It is likely that, in addition to general mental health stigma, fear of a negative impact on career goals may contribute to not accepting treatment.

The President's New Freedom Commission on Mental Health has set a goal to use technology to access mental health care and information.[27] All VHA medical facilities use a fully integrated electronic medical record that assists with direct patient care. Although data in this system can be analyzed, extraction of data for a study such as this is still very labor intensive. To enhance the ease of data selection and extraction, particularly at the local level, we are currently developing software that can complement the current computerized patient information. Combining current computerized patient information with data on assessment and treatment variables will allow monitoring and evaluation of processes and outcomes across a large health care system.

In conclusion, our findings illustrate the importance of close, continual monitoring of clinical process data to improve care for veterans. Our results demonstrate the benefits of screening for mental health difficulties in primary care and the advantages of integrated care. The data demonstrate similarities in rates of acceptance and initial adherence to care between OEF/OIF and other era veterans, but suggests different factors may be affecting these patterns in the two groups. Further improvements in medical information technology would allow for easier access to more process and outcome data for continued system redesign improvements.

Conflicts of interest

The authors declare no conflicts of interest.

References

1. Rosenheck, R.A. & A.F. Fontana. 2007. Recent trends in VA treatment of post-traumatic stress disorder and other mental disorders. *Health Aff. (Millwood)* **26:** 1720–1727.
2. Office of Patient Care Services. 2008. Uniform mental health services in VA medical centers and clinics. *VHA Handbook 1160.01.* Department of Veterans Affairs. Washington, DC.
3. Hoge, C.W., C.A. Castro, S.C. Messer, *et al.* 2004. Combat duty in Iraq and Afghanistan, mental health problems, and barriers to care. *N. Engl. J. Med.* **351:** 13–22.
4. Garvey Wilson, A.L., S.C. Messer & C.W. Hoge. 2009. U.S. military mental health care utilization and attrition prior to the wars in Iraq and Afghanistan. *Soc. Psychiatry Psychiatr. Epidemiol.* **44:** 473–481.
5. Erbes, C.R., K.T. Curry & J. Leskela. 2009. Treatment presentation and adherence of Iraq/Afghanistan Era veterans in outpatient care for posttraumatic stress disorder. *Psychol. Serv.* **6:** 175–183.
6. Hoge, C.W., J.L. Auchterlonie & C.S. Milliken. 2006. Mental health problems, use of mental health services, and attrition from military service after returning from deployment to Iraq or Afghanistan. *JAMA* **295:** 1023–1032.
7. Erbes, C., J. Westermeyer, B. Engdahl & E. Johnsen. 2007. Post-traumatic stress disorder and service utilization in a sample of service members from Iraq and Afghanistan. *Mil. Med.* **172:** 359–363.
8. Spoont, M.R., M. Murdoch, J. Hodges & S. Nugent. 2010. Treatment receipt by veterans after a PTSD diagnosis in PTSD, mental health, or general medical clinics. *Psychiatr. Serv.* **61:** 58–63.
9. Kessler, R.C. *et al.* 2001. The prevalence and correlates of untreated serious mental illness. *Health Serv. Res.* **36:** 987–1007.
10. Kessler, R.C. *et al.* 2005. Prevalence and treatment of mental disorders, 1990 to 2003. *N. Engl. J. Med.* **352:** 2515–2523.
11. Regier, D.A., W.E. Narrow, D.S. Rae, *et al.* 1993. The de facto US mental and addictive disorders service system: epidemiologic catchment area prospective 1-year prevalence

rates of disorders and services. *Arch. Gen. Psychiatry.* **50:** 85–94.

12. Greene-Shortridge, T.M., T.W. Britt & C.A. Castro. 2007. The stigma of mental health problems in the military. *Mil. Med.* **172:** 157–161.

13. Kroenke, K., R.L. Spitzer & J.B. Williams. 2003. The Patient Health Questionnaire-2: validity of a two-item depression screener. *Med. Care* **41:** 1284–1292.

14. Kroenke, K., R.L Spitzer & J.B. Willaims. 2001. The PHQ-9: validity of a brief depression severity measure. *J. Gen. Intern. Med.* **16:** 606–613.

15. Ouimette, P., M. Wade, A. Prins & M. Schohn. 2008. Identifying PTSD in primary care: comparison of the Primary Care-PTSD screen (PC-PTSD) and the General Health Questionnaire-12 (GHQ). *J. Anxiety Disord.* **22:** 337–343.

16. Weathers, F., B. Litz, D. Herman, *et al.* 1993. The PTSD checklist (PCL): reliability, validity, and diagnostic utility. Presented at Annual Convention of the International Society for Traumatic Stress Studies, San Antonio, TX.

17. Hankin, C.S., A. Spiro, III, D.R. Miller & L. Kazis. 1999. Mental disorders and mental health treatment among U.S. Department of Veterans Affairs outpatients: the Veterans Health Study. *Am. J. Psychiatry.* **156:** 1924–1930.

18. Seal, K.H. *et al.* 2010. VA mental health services utilization in Iraq and Afghanistan veterans in the first year of receiving new mental health diagnoses. *J Trauma Stress* **23:** 5–16.

19. Pietrzak, R.H., D.C. Johnson, M.B. Goldstein, *et al.* 2009. Psychosocial buffers of traumatic stress, depressive symptoms, and psychosocial difficulties in veterans of Operations Enduring Freedom and Iraqi Freedom: the role of resilience, unit support, and postdeployment social support. *J. Spec. Oper. Med.* **9:** 74–78.

20. Telemental Health Work Group. 2009. Telemental Health Standards and Guidelines Working Group. American Telemedicine Association.

21. Smith, H.A. & R.A. Allison. 2001. Telemental Health: Delivering Mental Health Care at a Distance: A Summary Report. U.S. Department of Health and Human Services; Substance Abuse and Mental Health Services Administration Center for Mental Health Services. Rockville, MD.

22. Unutzer, J. *et al.* 2002. Collaborative care management of late-life depression in the primary care setting: a randomized controlled trial. *JAMA* **288:** 2836–2845.

23. Bruce, M.L. *et al.* 2004. Reducing suicidal ideation and depressive symptoms in depressed older primary care patients: a randomized controlled trial. *JAMA* **291:** 1081–1091.

24. Ouimette, P., D. Coolhart, D. Sugarman, *et al.* 2008. A pilot study of posttraumatic stress and associated functioning of army national guard following exposure to Iraq Warzone Trauma. *Traumatology* **15:** 51–56.

25. Bruffaerts, R. *et al.* 2008. The relation between body mass index, mental health, and functional disability: a European population perspective. *Can. J. Psychiatry.* **53:** 679–688.

26. McLaren, L., C.A. Beck, S.B. Patten, *et al.* 2008. The relationship between body mass index and mental health. A population-based study of the effects of the definition of mental health. *Soc. Psychiatry Psychiatr. Epidemiol.* **43:** 63–71.

27. New Freedom Commission on Mental Health. 2003. Achieving the promise: transforming mental health care in America. Final Report. Department of Health and Human Services. DHHS Publication No. SMA-03-3832. Rockville, MD.

Ann. N.Y. Acad. Sci. ISSN 0077-8923

ANNALS OF THE NEW YORK ACADEMY OF SCIENCES
Issue: *Psychiatric and Neurologic Aspects of War*

Development and early evaluation of the *Virtual Iraq/Afghanistan* exposure therapy system for combat-related PTSD

Albert "Skip" Rizzo,[1] JoAnn Difede,[2] Barbara O. Rothbaum,[3] Greg Reger,[4] Josh Spitalnick,[3] Judith Cukor,[2] and Rob Mclay[5]

[1]Institute for Creative Technologies, Department of Psychiatry and School of Gerontology, University of Southern California, Playa Vista, California. [2]Department of Psychiatry, Weill Cornell Medical College, New York, New York. [3]Department of Psychiatry, Emory University, Atlanta, Georgia. [4]Department of Psychology, Madigan Army Medical Center, Tacoma, Washington. [5]Department of Psychiatry, Naval Medical Center, San Diego, California

Address for correspondence: Albert Rizzo, Ph.D., Institute for Creative Technologies, Department of Psychiatry and School of Gerontology, University of Southern California, 12015 Waterfront Drive, Playa Vista, California 90094. arizzo@usc.edu

Numerous reports indicate that the growing incidence of posttraumatic stress disorder (PTSD) in returning Operation Enduring Freedom (OEF)/Operation Iraqi Freedom (OIF) military personnel is creating a significant health care and economic challenge. These findings have served to motivate research on how to better develop and disseminate evidence-based treatments for PTSD. Virtual reality-delivered exposure therapy for PTSD has been previously used with reports of positive outcomes. The current paper will detail the development and early results from use of the *Virtual Iraq/Afghanistan* exposure therapy system. The system consists of a series of customizable virtual scenarios designed to represent relevant Middle Eastern contexts for exposure therapy, including a city and desert road convoy environment. The process for gathering user-centered design feedback from returning OEF/OIF military personnel and from a system deployed in Iraq (as was needed to iteratively evolve the system) will be discussed, along with a brief summary of results from an open clinical trial using *Virtual Iraq* with 20 treatment completers, which indicated that 16 no longer met PTSD checklist-military criteria for PTSD after treatment.

Keywords: virtual reality; exposure therapy; PTSD; behavior therapy; veterans; service members; military; invisible wounds of war

Introduction

War is one of the most challenging environments that a human can experience. The cognitive, emotional, and physical demands of a combat environment place enormous stress on even the best-prepared military personnel: the human costs are high. Since the start of the Operation Enduring Freedom (OEF)/ Operation Iraqi Freedom (OIF) conflicts in Afghanistan and Iraq, 1.6 million troops have been deployed. As of March 2009, there have been 4,923 deaths and 33,856 service members (SMs) wounded in action (WIA).[1] Of the WIA, the total includes 935 major limb amputations and 351 minor amputations and as of 2008, traumatic brain injury (TBI) has been diagnosed in 43,779 patients

(many of which are not included in the WIA statistics as mild TBI is often reported retrospectively, upon redeployment home). Moreover, the stressful experiences that are characteristic of the OIF/OEF warfighting environments have been seen to produce significant numbers of returning SMs at risk for developing posttraumatic stress disorder (PTSD). In the first systematic study of OIF/OEF mental health problems, the results indicated that "... The percentage of study subjects whose responses met the screening criteria for major depression, generalized anxiety, or PTSD was significantly higher after duty in Iraq (15.6–17.1%) than after duty in Afghanistan (11.2%) or before deployment to Iraq (9.3%)" (p. 13).[2] Reports since that time on OIF/OEF PTSD and psychosocial disorder rates suggest even higher

doi: 10.1111/j.1749-6632.2010.05755.x

 Ann. N.Y. Acad. Sci. 1208 (2010) 114–125 © 2010 Association for Research in Nervous and Mental Disease.

incidence statistics.[1,3,4] For example, as of 2008, the Military Health System has recorded 39,365 active duty patients who have been diagnosed with PTSD[1] and the Rand Analysis on PTSD[4] estimated that more than 300,000 active duty and discharged veterans will suffer from the symptoms of PTSD and major depression. These figures are troubling and make a strong case for continued efforts at developing and enhancing the availability of evidence-based treatments to address a mental health care challenge that will have significant impact for many years to come.

At the same time, a revolution has occurred in the development of virtual reality (VR) systems for enhancing therapeutic practice. Technological advances in the areas of computation speed and power, graphics and image rendering, display systems, tracking, interface technology, authoring software, and artificial intelligence have supported the creation of low-cost and usable PC-based VR systems. As well, a determined and expanding cadre of researchers and clinicians have not only recognized the potential impact of VR technology but have also now generated a significant research literature that documents the many clinical targets where VR can add value over traditional assessment and intervention approaches.[5–9] This convergence of the exponential advances in underlying VR enabling technologies with a growing body of clinical research and experience has fueled the evolution of the discipline of "Clinical Virtual Reality." And this state of affairs now stands to transform the vision of future clinical practice and research in the disciplines of psychology, medicine, neuroscience, physical, and occupational therapy, and in the many allied health fields that address the therapeutic needs of those with clinical disorders.

This paper will detail the development process and briefly summarize an early open clinical test of a VR exposure therapy (VRET) application designed for the treatment of PTSD related to OIF/OEF combat exposure in active duty and veteran populations. Although randomized controlled trials are currently under way to compare VRET with traditional imaginal exposure approaches to determine its relative efficacy, encouraging results thus far suggest that VRET may be a viable treatment alternative. Moreover, the use of VR for clinical care may have some appeal to a generation of SMs and veterans who have grown up "digital" and are comfortable with treatment delivered within this computer and information technology format.

Clinical VR applications for psychological health

The unique match between VR technology assets and the needs of various clinical treatment approaches has been recognized by a number of authors and an encouraging body of research has emerged, particularly in the area of exposure therapy for anxiety disorders.[6,7,10–17] Whereas in the mid-1990s, VR was generally seen as "a hammer looking for a nail," it soon became apparent to some scientists in both the engineering and clinical communities that VR could bring something to clinical care that was not possible before its advent. The capacity of VR technology to create controllable, multisensory, interactive three-dimensional (3D) stimulus environments, within which human behavior could be motivated and measured, offered clinical assessment and treatment options that were not possible using traditional methods. As well, a long and rich history of encouraging findings from the aviation simulation literature lent support to the concept that testing, training, and treatment in highly proceduralized VR simulation environments would be a useful direction for psychology and rehabilitation to explore. Much like an aircraft simulator serves to test and train piloting ability under a variety of controlled conditions, VR could be used to create relevant simulated environments where assessment and treatment of cognitive, emotional, and motor problems could take place.

A short list of areas where "Clinical VR" has been usefully applied includes fear reduction in persons with simple phobias,[6,7] treatment for PTSD,[14,17–19] stress management in cancer patients,[20] acute pain reduction during wound care and physical therapy with burn patients,[21] body image disturbances in patients with eating disorders,[9] navigation and spatial training in children and adults with motor impairments,[11,22] functional skill training and motor rehabilitation with patients having central nervous system dysfunction (e.g., stroke, TBI, spinal cord injury cerebral palsy, multiple sclerosis, etc.),[5,23] and in the assessment and rehabilitation of attention, memory, spatial skills, and executive cognitive functions in both clinical and unimpaired populations.[8,24] To do this, VR scientists have constructed virtual airplanes, skyscrapers, spiders, battlefields, social settings, beaches, fantasy worlds, and the mundane (but highly relevant) functional environments of the schoolroom, office, home, street, and supermarket. In essence, clinicians can now use VR as an "ultimate skinner box" that allows them to bring simulated elements from the outside world into the treatment setting and immerse patients in simulations that support the aims and mechanics of a specific therapeutic approach.

Concurrent with the emerging acknowledgment of the unique value of Clinical VR by scientists and clinicians, has come a growing awareness of its potential relevance and impact by the general public. Although much of this recognition may be due to the high visibility of digital 3D games, the Nintendo Wii, and massive shared internet-based virtual worlds (World of Warcraft, Halo, and 2nd Life), the public consciousness is also routinely exposed to popular media reports on clinical and research VR applications. Whether this should be viewed as "hype" or "help" to a field that has had a storied history of alternating periods of public enchantment and disregard still remains to be seen. Regardless, growing public awareness coupled with the solid scientific results has brought the field of Clinical VR past the point where skeptics can be taken seriously when they characterize VR as a "fad technology." A description of the technology required for VRET and a review of the literature on its use with anxiety disorders is presented elsewhere in this issue.[25]

Development of the *Virtual Iraq/Afghanistan* exposure therapy system

In 2004, the University of Southern California's Institute for Creative Technologies (ICT), in collaboration with the authors of this paper, partnered on a project funded by the Office of Naval Research (ONR) to develop a series of VRET environments known as *Virtual Iraq*. The initial prototype system was constructed by recycling virtual art assets that were originally designed for the commercially successful X-Box game and U.S. Army-funded combat tactical simulation trainer, *Full Spectrum Warrior*. The first prototype was then continually evolved with specifically created art and technology assets available to ICT in a process that was highly informed by feedback from both clinicians and SMs with combat experience in Iraq and Afghanistan.

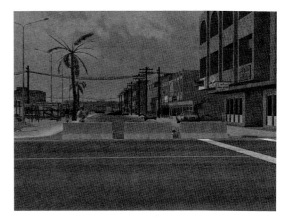

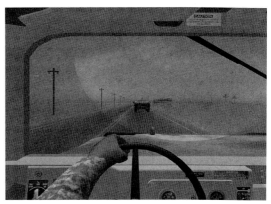

Figure 1. Scenes from *Virtual Iraq* City and Desert Road high-mobility multipurpose wheeled vehicle (HUMVEE) interior. (In color in *Annals* online.)

Virtual Iraq *content and clinician interface*

Virtual Iraq consists of Middle Eastern themed city and desert road environments (see Fig. 1) and was designed to resemble the general contexts that most SMs experience during deployment to Iraq. The 24 square block "City" setting has a variety of elements including a marketplace, desolate streets, checkpoints, ramshackle buildings, warehouses, mosques, shops, and dirt lots strewn with junk. Access to building interiors and rooftops is available and the backdrop surrounding the navigable exposure zone creates the illusion of being embedded within a section of a sprawling densely populated desert city. Vehicles are active in streets and animated virtual pedestrians (civilian and military) can be added or eliminated from the scenes. The software has been designed such that users can be "teleported" to specific locations within the city, on the basis of a determination as to which components of the

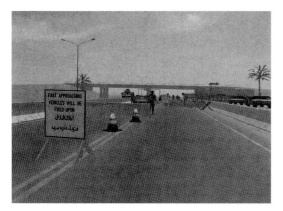

Figure 2. Desert road checkpoint. (In color in *Annals* online.)

environment most closely match the patient's needs, relevant to their individual trauma-related experiences.

The "Desert Road" scenario consists of a roadway through an expansive desert area with sand dunes, occasional areas of vegetation, intact and broken down structures, bridges, battle wreckage, a checkpoint, debris, and virtual human figures (see Fig. 2). The user is positioned inside of a high-mobility multipurpose wheeled vehicle (HUMVEE) that supports the perception of travel within a convoy or as a lone vehicle with selectable positions as a driver, passenger, or from the more exposed turret position above the roof of the vehicle. The number of soldiers in the cab of the HUMVEE can also be varied as well as their capacity to become wounded during certain attack scenarios (e.g., improvised explosive devices (IEDs), rooftop/bridge attacks).

Both the city and desert road HUMVEE scenarios are adjustable for time of day or night, weather conditions, illumination, night vision (see Fig. 3), and ambient sound (wind, motors, city noise, prayer call, etc.). Users can navigate in both scenarios via the use of a standard gamepad controller, although we have recently added the option for a replica M4 weapon with a "thumb-mouse" controller that supports movement during the city foot patrol. This was based on repeated requests from Iraq-experienced SMs who provided frank feedback indicating that to walk within such a setting without a weapon in hand was completely unnatural and distracting! However, there is no option for firing a weapon within the VR scenarios. It is our firm belief that the principles of exposure therapy are incompatible with the cathartic acting out of a revenge fantasy that a responsive weapon might encourage.

In addition to the visual stimuli presented in the VR head-mounted display (HMD), directional 3D audio, vibrotactile, and olfactory stimuli can be delivered into the *Virtual Iraq* scenarios in real time by the clinician. The presentation of additive, combat-relevant stimuli into the VR scenarios can be controlled in real time via a separate "Wizard of Oz" clinician's interface (see Fig. 4), while the clinician is in full audio contact with the patient. The clinician's interface is a key feature that provides a clinician with the capacity to customize the therapy experience to the individual needs of the patient. This interface allows a clinician to place the patient in VR scenario locations that resemble the setting in which the trauma-relevant events occurred and ambient light and sound conditions can be modified to match the patients description of their experience. The clinician can then gradually introduce and control real-time trigger stimuli (visual, auditory,

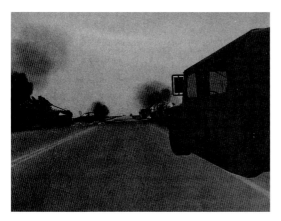

Figure 3. Night vision setting. (In color in *Annals* online.)

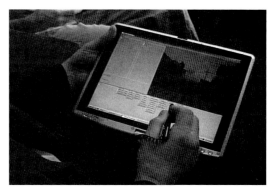

Figure 4. Clinician's interface (wireless version). (In color in *Annals* online.)

olfactory, and tactile), *via* the clinician's interface, as required to foster the anxiety modulation needed for therapeutic habituation and emotional processing in a customized fashion according to the patient's past experience and treatment progress. The clinician's interface options have been designed with the aid of feedback from clinicians with the goal to provide a usable and flexible control panel system for conducting thoughtfully administered exposure therapy that can be readily customized to address the individual needs of the patient. Such options for real-time stimulus delivery flexibility and user experience customization are key elements for these types of VRET applications.

The specification, creation, and addition of trigger stimulus options into the *Virtual Iraq* system has been an evolving process throughout the development of the application on the basis of continually solicited patient and clinician feedback. We began this part of the design process by including options that have been reported to be relevant by returning soldiers and military subject matter experts. For example, the Hoge *et al.* [2] study of Iraq/Afghanistan SMs presented a listing of combat-related events that were commonly experienced in their sample. These events provided a useful starting point for conceptualizing how relevant trigger stimuli could be presented in a VR environment. Such commonly reported events included: "*Being attacked or ambushed. . .receiving incoming artillery, rocket, or mortar fire. . . being shot at or receiving small-arms fire. . .seeing dead bodies or human remains. . .*" (p. 18). From this and other sources, we began our initial effort to conceptualize what was both functionally relevant and technically possible to include as trigger stimuli.

Thus far, we have created a variety of auditory trigger stimuli (e.g., incoming mortars, weapons fire, voices, wind, etc.) that are actuated by the clinician via mouse clicks on the clinician's interface. Clinicians can also similarly trigger dynamic audiovisual events, such as helicopter flyovers, bridge attacks, exploding vehicles, and IEDs. The creation of more complex events that can be intuitively delivered in *Virtual Iraq* from the clinician's interface while providing a patient with options to interact or respond in a meaningful manner is one of the ongoing focuses in this project. However, such trigger options require not only interface design expertise but also clinical wisdom as to how much and what type of exposure is needed to produce a positive clinical effect. These issues have been keenly attended to in our initial nonclinical user-centered tests with Iraq-experienced SMs and in the current clinical trials with patients. This expert feedback is essential for informed VR combat scenario design and goes beyond what is possible to imagine from the "Ivory Tower" of the academic world.

Virtual Iraq *hardware and software*

Whenever possible, *Virtual Iraq* was designed to use off-the-shelf equipment in order to minimizes costs and maximize the access and availability of the finished system. The minimum computing requirements for the current application are two Pentium 4 computers each with 1 GB RAM, and a 128 MB DirectX 9-compatible *NVIDIA* 3D graphics card. The two computers are linked using a null Ethernet cable (or wireless network option) with one running the clinician's interface, whereas the second one drives the simulation via the user's HMD and navigation interface (gamepad or gun controller). The HMD that was chosen was the *eMagin z800*, with displays capable of 800×600 resolution within a $40°$ diagonal field of view (http://www.emagin.com/). The major selling point for using this HMD was the presence of a built-in head tracking system. At under U.S. \$1,500 per unit with built-in head tracking, this integrated display/tracking solution was viewed as the best option to minimize costs and maximize the access to this system. The simulation's real-time 3D scenes are presented using the FlatWorld Simulation Control Architecture with Emergent's *Gamebryo* used as a rendering engine. Preexisting art assets were integrated using *Alias' Maya 6* and *AutoDesk 3D Studio Max 7* with new art created primarily in *Maya*.

Olfactory and tactile stimuli can be delivered into the simulation to further augment the experience of the environment. Olfactory stimuli are produced by the *EnviroScent, Inc. Scent Palette*. This is a USB-driven device that contains eight pressurized chambers, within which individual smell cartridges can be inserted, a series of fans and a small air compressor to propel the customized scents to participants. The scent delivery is controlled by mouse clicks on the clinician's interface. Scents may be employed as direct stimuli (e.g., scent of smoke as a user walks by a burning vehicle) or as cues to help immerse users in the world (e.g., ethnic food cooking). The scents selected for this application include burning rubber, cordite, garbage, body odor, smoke, diesel fuel, Iraqi food spices, and gunpowder. Vibration is also used as an additional user sensory input. Vibration is generated through the use of a *Logitech* force-feedback game control pad and through low-cost (<U.S. $120) audio-tactile sound transducers from *Aura Sound Inc.* located beneath the patient's floor platform and seat. Audio files are customized to provide vibration consistent with relevant visual and audio stimuli in the scenario. For example, in the HUMVEE desert road scenario, the user experiences engine vibrations as the vehicle moves across the virtual terrain and a shaking floor can accompany explosions. This package of controllable multi-sensory stimulus options was included in the design of *Virtual Iraq* to allow a clinician the flexibility to engage users across a wide range of unique and highly customizable levels of exposure intensity. As well, these same features have broadened the applicability of *Virtual Iraq* as a research tool for studies that require systematic control of stimulus presentation within combat relevant environments.[26]

Preliminary user-centered design phase

The *Virtual Iraq* scenario is currently being implemented as an exposure therapy tool with active duty SMs and veterans at Madigan Army Medical Center (MAMC) at Ft. Lewis, WA, the Naval Medical Center-San Diego (NMCSD), Camp Pendleton, Emory University, Walter Reed Army Medical Center, the Weill Medical College of Cornell University, and at approximately 35 other VA, Military, and University Laboratory sites for VRET research and a variety of other PTSD-related investigations. However, the user-centered design process for optimizing *Virtual Iraq* for clinical use is noteworthy and will be described before briefly summarizing the VRET treatment protocol and results from the initial open clinical trial.

User-centered feedback from non-PTSD SMs

User-centered tests with early prototypes of the *Virtual Iraq* application were conducted at the NMCSD and within an Army Combat Stress Control Team in Iraq (see Fig. 5). This formative feedback from nondiagnosed Iraq-experienced military personnel provided essential information that fed an iterative design process on the content, realism, and usability of the initial "intuitively designed" system.

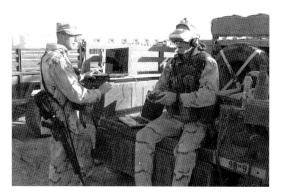

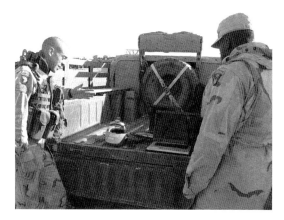

Figure 5. User-centered feedback from Iraq stress control team. (In color in *Annals* online.)

More formal evaluation of the system took place at MAMC from late 2006 to early 2007.[27] Ninety-three screened SMs (all non-PTSD) evaluated the *Virtual Iraq* scenarios shortly after returning from deployment in Iraq. SMs experienced the city and HUMVEE environments while exposed to scripted researcher-initiated VR trigger stimuli to simulate an actual treatment session. SMs then completed standardized questionnaires to evaluate the realism, sense of "presence" (the feeling of being in Iraq), sensory stimuli, and overall technical capabilities of *Virtual Iraq*. Items were rated on a scale from 0 (poor) to 10 (excellent). Qualitative feedback was also collected to determine additional required software improvements. The results suggested that the *Virtual Iraq* environment in its form at the time was realistic and provided a good sense of "being back in Iraq."

Average ratings across environments were between adequate and excellent for all evaluated aspects of the virtual environments. Auditory stimuli realism (M = 7.9, SD = 1.7) and quality (M = 7.9, SD = 1.8) were rated higher than visual realism (M = 6.7, SD = 2.1) and quality (M = 7.0, SD = 2.0). Soldiers had high ratings of the computer's ability to update visual graphics during movement (M = 8.4, SD = 1.7). The *eMagin* HMD was reportedly very comfortable (M = 8.2, SD = 1.7), and the average ratings for the ability to move within the virtual environment was generally adequate or above (M = 6.1, SD = 2.5). These data, along with the collected qualitative feedback, were used to inform upgrades to the current version of *Virtual Iraq* that is now in clinical use and this "design-collect feedback-redesign" cycle will continue throughout the lifecycle of this project.

SM acceptance of VR in treatment

The user-centered results indicated that *Virtual Iraq* was capable of producing the level of engagement in Iraq-experienced SMs that was believed to be required for exposure therapy. However, successful clinical implementation also requires patients to accept the approach as a useful and credible behavioral health treatment. To address this issue, a survey study with 325 Army SMs from the MAMC/Fort Lewis deployment screening clinic was conducted to assess knowledge of current technologies and attitudes toward the use of technology in behavioral health care.[28] One section of the survey asked these active duty SMs to rate on a five-point scale how willing they would be to receive mental health treatment ("Not Willing at All" to "Very Willing") via traditional approaches (e.g., face-to-face counseling) and a variety of technology-oriented delivery methods (e.g., website, video teleconferencing, and use of VR). Eighty-three percent of participants reported that they were neutral-to-very willing to use some form of technology as part of their behavioral health care, with 58% reporting some willingness to use a VR treatment program. Seventy-one percent of SMs were equally or more willing to use some form of technological treatment than solely talking to a therapist in a traditional setting. Most interesting is that 20% of SMs who stated they were not willing to seek traditional psychotherapy rated their willingness to use a VR-based treatment as neutral to very willing. One possible interpretation of this finding is that a subgroup of this sample of SMs with a significant disinterest in traditional mental

health treatment would be willing to pursue treatment with a VR-based approach. It is also possible that these findings generalize to SMs who have disengaged from or terminated traditional treatment.

VRET open clinical trial protocol and results

Participants

The ONR funding for the *Virtual Iraq* system development also supported an initial open clinical trial to evaluate the efficacy of VRET for use with active duty participants at NMCSD and Camp Pendleton. The participants were 20 active duty SMs (19 male, one female, mean age = 28 years, age range 21–51 years) who recently redeployed from Iraq and who had engaged in previous PTSD treatments (e.g., group counseling, medications, etc.) without benefit. However, in this initial open clinical trial, elements of the protocol were occasionally modified (i.e., adjusting the number and timing of sessions) to meet patients' needs and thus these data represent outcomes from an uncontrolled feasibility trial.

Clinical protocol

The standard VRET exposure therapy protocol consisted of 2× weekly, 90–120 min sessions over 5 weeks that also included physiological monitoring (heart rate (HR), galvanic skin response (GSR), and respiration) as part of the data collection. The VRET protocol followed the principles of graded prolonged behavioral exposure[29] and the pace was individualized and patient driven. The first VRET session consisted of a clinical interview that identified the index (or most significant) trauma experience, provided psychoeducation on trauma and PTSD, and instruction on a deep breathing technique for general stress management purposes. The second session provided instruction on the use of subjective units of distress (SUDS; a 1–100 self-rating of current distress), the rationale for prolonged exposure, including imaginal exposure and *in vivo* (i.e., real-world) exposure. The participants also engaged in their first experience of imaginal exposure of a significant trauma event and an *in vivo* hierarchical exposure list was constructed, with the first item assigned as homework. Session three introduced the rationale for VRET and the participant experienced the *Virtual Iraq* environment without recounting any trauma narrative for approximately 25 min with no provocative trigger stimuli introduced.

The purpose of not recounting any trauma events was to allow the participant to learn how to navigate in *Virtual Iraq* in an exploratory manner and to function as a "bridge session" from imaginal alone to imaginal exposure combined with virtual reality (VRET). Sessions 4–10 are when the VRET proper was conducted with the participant engaging in the VR while recounting the trauma narrative.

During the VRET sessions, participants were asked to recount their trauma experiences in the first person, as if it were happening again with as much attention to sensory detail as they could provide. Using clinical judgment, the therapist might prompt the patient with questions about their experience or provide encouraging remarks as deemed necessary to facilitate the recounting of the trauma narrative. The treatment included homework, such as requesting the participant to listen to the audiotape of their exposure narrative from the most recent session. Listening to the audiotape several times over a week functioned as a source of continual exposure to promote processing of the trauma events with the aim to further enhance the process of therapeutic habituation outside of the therapy office. *In vivo* hierarchy exposure items were assigned in a sequential fashion, starting with the lowest rated item. A new item was assigned once the participant demonstrated approximately a 50% reduction of SUDs ratings on the previous item. Self-report measures were obtained at baseline, prior to sessions 3, 5, 7, 9, 10, and at 1 week and 3 months after treatment to assess in-treatment and follow-up symptom status. The measures used were the PTSD Checklist-Military Version (PCL-M),[30] Beck Anxiety Inventory (BAI),[31] and Patient Health Questionnaire (PHQ-9) (Depression).[32]

Results

A paper that fully details the results from this project is currently under review.[33] Analyses from the first 20 *Virtual Iraq* treatment completers have suggested positive clinical outcomes. The average number of VRET sessions for this sample was just under 11. For this sample, mean pre-/post-PCL-M scores decreased in a statistical and clinically meaningful fashion; mean (SD) values went from 54.4 (9.7) to 35.6 (17.4). Paired pre-/post-*t*-test analysis showed these differences to be significant ($t = 5.99$, df $= 19$, $P < 0.001$). Correcting for the PCL-M no-symptom baseline of 17 indicated a greater than 50% decrease

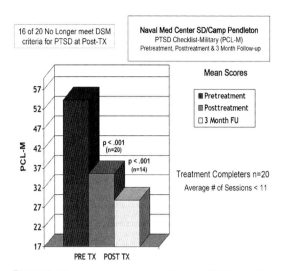

Figure 6. Mean posttraumatic stress disorder (PTSD) checklist scores across treatment.

in symptoms and 16 of the 20 completers no longer met Diagnostic and Statistical Manual of Mental Disorders criteria for PTSD at posttreatment. Five participants in this group with PTSD diagnoses had pretreatment baseline scores below the conservative PCL-M cutoff value of 50 (prescores $= 49, 46, 42, 36$, and 38) and reported decreased values at posttreatment (postscores $= 23, 19, 22, 22$, and 24, respectively). Mean and individual participant PCL-M scores at baseline, after treatment, and 3-month follow-up are graphed in Figures 6 and 7. For this same group, mean BAI scores significantly decreased

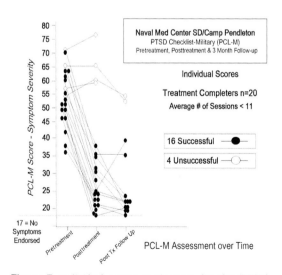

Figure 7. Individual posttraumatic stress disorder (PTSD) Checklist scores across treatment.

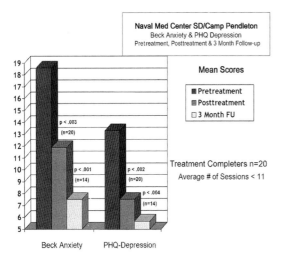

Figure 8. Beck Anxiety Scale and Patient Health Questionnaire-Depression scores across treatment.

33% from 18.6 (10.7) to 11.9 (13.3), ($t = 3.67$, df $= 19$, $P < 0.003$) and mean PHQ-9 (Depression) scores decreased 49% from 13.3 (5.4) to 7.1 (6.7) ($t = 3.68$, df $= 19$, $P < 0.002$) (see Fig. 8). Also, two of the successful treatment completers had documented mild and moderate TBIs, which suggest that this form of exposure can be usefully applied with this population.

Conclusions and future research

Results from uncontrolled trials and case reports are difficult to generalize from, and we are cautious not to make excessive claims on the basis of these early results. However, in the summary of results from an open clinical trial using accepted diagnostic measures, 80% of the treatment completers in this VRET sample showed both statistically and clinically meaningful reductions in PTSD, anxiety, and depression symptoms, and anecdotal evidence from patient reports suggested that they saw improvements in their everyday life situations. These improvements were also maintained at 3-month posttreatment follow-up. Similar findings are about to be reported by Reger *et al.*[34] with another active duty sample of U.S. Army participant. On the basis of these initial open clinical trial results and single case reports by Reger & Gahm[35] and Gerardi *et al.*,[36] we are encouraged by these early successes and continue to gather feedback from patients regarding the therapy and the *Virtual Iraq* environment. The system is currently being updated with added

functionality that has its design "roots" from feedback acquired from these initial patients and the clinicians who have used the system thus far. These findings will be used to develop, explore, and test hypotheses as to how we can improve treatment and also determine what patient characteristics may predict who will complete and benefit from VRET and who may be best served by other approaches. As well, three randomized controlled trials are currently in progress that will compare the efficacy of VR exposure with the traditional imaginal approach, and in one study, provide a test of the additive value of conducting both forms of exposure therapy with the adjunctive use of a cognitive enhancer medication (D-cycloserine).

It should be noted that in spite of these initial positive results for treatment completers, challenges exist with treatment attrition in active duty populations. Seven participants who were assessed and approved for the result described above failed to appear at the first session, six attended the first session and dropped out prior to formal commencement of VRET, and seven dropped out at various points following the start of VRET proper in session 4. Although some of these active duty participants left owing to transfers and other reasons beyond their control, these dropout numbers are concerning and we are in the process of examining all data gathered from this subset of the total sample to search for discriminating factors.

Such treatment attrition rates need to be viewed in the context of research that suggests there is an urgent need to reduce the stigma of seeking mental health treatment in military populations. For example, one of the more foreboding findings in the Hoge *et al.*[2] report was the observation that among Iraq/Afghanistan War veterans, "*. . . those whose responses were positive for a mental disorder, only 23 to 40 percent sought mental health care. Those whose responses were positive for a mental disorder were twice as likely as those whose responses were negative to report concern about possible stigmatization and other barriers to seeking mental health care*" (p. 13). Although military training methodology has better-prepared soldiers for combat in recent years, such hesitancy to seek treatment for difficulties that emerge upon return from combat, especially by those who may need it most, suggests an area of military mental health care that is in need of attention. To address this concern, a VR system for

PTSD treatment could serve as a component within a reconceptualized approach to how treatment is accessed by SMs and veterans returning from combat. Perhaps VR exposure could be embedded within the context of "postdeployment *reset* training" whereby the perceived stigma of seeking treatment could be lessened as the soldier would simply be involved in this "training" in similar fashion to other designated duties upon redeployment stateside. VRET therapy may also offer an additional attraction and promote treatment seeking by certain demographic groups in need of care. The current generation of young military personnel, having grown up with digital game technology, may actually be more attracted to and comfortable with participation in VRET as an alternative to what is perceived as traditional "talk therapy."

The current clinical research and development program with the *Virtual Iraq* application is also providing important knowledge for determining the feasibility of expanding the range of applications that can be created from this system to address other scientific questions. For example, following a similar design process, we have now created a *Virtual Afghanistan* themed scenario (see Fig. 6) that has more mountainous terrain and relevant building architecture. During the course of the ongoing research and development evolution of this application, our design approach has always focused on the creation of a flexible VR system/tool that could address *both* clinical and scientific PTSD research questions in a more comprehensive fashion. In this regard, we aim to repurpose the *Virtual Iraq* and *Virtual Afghanistan* applications as tools to investigate a variety of clinical and scientific questions including:

- The feasibility of assessing soldiers prior to deployment to predict potential risk for developing PTSD or other mental health difficulties on the basis of physiological reactivity to a series of virtual combat engagements.
- The creation of a stress resilience training tool where users are put in standardized simulations of emotionally challenging situations that may provide a more meaningful context in which to learn and practice cognitive coping strategies and psychologically prepare for what might occur in real combat situations.
- The effectiveness of using VR as an assessment tool immediately upon redeployment home to

determine who may be "at risk" for developing PTSD after an incubation period. Physiological reactivity could figure well as a marker variable for this project and a prospective longitudinal study is needed in this area. This is particularly important for maximizing the probability that a soldier at risk would be directed into a "reset" program before being sent on a second or third deployment.

- The comparison of National Guard, reservist personnel, Army/Navy/Marine/Air Force standing military SMs and veterans in terms of their susceptibility for developing PTSD and if variations in the course of treatment would be required. This is also relevant for the study of PTSD treatment response differences due to multiple deployments, age, gender, education, family support, and previous civilian exposure to trauma.
- The neuroscience of PTSD via the use of brain imaging (e.g., functional magnetic resonance imaging and diffusion tensor imaging), traditional physiological measurement (e.g., electroencephalography, electrocardiography, and GSR), and other responses (e.g., eyeblink and startle response) by leveraging the high controllability of stimulus presentation that is available within the *Virtual Iraq/Afghanistan* applications.
- The interaction effects of the use of VR exposure in combination with pharmacological treatments. Randomized controlled trials comparing VRET alone and VRET + D-cycloserine are in progress at Emory University, the Weill Cornell Medical College, and University of Southern California, instigated by successful results, were reported with VRET + D-cycloserine for treating fear of heights.[37]
- The expansion of the functionality of the existing *Virtual Iraq* system based on the results of ongoing and future research. This will involve refining the system in terms of the breadth of scenarios/trigger events, the stimulus content, and the level of artificial intelligence of virtual humans that "inhabit" the system.

Finally, a guiding principle in the development of *Virtual Iraq* concerns how novel VR systems can extend the skills of a well-trained clinician. VRET is not intended to be an automated treatment or administered in a "self-help" format. The presentation of such emotionally evocative VR combat-related scenarios, while providing treatment options not possible until recently, will most likely produce therapeutic benefits when administered with a professional appreciation of the complexity and impact of this disorder.

Acknowledgments

The project described here has been sponsored by the ONR; Telemedicine and Advanced Technology Research Center; and U.S. Army Research, Development, and Engineering Command. Statements and opinions expressed do not necessarily reflect the position or the policy of the United States Government, and no official endorsement should be inferred.

Conflicts of interest

The authors declare no conflicts of interest.

References

1. Fischer, H. 2009. United States Military casualty statistics: Operation Iraqi Freedom and Operation Enduring Freedom. *Congressional Research Service* **7-5700:** RS22452. www.fas.org/sgp/crs/natsec/RS22452.pdf (accessed September 7, 2010).

2. Hoge, C.W., C.A. Castro, S.C. Messer, *et al.* 2004. Combat duty in Iraq and Afghanistan, mental health problems, and barriers to care. *N. Engl. J. Med.* **351:** 13–22.

3. Seal, K.H., D. Bertenthal, C.R. Nuber, *et al.* 2007. Bringing the war back home: mental health disorders among 103,788 US veterans returning from Iraq and Afghanistan seen at Department of Veterans Affairs facilities. *Arch. Intern. Med.* **167:** 476–482.

4. Tanielian, T., L.H. Jaycox, T.L. Schell, *et al.* 2008. Invisible wounds of war: summary and recommendations for addressing psychological and cognitive injuries. *Rand Report.* http://veterans.rand.org/ (accessed April 18, 2008).

5. Holden, M.K. 2005. Virtual environments for motor rehabilitation: review. *CyberPsychol. Behav.* **83:** 187–211.

6. Parsons, T.D. & A.A. Rizzo. 2008. Affective outcomes of virtual reality exposure therapy for anxiety and specific phobias: a meta-analysis. *J. Behav. Ther. Exp. Psychiatry* **39:** 250–261.

7. Powers, M.B. & P.M. Emmelkamp. 2008. Virtual reality exposure therapy for anxiety disorders: a meta-analysis. *J. Anxiety Disord.* **22:** 561–569.

8. Rose, F.D., B.M. Brooks & A.A. Rizzo. 2005. Virtual reality in brain damage rehabilitation: review. *CyberPsychol. Behav.* **83:** 241–262.

9. Riva, G. 2005. Virtual reality in psychotherapy: review. *CyberPsychol. Behav.* **83:** 220–230.

10. Glantz, K., A.A. Rizzo & K. Graap. 2003. Virtual reality for psychotherapy: current reality and future possibilities. *Psychother. Res. Theory Pract. Training* **40:** 55–67.

11. Rizzo, A.A., M.T. Schultheis, K. Kerns & C. Mateer. 2004. Analysis of assets for virtual reality applications in neuropsychology. *Neuropsychol Rehabil.* **141:** 207–239.

12. Rothbaum, B.O., L. Hodges, R. Alarcon, *et al.* 1999. Virtual reality exposure therapy for PTSD Vietnam Veterans: a case study. *J. Trauma. Stress* **122:** 263–271.

13. Rothbaum, B.O., E.A. Meadows, P. Resick, *et al.* 2000. Cognitive behavioral therapy. In *Effective Treatments for PTSD: Practice Guidelines from the International Society for Traumatic Stress Studies.* E.B. Foa, T.M. Keane, & M.J. Friedman, Eds.: 60–83. Guilford Press. New York.

14. Rothbaum, B.O., L. Hodges, D. Ready, *et al.* 2001. Virtual reality exposure therapy for Vietnam Veterans with posttraumatic stress disorder. *J. Clin. Psychiatry* **62:** 617–622.

15. Rothbaum, B.O., L. Hodges, P.L. Anderson, *et al.* 2002. Twelve month follow-up of virtual reality exposure therapy for the fear of flying. *J. Consult. Clin. Psychol.* **70:** 428–432.

16. Zimand, E., P. Anderson, G. Gershon, *et al.* 2003. Virtual reality therapy: innovative treatment for anxiety disorders. *Prim. Psychiatry* **97:** 51–54.

17. Difede, J. & H. Hoffman. 2002. Virtual reality exposure therapy for PTSD following the WTC: a case report. *Cyberpsychol. Behav.* **56:** 529–535.

18. Difede, J., J. Cukor, N. Jayasinghe, *et al.* 2007. Virtual reality exposure therapy for the treatment of posttraumatic stress disorder following September 11, 2001. *J. Clin. Psychiatry* **68:** 1639–1647.

19. Rizzo, A.A., G. Reger, G. Gahm, *et al.* 2009. Virtual reality exposure therapy for combat related PTSD. In *Post-Traumatic Stress Disorder: Basic Science and Clinical Practice.* P. Shiromani, T. Keane & J. LeDoux, Eds.: 375–399. Springer. New York.

20. Schneider, S.M., M. Prince-Paul, M.J. Allen, *et al.* 2004. Virtual reality as a distraction intervention for women receiving chemotherapy. *Oncol. Nurs. Forum* **31:** 81–88.

21. Hoffman, H.G. *et al.* 2004. Water-friendly virtual reality pain control during wound care. *J. Clin. Psychol.* **60:** 189–195.

22. Stanton, D., N. Foreman & P. Wilson. 1998. Uses of virtual reality in clinical training: developing the spatial skills of children with mobility impairments. In *Virtual Reality in Clinical Psychology and Neuroscience.* G. Riva, B. Wiederhold & E. Molinari, Eds.: 219–232. IOS Press. Amsterdam, the Netherlands.

23. Weiss, P.L., R. Kizony, U. Feintuch & N. Katz. 2006. Virtual reality in neurorehabilitation. In *Textbook of Neural Repair and Neurorehabilitation,* vol. 2. M.E. Selzer, S. Clarke, L. Cohen, P.W. Duncan & F.H. Gage, Eds.: 182–197. Cambridge University Press. Cambridge, UK.

24. Rizzo, A.A. & G. Kim. 2005. A SWOT analysis of the field of Virtual Rehabilitation and Therapy. *Presence: Teleoperators Virtual Environ.* **14:** 119–146.

25. Rothbaum, B.O., A.A. Rizzo & J. Difede. 2010. Virtual reality exposure therapy for combat-related posttraumatic stress disorder. *Ann. N.Y. Acad. Sci.* **1208:** 126–132.

26. Parsons, T.D. & A.A. Rizzo. 2008. Initial validation of a virtual environment for assessment of memory functioning: virtual reality cognitive performance assessment test. *Cyberpsychol. Behav.* **11:** 17–25.

27. Reger, G.M., G.A. Gahm, A.A. Rizzo, *et al.* 2009. Soldier evaluation of the virtual reality Iraq. *Telemed. J. E Health* **15:** 101–104.

28. Wilson, J., K. Onorati, M. Mishkind, *et al.* 2008. Soldier attitudes about technology-based approaches to mental healthcare. *Cyberpsychol. Behav.* **11:** 767–769.

29. Foa, E.B., R.T. Davidson & A. Frances. 1999. Expert consensus guideline series: treatment of posttraumatic stress disorder. *Am. J. Clin. Psychiatry* **60:** 5–76.

30. Blanchard, E.B., J. Jones-Alexander, T.C. Buckley & C.A. Forneris. 1996. Psychometric properties of the PTSD checklist (PCL). *Behav. Res. Ther.* **34:** 669–673.

31. Beck, A.T., N. Epstein, G. Brown & R.A. Steer. 1988. An inventory for measuring clinical anxiety: psychometric properties. *J. Consult. Clin. Psychol.* **56:** 893–897.

32. Kroenke, K. & R.L. Spitzer. 2002. The PHQ-9: a new depression and diagnostic severity measure. *Psychiatr. Ann.* **32:** 509–521.

33. McLay, R.N., A.A. Rizzo, K. Graap, *et al.* Development and testing of virtual reality exposure therapy for post traumatic stress disorder in active duty service members who served in Iraq and Afghanistan. *Mil. Med.* In press.

34. Reger, G.M., K.M. Holloway, P. Koenen-Woods, *et al.* Effectiveness of virtual reality exposure therapy for active duty soldiers in a military mental health clinic. *J. Trauma. Stress.* In press.

35. Reger, G.M. & G.A. Gahm. 2008. Virtual reality exposure therapy for active duty soldiers. *J. Clin. Psychol.* **64:** 940–946.

36. Gerardi, M., B.O. Rothbaum, K. Ressler, *et al.* 2008. Virtual reality exposure therapy using a virtual Iraq: case report. *J. Trauma. Stress* **21:** 209–213.

37. Ressler, K.J., B.O. Rothbaum, L. Tannenbaum, *et al.* 2004. Facilitation of psychotherapy with D-cycloserine, a putative cognitive enhancer. *Arch. Gen. Psych.* **61:** 1136–1144.

Ann. N.Y. Acad. Sci. ISSN 0077-8923

ANNALS OF THE NEW YORK ACADEMY OF SCIENCES
Issue: *Psychiatric and Neurologic Aspects of War*

Virtual reality exposure therapy for combat-related posttraumatic stress disorder

Barbara O. Rothbaum,[1] Albert "Skip" Rizzo,[2] and JoAnn Difede[3]

[1]Emory University, Atlanta, Georgia. [2]University of Southern California, Los Angeles, California. [3]Weill Cornell Medical College, New York, New York

Address for correspondence: Barbara O. Rothbaum, Emory University, 1256 Briarcliff Road, Atlanta, Georgia 30306. brothba@emory.edu

Posttraumatic stress disorder (PTSD) is a chronic, debilitating, psychological condition that occurs in a subset of individuals who experience or witness life-threatening traumatic events. PTSD is highly prevalent in those who served in the military. In this paper, we present the underlying theoretical foundations and existing research on virtual reality exposure therapy, a recently emerging treatment for PTSD. Three virtual reality scenarios used to treat PTSD in active duty military and combat veterans and survivors of terrorism are presented: Virtual Vietnam, Virtual Iraq, and Virtual World Trade Center. Preliminary results of ongoing trials are presented.

Keywords: virtual reality; exposure therapy; PTSD; behavior therapy; veterans; military

Introduction

Posttraumatic stress disorder (PTSD) is a chronic condition that occurs in a significant minority of persons who experience life-threatening traumatic events. PTSD is characterized by reexperiencing, avoidance, and hyperarousal symptoms.[1] PTSD has been estimated to affect up to 18% of returning Operation Iraqi Freedom (OIF) Veterans.[2] In addition to the specific conditions in Iraq and Afghanistan, an unprecedented number are now surviving serious wounds.[3] The stigma of treatment often prevents service members and veterans from seeking help,[2] so finding an acceptable form of treatment to military personnel is a priority. The current generation of military personnel may be more comfortable participating in a virtual reality (VR) treatment approach than traditional talk therapy, as they are likely familiar with gaming and training simulation technology.

Exposure to traumatic events is a common experience with estimates ranging between 37% and 92% of individuals.[4] The symptoms of PTSD should be considered part of the normal reaction to trauma, as they occur almost universally following severe enough traumas. In a prospective study of rape vic-

tims, 94% met symptomatic criteria for PTSD in the first week following the assault.[5] Those who did not end up with chronic PTSD showed steadily decreasing PTSD symptoms over time beginning soon after the assault, but those who ended up with chronic PTSD showed a slightly different pattern: their PTSD symptoms declined in the first 4 weeks following the assault then remained fairly steady across time. They did not get worse, but they did not get better. We concluded that PTSD can be viewed as a failure of recovery caused in part by a failure of fear extinction following trauma.[5,6]

Cognitive behavioral therapy (CBT) includes a variety of treatment programs, including exposure procedures, cognitive restructuring procedures, anxiety management programs, and their combinations that have been found useful for treating anxiety, and PTSD in particular.[7,8] One form of CBT employed with PTSD sufferers is exposure therapy, which assists patients in confronting their feared memories and situations in a therapeutic manner. A comprehensive review of CBT studies for PTSD found the strongest evidence for exposure therapy.[9] Prolonged exposure (PE) therapy, developed by Foa and Rothbaum and their colleagues incorporates imaginal exposure in which the patient

doi: 10.1111/j.1749-6632.2010.05691.x

Ann. N.Y. Acad. Sci. 1208 (2010) 126–132 © 2010 Association for Research in Nervous and Mental Disease.

is asked to return to the time of the trauma in his or her mind and to relive it in imagination repeatedly and until anxiety decreases and in *in vivo* exposure to safe trauma reminders.[10,11] The idea underlying this treatment approach is that the traumatic memory needs to be emotionally processed to become less painful.[12,13] Procedures consist of confronting the patient with trauma-related information to activate the trauma memory. This activation provides an opportunity for the patient to integrate corrective information and modify pathological components of the trauma memory. Detailed instructions for conducting exposure therapy with PTSD patients can be found in Foa *et al.*[11]

VR exposure therapy

VR offers a human–computer interaction system in which users are no longer simply external observers of images on a screen but are active participants within a computer-generated three-dimensional virtual world. The most common approach to the creation of a virtual environment is to outfit the user in a head-mounted display. Head-mounted displays consist of separate display screens for each eye, display optics, stereo earphones, and a head-tracking device. The user is presented with a computer-generated view of a virtual world that changes in a natural way with head and body motion. For some environments, users also hold a second position sensor or interface controller that allows them to manipulate their environment and allow the user to navigate throughout the virtual world. VR environments presented here differ from traditionally displayed programs in that computer graphics displayed in the head mounted display are augmented with motion tracking; vibration platforms; localizable three-dimensional sounds within the VR space; and, in some scenarios, scent delivery technology to facilitate an immersive experience for participants.

The immersive nature of the VR environments typically leads to a strong sense of presence (i.e., "being there") reported by those immersed in the virtual environment. A sense of presence is also essential for conducting exposure therapy.[11] A specific form of exposure therapy, VR exposure (VRE) therapy immerses patients in a virtual environment to provide a sense of presence to facilitate emotional engagement with the traumatic memory. In this way, VRE is proposed to effectively elicit the fear structure and aid the emotional processing of fears.[14] The VR

simulation also allows for the precise delivery and control of trauma relevant exposure stimuli within a safe virtual environment.

VR has emerged as a viable therapeutic tool in the areas of assessment and intervention, especially for anxiety disorders, with the bulk of early research focusing on its efficacy in treating specific phobias. Several controlled studies over the last 10 years and two recent meta-analyses have documented its clinical efficacy as an exposure therapy treatment for anxiety disorders. In their investigation of 13 studies comparing VR treatment to *in vivo* exposure, Powers and Emmelkamp[15] found a large effect size for VRE compared to controls ($d = 1.1$, $P < 0.05$) and a small effect size for VRE over *in vivo* treatments ($d = 0.35$, $P < 0.05$). Similarly, Parsons and Rizzo located 52 studies using VR and evaluated 21 with over 300 total participants and concluded that, overall, VR therapy appears to be well supported.[16]

The first use of VR for a Vietnam Veteran with PTSD was reported in a case study of a 50-year-old, Caucasian male Veteran meeting Diagnostic and Statistical Manual of Mental Disorders, Fourth Edition (DSM-IV) criteria for PTSD.[17] Results indicated posttreatment improvement on all measures of PTSD and maintenance of these gains were seen at a 6-month follow-up. This case study was followed by an open clinical trial of VR for Vietnam Veterans.[18] In this study, 16 male Vietnam Veterans with PTSD were exposed to two virtual environments delivered in a head-mounted display, a virtual clearing surrounded by jungle, and a virtual Huey helicopter, in which the therapist controlled various visual and auditory effects (e.g., helicopter fly bys, explosions, day/night effects, men yelling) (see Fig. 1, for scenes from Virtual Vietnam). After an average of 13 exposure therapy sessions over 5–7 weeks, there was a significant reduction in PTSD and related symptoms in the treatment completers. After VRE, the majority of patients' ratings of their global improvement indicated improvement. Clinician's ratings of patients' global improvement as measured by the Clinical Global Improvement Scale indicated that five of six showed improvement immediately after the study while one appeared unchanged. At 6 months, seven of eight were rated as demonstrating some improvement. Clinician-rated PTSD symptoms as measured by the Clinician-Administered

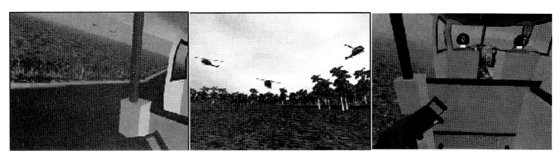

Figure 1. Virtual Vietnam scenarios (courtesy Virtually Better, www.virtuallybetter.com). (In color in *Annals* online.)

PTSD Scale (CAPS), the primary outcome measure, at 6-month follow-up indicated an overall statistically significant reduction from baseline in symptoms associated with specific reported traumatic experiences. Eight of eight participants at the 6-month follow-up reported reductions in PTSD symptoms ranging from 15% to 67%. Significant decreases were seen in all three symptom clusters. Patient self-reported intrusion and avoidance symptoms as measured by the impact of events scale were significantly lower at 3 months than at baseline but not at 6 months, although there was a clear trend toward fewer intrusive thoughts and somewhat less avoidance. VRE therapy was associated with significant reductions in PTSD and related symptoms and was well tolerated. This preliminary evidence suggested that VRE could be a promising component of a comprehensive treatment approach for Veterans with combat-related PTSD.

In the aftermath of the September 11 terrorist attacks on New York City, many thousands of World Trade Center (WTC) survivors, including first responders and disaster recovery workers as well as civilians, were deemed to be at high-risk for developing PTSD. In response to this, Difede and Hoffman developed a virtual WTC for treating survivors that gradually, yet systematically exposes the client to a simulated attack on the WTC.[19,20] A wait-list controlled study, composed of firefighters, disaster recovery workers and civilians, some of whom were not successful in previous imaginal therapy, found positive results from VR treatment.[21] The VR group showed both statistically and clinically significant improvement in the CAPS compared to the wait-list comparison group.

VR environments have been used worldwide to facilitate PTSD treatment in civilians. In Portugal, Gamito *et al.* developed a VR application in re-

sponse to the estimated 25,000 survivors with PTSD from their 1961–1974 wars in Mozambique, Angola, and Guiné. This research group constructed a single VR "ambush" scenario by modifying a common PC-based combat game.[22] They report having recently conducted an initial user-centered test with one PTSD patient who provided feedback suggesting the need for a system that provides more graduated delivery of anxiety provoking trigger stimuli. Josman *et al.* are currently implementing a virtual bus bombing PTSD treatment scenario for civilian survivors of terrorist attacks in Israel.[23]

Finally, in response to the growing numbers of veterans returning with PTSD from OIF, development of a Virtual Iraq scenario was commenced in 2005 at the University of Southern California,[24] and is currently the focus of on-going research being conducted at several civilian sites at Emory University[25] and Cornell University,[26] in addition to several active duty military sites including Walter Reed Medical Center,[27] Madigan Army Hospital,[28] and Naval Medical Center.[24]

Virtual Iraq

The Virtual Iraq environment was developed using input from Veterans returning from Iraq and Afghanistan and from military information experts. It allows for the simultaneous delivery of visual, audio, vibrotactile, and olfactory stimuli to create an immersive and multisensory experience for the user. The environment includes two general scenario settings with different first person user perspective options: a Middle Eastern city and Humvee driving down a desert highway alone or in a convoy (see Fig. 2, for scenes from Virtual Iraq). All scenario settings are adjustable for time of day or night, lighting illumination and weather conditions. The current environment includes different trigger stimuli:

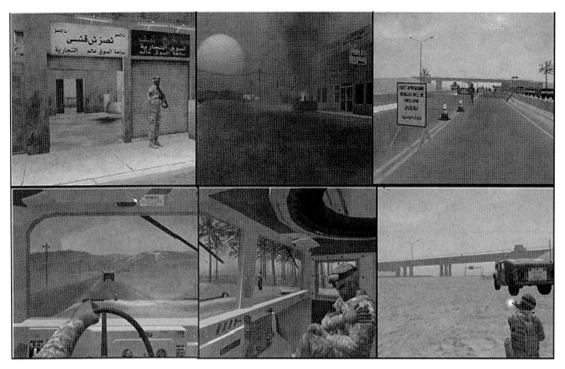

Figure 2. *Virtual Iraq/Afghanistan* city and desert humvee scenarios (courtesy of USC Institute for Creative Technologies and Virtually Better, www.virtuallybetter.com). (In color in *Annals* online.)

auditory (e.g., weapons fire, explosions, vehicle noise, wind, human voices, helicopter flying overhead), static visual (e.g., wrecked vehicles), dynamic visual (e.g., distant views of vehicle movement), and dynamic audiovisual (e.g., nearby human and vehicle movement, explosions, insurgent attacks).

Olfactory and tactile stimuli may be delivered simultaneously with the audiovisual content as a means to further customize the virtual environment and create a multimodal sensory experience. Scents may be employed as direct stimuli (e.g., scent of burning rubber) or as cues to help generally immerse users in the world (e.g., ethnic food cooking). When activated, the scent is released from an airtight chamber into an air stream provided by four electric fans so that it moves past the user and diffuses throughout the room. Scents currently in use include: burning rubber, cordite, garbage, body odor, smoke, diesel fuel, Iraqi spices, and gunpowder. Vibration adds another sensory component to augment the user's sense of presence in the virtual environment. The sound files embedded in the software provide vibrations, via a bass-shaker platform that the user sits or stands upon, that are consis-

tent with relevant visual and audio stimuli in the scenario. For example, gunfire and explosions can be accompanied by this sensation and the vibration can be varied as when a virtual vehicle moves across uneven terrain.

These features are delivered through a "Wizard of Oz" type clinical interface that provides the clinician with a tool for selecting and placing the patient in VR scenarios that are customized to approximate the traumatic content that is clinically relevant for graduated exposure. Patients are exposed to specific scenario settings based on an assessment of which environments most closely match the patient's needs, relevant to their individual combat-related experiences. Once the scenario is selected, different user perspectives and navigation options allow the clinician to further customize the interaction. The clinical interface allows the therapist the capacity to administer relevant stimuli to modulate patient anxiety as is required for a therapeutic exposure. As with traditional imaginal exposure therapy, sound clinical judgment is required to determine how much and what type of exposure is needed to produce a therapeutic effect.

Initial analyses of results from the first 20 Virtual Iraq treatment completers in an open clinical trial at an active duty military base have produced clinically meaningful and statistically significant outcomes with the use of VRE on standard PTSD and related anxiety assessment measures. Sixteen of the 20 completers no longer met DSM criteria for PTSD at post-treatment on a self-report measure of PTSD.[29] Another ongoing study being conducted by Rothbaum *et al.* is combining a cognitive enhancing medication (D-cycloserine) with VRE for Iraq Veterans with PTSD. Treatment involves six sessions, five of which incorporate VRE, preceded by taking one pill of 50 mg D-cycloserine (an NMDA partial agonist that had been shown to facilitate extinction training with animals), placebo pill, or alprazolam (Xanax). Assessments include interviews, self-report measures, and a psychophysiological evaluation that includes startle assessment during blue screen ("baseline") and during three 2-min clips of the Virtual Iraq (humvee turret view, humvee in a convoy, foot patrol in a city). A case study of the first pilot patient treated with the Virtual Iraq indicated a 56% decrease in CAPS scores.[24]

Advantages and disadvantages of VRE

VR is employed at the point in therapy when exposure therapy would normally be introduced and has several advantages over other exposure approaches. First, VR introduces a shared experience between the therapist and participant that is practically impossible without VR. For example, it is impossible to bring clinicians on the battlefield with combat PTSD patients and it is currently impossible to share all PTSD patients' imagined scenes. Second, VR extends the range of options available to a clinician by allowing the opportunity for exposures to situations that are difficult or costly or time-consuming in real life. For instance, using the Virtual Airplane, the therapist can expose the patient to the airport and spend time on a virtual airplane taking off, flying in smooth and turbulent weather, and landing, repeatedly, without leaving the office, all within the typical therapy hour. Third, in VR, the therapist can titrate the situation to create the perfect exposure for the patient, for example, guaranteeing no turbulence until the patient is ready to confront turbulence therapeutically. Fourth, VRE augments the patient's imaginative capacities with visual, auditory, olfactory, and even haptic computer-generated

experiences. In this way, VR provides a sensory rich and evocative therapeutic environment that may be particularly helpful for patients who are reluctant to recall feared memories, have difficulty emotionally engaging in the traumatic memory, or are not very good at imagining situations.

VRE may have special appeal for members of the digital generation who may not otherwise participate in therapy. Wilson, Onorati, Mishkind, Reger, and Gahm recently found that one in five military personnel who reported not being interested in therapy would consider VRE.[30] This suggests that VRE may provide a means of reaching 20% of this particular population who may not otherwise seek or participate in treatment. The ability to repeat needed exposures, opportunities to monitor patients' responses in multiple domains, and less exposure of the patient to possible harm or embarrassment are other clinical benefits of using VR for exposure therapy.

Another advantage of VR is the control it offers can add methodological rigor to clinical studies. In VR, one can exactly control the dose of exposure to a specific stimulus and guarantee that each participant receives the exact same exposure to the exact same stimulus. This was a distinct advantage in translational research of the first clinical test of a treatment for a specific phobia in humans that combined D-cycloserine with exposure therapy. Participants underwent two VRE therapy sessions (suboptimal exposure) using a virtual elevator and were instructed to take a single pill before the therapy session, for a total of two pills during the course of the study. Participants who received D-cycloserine in conjunction with VRE had significantly less fear within the virtual environment, reported significantly more improvement in their overall acrophobic symptoms at the 3-month follow-up, and displayed significantly more improvements in psychophysiological measures of anxiety than the placebo group.[31]

There are limitations to VRE as well. First, virtual environments are costly to develop, and the required hardware is more expensive than treatment in an office without VR. Second, as with any form of technology, there can be malfunctions in the software or hardware that interrupt session flow. Clinicians using VR require extra training in using the VR equipment and program and must be able to use it seamlessly with patients. Third, VR patients can sometimes get distracted by the technology ("this isn't real") when it does not exactly simulate their experience and use this discrepancy to avoid emotionally engaging in their traumatic memory. Therapists administering VRE must manage technological difficulties and avoidance while facilitating the patient's emotional processing of their traumatic memory.

An additional limitation is that sensory stimuli used in VR are restricted to those available through existing software and may omit sights, sounds, smells, and tactile sensations that are salient for a particular individual. It is important for the therapist to use VR to invoke the trauma memory in its entirety and encourage the participant to describe the traumatic memory with as much detail as possible. For these reasons, it is important to only use VR applications where they afford some advantages and not just because they are sensational or available.

Disclosure

Dr. Rothbaum is a consultant to, and owns equity in, Virtually Better Inc., which is developing products related to the VR research described in this paper. The terms of this arrangement have been reviewed and approved by Emory University in accordance with its conflict of interest policies.

References

1. American Psychiatric Association. 1994. Diagnostic and statistical manual for mental disorders version four (DSM-IV). Washington, DC.
2. Hoge, C.W., C.A. Castro, S.C. Messer, *et al.* 2004. Combat duty in Iraq and Afghanistan, mental health problems, and barriers to care. *N. Engl. J. Med.* **351:** 1798–1800.
3. Blimes, L. 2007. Soldiers returning from Iraq and Afghanistan: the long-term costs of providing Veterans medical care and disability benefits. John F. Kennedy School of Government Faculty Research Working Paper Series, No. RWP07–001.
4. Breslau, N., G.C. Davis, P. Andreski & E. Peterson. 1991. Traumatic events and posttraumatic stress disorder in an urban population of young adults. *Arch. Gen. Psychiatry* **48:** 216–222.
5. Rothbaum, B.O., E.B. Foa, D. Riggs, *et al.* 1992. A prospective examination of post-traumatic stress disorder in rape victims. *J. Trauma. Stress* **5:** 455–475.
6. Rothbaum, B.O. & M. Davis. 2003. Applying learning principles to the treatment of post-trauma reactions. *Ann. N.Y. Acad. Sci.* **1008:** 112–121.
7. Bisson, J. & M. Andrew. 2007. Psychological treatment of posttraumatic stress disorder (PTSD). *Cochrane Database Syst. Rev.* **3:** CD00338.
8. Institute of Medicine. 2008. *Treatment of Posttraumatic Stress Disorder: An Assessment of the Evidence.* National Academies Press. Washington, DC.
9. Rothbaum, B.O., E.A. Meadows, P. Resick & D.W. Foy. 2000. Cognitive behavioral therapy. In *Effective Treatments for PTSD: Practice Guidelines from the International Society for Traumatic Stress Studies.* E.B. Foa, T.M. Keane & M.J. Friedman, Eds.: 60–83. Guilford Press. New York.
10. Foa, E. & B. Rothbaum. 1998. *Treating the Trauma of Rape: Cognitive-Behavioral Therapy for PTSD.* Guilford Press. New York, N.Y.
11. Foa, E.B., E.A. Hembree & B.O. Rothbaum. 2007. *Prolonged Exposure Therapy for PTSD: Emotional Processing of Traumatic Experiences, Therapist Guide.* Oxford University Press. New York.
12. Foa, E.B. & M.J. Kozak. 1986. Emotional processing of fear: exposure to corrective information. *Psychol. Bull.* **99:** 20–35.
13. Foa, E.B., G. Steketee & B.O. Rothbaum. 1989. Behavioral/cognitive conceptualizations of post-traumatic stress disorder. *Behav. Ther.* **20:** 155–176.
14. Rothbaum, B.O., L.F. Hodges, R. Kooper, *et al.* 1995. Effectiveness of computer-generated (virtual reality) graded exposure in the treatment of acrophobia. *Am. J. Psychiatry* **152:** 626–628.
15. Powers, M.B. & P.M. Emmelkamp. 2008. Virtual reality exposure therapy for anxiety disorders: a meta-analysis. *J. Anxiety Disord.* **22:** 561–569.
16. Parsons, T.D. & A.A. Rizzo. 2008. Affective outcomes of virtual reality exposure therapy for anxiety and specific phobias: a meta-analysis. *J. Behav. Ther. Exp. Psychiatry* **39:** 250–261.
17. Rothbaum, B.O., L. Hodges, R. Alarcon, *et al.* 1999. Virtual reality exposure therapy for PTSD Vietnam Veterans: a case study. *J. Trauma. Stress* **12:** 263–271.
18. Rothbaum, B.O., L. Hodges, D. Ready, *et al.* 2001. Virtual reality exposure therapy for Vietnam Veterans with posttraumatic stress disorder. *J. Clin. Psychiatry* **62:** 617–622.
19. Difede, J. & H. Hoffman. 2002. Virtual reality exposure therapy for World Trade Center posttraumatic stress disorder. *Cyberpsychology Behav.* **5:** 529–535.
20. Difede, J., J. Cukor, I. Patt, *et al.* 2006. The application of virtual reality to the treatment of PTSD following the WTC attack. *Ann. N.Y. Acad. Sci.* **1071:** 500–501.
21. Difede, J., J. Cukor, N. Jayasinghe, *et al.* 2007. Virtual reality exposure therapy for the treatment of posttraumatic stress disorder following September 11, 2001. *J. Clin. Psychiatry* **68:** 1639–1647.
22. Gamito, P., C. Ribeiro, L. Gamito, *et al.* 2005. Virtual war PTSD: a methodological thread. Paper presented at the 10th Annual Cybertherapy Conference, Basel Switzerland.
23. Josman, N., E. Somer, A. Reisberg, *et al.* 2006. BusWorld: designing a virtual environment for post-traumatic stress disorder in Israel: a protocol. *CyberPsychol. Behav.* **9:** 241–244.
24. Rizzo, A.A., G. Reger, G. Gahm, *et al.* 2009. Virtual reality exposure therapy for combat related PTSD. In *Post-Traumatic Stress Disorder: Basic Science and Clinical Practice.* P. Shiromani, T. Keane & J. LeDoux, Eds.: 375–399. Humana Press. New York.

25. Gerardi, M., B.O. Rothbaum, K. Ressler, *et al.* 2008. Virtual reality exposure therapy using a virtual Iraq: case report. *J. Trauma. Stress* **21:** 209–213.

26. Difede, J., J. Cukor & K. Wyka. 2009. The use of virtual reality technology in the treatment of PTSD in at-risk occupations. In Reger G (Chair) Virtual Reality Exposure Therapy for PTSD. Symposium at the International Society for Traumatic Stress Studies 25th Silver Anniversary Annual Meeting, Atlanta, GA, November 6.

27. Roy, M.J., J. Francis, J. Friedlander, *et al.* 2010. Improvement in cerebral function with treatment of posttraumatic stress disorder. *Ann. N.Y. Acad. Aci.* **1208:** 142–149.

28. Reger, G.M. & G.A. Gahm. 2008. Virtual reality exposure therapy for active duty soldiers. *J. Clin. Psychol.* **64:** 940–946.

29. Rizzo, A.A., G. Reger, J. Difede, *et al.* 2009. Development and clinical results from the virtual Iraq exposure therapy application for PTSD. IEEE Explore: Virtual Rehabilitation 2009.

30. Wilson, J.A.B., K. Onorati, M. Mishkind, *et al.* 2008. Soldier attitudes about technology-based approaches to mental healthcare. *Cyberpsychol. Behav.* **11:** 767–769.

31. Ressler, K., B.O. Rothbaum, L. Tannenbaum, *et al.* 2004. Cognitive enhancers as adjuncts to psychotherapy: use of d-cycloserine in phobic individuals to facilitate extinction to fear. *Arch. Gen. Psychiatry* **61:** 1136–1144.

Ann. N.Y. Acad. Sci. ISSN 0077-8923

ANNALS OF THE NEW YORK ACADEMY OF SCIENCES

Issue: *Psychiatric and Neurologic Aspects of War*

House calls revisited: leveraging technology to overcome obstacles to veteran psychiatric care and improve treatment outcomes

Megan Olden,[1] Judith Cukor,[1] Albert "Skip" Rizzo,[2] Barbara Rothbaum,[3] and JoAnn Difede[1]

[1]Department of Psychiatry, Weill Cornell Medical College of Cornell University, New York, New York. [2]Institute for Creative Technologies, Department of Psychiatry and School of Gerontology, University of Southern California, Playa Vista, California. [3]Department of Psychiatry and Behavioral Science, Emory University, Atlanta, Georgia

Address for correspondence: Megan Olden, Ph.D., Weill Cornell Medical College of Cornell University, 525 East 68th Street, Box 200, New York, New York 10065. meo9011@med.cornell.edu

Despite an increasing number of military service members in need of mental health treatment following deployment to Iraq and Afghanistan, numerous psychological and practical barriers limit access to care. Perceived stigma about admitting psychological difficulties as well as frequent long distances to treatment facilities reduce many veterans' willingness and ability to receive care. Telemedicine and virtual human technologies offer a unique potential to expand services to those in greatest need. Telemedicine-based treatment has been used to address multiple psychiatric disorders, including posttraumatic stress disorder, depression, and substance use, as well as to provide suicide risk assessment and intervention. Clinician education and training has also been enhanced and expanded through the use of distance technologies, with trainees practicing clinical skills with virtual patients and supervisors connecting with clinicians via videoconferencing. The use of these innovative and creative vehicles offers a significant and as yet unfulfilled promise to expand delivery of high-quality psychological therapies, regardless of clinician and patient location.

Keywords: telemedicine; virtual reality; videoconferencing; OIF/OEF veterans; barriers to care

Introduction

In this age of Facebook, MySpace, YouTube, and Twitter, computers are accessed and used at increasingly frequent rates. Technological advances have opened new vistas of possibility. Special issues of psychology and psychiatry journals have been devoted to the incorporation of technology into clinical practice, cautioning that in an ever-changing world, the field can not stand still.[1] Virtual reality (VR), telemedicine, and virtual humans (VHs) may offer the opportunity to address the many barriers to mental health treatment for U.S. service personnel. As strides are made to enhance current clinical practice, new hope may be offered to those with combat-related psychiatric problems.

Barriers to care

Despite high rates of reported distress, soldiers struggling with psychological problems demonstrate a reluctance to seek care. One large-scale study examining mental health engagement in 2,530 Marines and Army personnel found that only 23–40% of soldiers who screened positive for a mental disorder following deployment to Iraq or Afghanistan sought mental health care.[2] Those who screened positive for mental disorders were also much more likely to endorse fears of stigma and other barriers to care.

Barriers to care can be both practical and emotional. Studies point to distance from Veterans Affairs (VA) facilities and lower priority status after returning from combat as likely deterrents to treatment for returning soldiers.[3] In addition, some younger soldiers have reported discomfort with VA hospitals and a tendency to associate those facilities with treatment of older and chronically ill patients.[4] Skepticism and cynicism about the potential benefits of treatment and side effects of medications are common among service members,[4] adding another barrier to care.

doi: 10.1111/j.1749-6632.2010.05756.x

Perceived stigma about admitting psychological difficulties also inhibits treatment seeking in U.S. service members needing mental health care. Soldiers who anticipate a negative societal reaction to revelations of emotional distress may be reluctant to disclose these problems, even to a mental health professional. Similarly, individuals who view themselves as responsible for their disorders or perceive their distress as an indication of weakness may also be reluctant to seek care.[5]

Military culture has been implicated in reinforcing the idea that soldiers should persist in spite of ailments or injuries, which may fuel soldiers' hesitance to admit psychological difficulties to peers or, at times, even to themselves.[6] This ethos of pride in inner strength appears to persist across ranks. One study examined U.S. Armed Forces commanders' attitudes toward stress-related problems and found that although commanders accepted the existence of mental health issues, they were reluctant to disclose their own stress-related problems or seek help out of concern for negative professional or personal consequences, such as fears that they might be considered weak or be overlooked for promotions.[7] These concerns mirror those reported by soldiers across ranks who also report fears of negative perceptions by leaders and fellow unit members, fears of being considered weak,[8,9] concerns that seeking mental health treatment will harm their careers,[9] and fears of stigma in general[10] as key deterrents to seeking care.

Research also indicates that it may be soldiers most in need of treatment who fear reprisals the most. In a study of Operation Iraqi Freedom/Operation Enduring Freedom (OIF/OEF) veterans, those who meet screening criteria for a psychiatric disorder were more likely than those who did not to endorse fears of increased stigma and other barriers to care.[11] This study additionally found that lower sense of unit support and negative beliefs about the usefulness of psychotherapy were also associated with lowered rates of seeking psychological treatment and medication services.

Telemedicine

Videoconferencing offers one avenue to address the challenges of perceived stigma and limited accessibility. Soldiers can seek care from the safety and comfort of their homes or communities, with a sense of increased confidentiality and privacy than

they might experience having to seek care in person. In addition, because state-of-the-art psychological treatments are often unavailable to those living in rural areas, where there may be a lack of access to specialized care, the use of telemedicine can allow soldiers to seek care regardless of the remoteness of their geographic location. Given the multiple barriers to care and significant stigma associated with seeking treatment, psychotherapy utilizing a videoconferencing format offers a promising and novel option to increase access to, and potentially acceptability of, care. This paper will discuss videoconferencing-based interventions for posttraumatic stress disorder (PTSD) as well as for other clinical areas relevant to veteran populations.

Posttraumatic stress disorder

Treatment efficacy research in PTSD has proliferated in the past decade, with numerous treatment approaches proposed, implemented, and analyzed. Exposure-based treatments, including prolonged exposure, cognitive processing therapy, and eye movement desensitization and reprocessing, have yielded especially promising results and are considered the first line of treatment for PTSD.[12,13] Yet, despite significant advances, treatment failures persist.[14] More compelling, treatment is not being accessed by those with symptoms of PTSD, a problem especially prominent in the veteran population.[2] Even when it is sought out, providers are often hesitant to employ exposure-based therapies.[15,16]

Preliminary research has been conducted in investigating the treatment of individuals with PTSD using videoconferencing modalities. Although only a few studies have investigated the feasibility and efficacy of conducting individual therapy with veterans with PTSD using telemedicine, this area is growing quickly. Tuerk *et al.* demonstrated the acceptability, feasibility, and safety of providing prolonged exposure therapy via videoconferencing in a pilot study of 12 veterans diagnosed with combat-related PTSD.[17] The authors encountered few technical problems throughout the treatment and patients demonstrated a large reduction in PTSD symptoms across a 10-session treatment. There were no emergencies requiring on-site staff to be contacted to ensure patient safety, and treatment completion rate was 75%, which was slightly lower than the completion rate of a comparison sample of veterans treated face-to-face (83%). In another study,

Shore and Manson describe their group's successful use of telepsychiatry to treat PTSD in Northern Plains American Indian Veterans in 50 clinic sessions over the course of 7 months, including individual, group, and medication management visits.[18]

Germain *et al.*[19] investigated treatment efficacy in 32 individuals with mixed traumas receiving cognitive behavioral therapy (CBT) in-person and 16 receiving treatment via videoconferencing. They found no differences in treatment effectiveness and significant symptom improvement in both groups after 16–25 weeks of treatment, providing preliminary support for the use of videoconferencing in PTSD treatment.

Investigators have also begun to investigate the feasibility and effectiveness of remote group treatments for combat veterans suffering from PTSD. Several studies demonstrate that videoconferenced group interventions are comparable to in-person group formats and are feasible to conduct.[20–23] A study of CBT treatment for combat-related PTSD randomized 17 patients into videoconferencing groups and 21 into in-person group treatment.[22] Each group received 14 weeks of social skills training and activities to increase social participation. No group differences were found on clinical outcomes at the end of treatment or at 3 months after treatment. Treatment satisfaction, dropout, and attendance did not differ between the two groups, although the in-person patients demonstrated better treatment adherence (e.g., higher rates of homework completion). Another randomized trial examining a 12-session manualized group therapy for treatment of anger symptoms for combat veterans with PTSD found that patients in the in-person ($n = 64$) and videoconferencing ($n = 61$) group treatments had equally significant reductions in anger symptoms, regardless of treatment modality.[23] Patients also demonstrated similar rates of attrition, adherence (e.g., homework completion), satisfaction with services, and treatment expectancy, although patients in the in-person modality reported higher levels of group therapy alliance.

Depression

A more extensive literature exists on assessment and treatment of depression. Studies have generally found videoconference-based assessment of depression to be acceptable and beneficial to patients. A randomized controlled equivalence trial of 495 pa-

tients with a range of diagnoses (296 diagnosed with depression) assigned patients to a videoconferencing or face-to-face psychiatric consultation and up to four monthly follow-up appointments.[24] Both groups showed equivalent clinical outcomes and levels of satisfaction. Another study explored the use of telemedicine-based interviews and assessments to diagnose and follow 45 primary care patients with symptoms of depression, panic, or generalized anxiety disorder.[25] Although study conclusions were limited due to the lack of a control group, patients demonstrated clinical improvement across diagnoses and reported satisfaction with the intervention. A study of the use of videoconference-based intake interviews of depressed veterans ($n = 31$) reported a high degree of satisfaction with the telemedicine modality and a willingness to recommend this method of treatment to others.[26]

Treatment of depression has also been widely investigated. A small study of veterans with cancer ($n = 25$) investigated telemedicine-based CBT treatment for anxiety and depression,[27] finding evidence for the acceptability and practicality of receiving services remotely. Ruskin *et al.* conducted a randomized controlled trial of 119 depressed veterans assigned to in-person or videoconference treatment.[28] The authors found no differences between groups in patients' depression levels, session attendance, or medication compliance. Dropout rates were also comparable between the two groups. Fortney *et al.* published a larger-scale randomized controlled trial of 395 veterans with depression assigned to either usual care or a stepped intervention with access to various off-site providers, including a depression nurse manager, pharmacologists, and a psychiatrist.[29] Intervention patients demonstrated greater adherence to treatment and medications at 6–12 months and larger gains in mental health status and health-related quality of life. One systematic review has been conducted on the use of videoconferencing and Internet-augmented interventions for depression.[30] This review identified 10 randomized controlled trials. Four of the nine studies that examined symptom reduction demonstrated greater improvements in patients receiving care via telemedicine, with the remaining five studies showing no significant differences between the study conditions. Only four studies examined treatment adherence, and of these, no significant differences were found between the telemedicine and control groups. All five studies that examined patient satisfaction reported equal satisfaction between the two conditions. Owing to limitations in the quality of studies, including issues with follow-up, definitions of control groups, and heterogeneity of patient populations and treatment interventions, the authors concluded that at this time, there is insufficient evidence to demonstrate the efficacy of telemedicine-based treatment for depression.

Suicide prevention

Recent epidemiological research has documented that veterans are twice as likely to die by suicide compared with nonveterans,[31] heightening interest in the use of telemedicine to increase access to suicide risk assessments. Researchers have begun to address the legal issues, licensing requirements, and best practices for remote suicide risk assessment.[32,33] The use of telemedicine to assess suicidal individuals has been documented in the literature.[34] In the single existing investigation, 71 patients living in Northern Canada were referred for suicide risk assessment with a psychiatrist, nurse, or mental health counselor via videoconference. Although no comparison group was included, patients and providers reported satisfaction with services, and the study demonstrated success in terms of cost-effectiveness.

Substance abuse

Substance abuse and dependence frequently co-occur in veterans and service members suffering from PTSD. Very few studies have examined the application of telemedicine to treat these disorders, but existing studies are encouraging. One study of intensified treatment for 37 patients on methadone maintenance who tested positive for an illicit substance found that patients randomized to counseling delivered via videoconferencing responded equally well to those receiving in-office group treatment, with 70% of videoconferencing patients achieving a minimum of 2 weeks of abstinence versus 71% of patients in the in-person treatment.[35] Treatment satisfaction was high and comparable across both groups. One case report also described the feasibility and effectiveness of exposure therapy delivered via videoconferencing to treat pathological gambling.[36]

Child and family therapy

The application of telemedicine may also be considered in the treatment of children of service members. Case studies, service descriptions, and nonrandomized trials of videoconferencing with children demonstrate feasibility in numerous areas including psychiatric consultation and management services,[37] diagnostic assessment,[38] behavioral assessment,[39] treatment of incarcerated youth,[40] American–Indian youth,[41] treatments for sleep difficulties,[42] and treatment of children with tics.[43] One randomized trial compared a manualized CBT intervention for children with depression delivered face-to-face to the same protocol delivered via televideo. Results showed similar rates of satisfaction and dropout between the two groups, demonstrating acceptability in the population.[44] Outcomes were also comparable, with 13 of 14 patients in the televideo group and 10 of 14 patients in the face-to-face group no longer meeting criteria for major depression at the end of the eight-session protocol.

A limited number of investigations have also demonstrated the feasibility of conducting family-based interventions using telemedicine. A study examining a family intervention for epileptic rural teenagers with social difficulties found no differences in outcomes between videoconferencing, telephone, and face-to-face groups.[45] Family interventions have also been conducted via videoconferencing for children and adolescents with traumatic brain injury.[46–48]

Caretaker interventions

Preliminary studies have evaluated a number of delivery mechanisms for the treatment and support of caregivers of individuals with a variety of diagnoses. Steffen compared the use of a video and telephone intervention ($n = 12$) to a face-to-face intervention ($n = 9$) and waitlist control ($n = 12$) for caregivers of patients with dementia.[49] Individuals in both treatment groups reported equally significant improvement in depressive affect, hostility, and confidence in their abilities to cope with the challenges of caregiving. Feasibility of a web-based videoconferencing training for caregivers of patients with mild-to-severe traumatic brain injury ($n = 15$) has also been demonstrated, with participants rating overall satisfaction and comfort with the videoconference-based training.[50] A small study also has explored the feasibility of offering a videoconferencing-based group program, consisting of psychoeducation and exercise self-management for patients and their caregivers.[51] In this study, five participants and their caregivers connected from two locations via video-conference and were compared to seven participants and their families who met in a live group format. Although attendance rates were slightly lower for the videoconference group as compared to the in-person group (70.4% versus 89.8%, respectively), all patients reported increased social support, improved ability to cope, and decreased loneliness.

Videoconferencing treatment and psychoeducational programs have also been piloted with support persons of individuals with schizophrenia[52] and parents of children with traumatic brain injury.[53] A home telehealth program was utilized to assess the needs of veterans who had a stroke and of their caregivers.[54] One randomized trial addressed needs of caregivers of spinal cord injury patients either through a monthly problem-solving intervention delivered via videoconferencing or via an education-only control group.[55] Despite high dropout rates, intent-to-treat analyses showed evidence for the efficacy of the problem-solving intervention delivered via videoconference on both the reduction of symptoms of depression and an increase in social activities.

Potential challenges in the use of telemedicine

Although telemedicine-delivered treatments have been used across multiple populations and disorders, the total number of studies thus far is relatively small. Despite the potential promise of telemedicine, many mental health professionals remain reluctant to use it as a tool for treatment. In a study of psychologists' attitudes toward using videoconferencing technology, psychologists reported the belief that therapy conducted via videoconferencing would be less effective than face-to-face therapy.[56] One study attempted to examine psychologists' perceptions of therapeutic alliance in psychotherapy conducted face-to-face versus via videoconferencing and found that in scripted, identical psychotherapy sessions (conducted by a psychologist with an actor), psychologists rated therapeutic alliance as higher in the face-to-face sessions as compared to videoconferenced sessions.[57] The authors concluded that psychologists tended to have negative beliefs regarding the use of videoconferencing for psychotherapy.

Psychologists also expressed concerns that crisis situations or complex patient presentations (e.g., suicidality, personality disorders, or psychosis) would be less manageable using telemedicine than in a face-to-face situation. Others have pointed out that in reality, as long as basic safety parameters are in place (e.g., an emergency plan), treatment delivered via telemedicine is not substantially different than in-room-delivered treatment. The therapist is present with a patient only for 1% of the time, whereas the patient is away from the therapist for the remaining 99% of the time, making risk substantially similar. In fact, patients are managed from a distance all but the single hour per week they appear in a psychologist's office.

Therapist adherence with telemedicine applications

Therapist adherence in providing CBT for PTSD either in-room or using videoconferencing technologies has also been examined.[58] Domains of therapist competence and adherence were found to be equal between videoconferencing and face-to-face group CBT sessions with combat veterans, including therapists' ability to structure sessions, implement session activities, provide feedback, deal with difficulties, develop rapport, and convey empathy.

Barriers to telemedicine training and implementation

One barrier to effective care is the paucity of specialists available to treat patients with PTSD. This appreciable shortage has led some researchers to issue a call to action[59] to draw attention to this nation-wide problem and propose solutions to increasing availability of high-quality trauma training. Limited availability of trained clinicians in many parts of the country has been cited as a significant obstacle to OIF/OEF veterans and their families receiving needed care.[60]

A survey of 217 licensed psychologists found that only 17% reported using exposure therapy to treat PTSD,[16] despite numerous reports naming it as the first-line treatment for this disorder.[12,13] The foremost reason cited for not using exposure was inadequate training. However, even among those who have been trained in exposure therapy, one-third (38–46%) were not utilizing it with patients, citing a reluctance to use manualized treatments and a concern that patients would decompensate during exposure, despite evidence to the contrary. Similar findings were reported among a group of psychologists trained to use prolonged exposure in the aftermath of the 9/11 attacks.[15]

An emphasis on training for providers is crucial. Moreover, a model has been proposed[15] and implemented[61] whereby the trainers provide ongoing supervision for the providers during the initial period of implementation of the techniques. Here, too, cutting-edge technology offers the means to enhance the acquisition of these goals, through enhanced training opportunities and means for more direct consultation.

Other technological applications

Virtual patients for training

The first clinical use of artificially intelligent virtual humans (VHs) dates back to 1966 when Joe Weizenbaum created a program (ELIZA) designed to emulate a Rogerian therapist. More current VH agents are designed to interact in a three-dimensional environment with real users and other VHs through face-to-face spoken dialogue and even emotional reactions. Recent technological advances have resulted in the ability to create VH agents that can engage in meaningful conversations, recognize nonverbal cues, and reason about social and emotional factors.[62]

The potential for applications to medical and psychological education is vast. Training in patient assessment, diagnosis, treatment, and general interaction typically relies upon classroom lectures, observation, and role-playing. Virtual patients can offer a means to rehearse clinician–patient interactions. The development of one virtual reality (VR) system for psychotherapy training is described in the literature whereby a virtual patient displays a predetermined problem and type of coping style.[63] External cueing is needed by an outside observer to determine how the patient responds at times in the interaction, but on a limited basis. Rizzo *et al.* developed a VH named "Justin," designed to simulate a teenage boy with conduct disorder.[62] Justin responds to questions voiced by the user, thereby enabling clinicians to practice designing interview questions to identify the diagnosis of the patient. They next created a female sexual assault victim named "Justina," a VH designed to train the interviewer in gleaning diagnostic information related to sensitive topics. In the initial trial, Justina was provided with 116 responses, which could serve as answers to 459 questions. The computer recognizes key words in the users' questions and the character responds accordingly. Her responses are accompanied by nonverbal cues, such as discomfort, indicated by a lowered head or halting response. This can teach new doctors to recognize the sensitivity of the material elicited when a patient who has been sexually assaulted is asked to recount her trauma, and to be conscious of the phrasing and tone of their questions. The initial trial also focused on how well users elicited answers regarding the major clusters of PTSD symptoms, teaching trainees to focus on diagnostic symptoms as described in the Diagnostic and Statistical Manual of Mental Disorders.[62]

Ongoing projects continue to expand the applications of VHs for the use of training in psychology. VHs with suicidal ideation are being designed to train users in identifying individuals at risk for suicidality. Military versions of these VHs are being created to address the growing problem of sexual assault in the military. Treatment applications are also in development whereby military patients are seen within environments designed for the administration of imaginal exposure or VR-enhanced exposure. The clinician is able to practice the skills necessary to help the patient engage in the exposure and to simultaneously utilize the VR setup. This enables the clinician to become accustomed to the basic principles of exposure and their implementation, and to practice the juggling of the clinical and technological pieces necessary for VR exposure, before utilizing the technique with patients.[62] This may address the hesitancy of some newly trained clinicians who cite unfamiliarity with the techniques and the technology as barriers to employing these evidence-based treatments.

Feedback and supervision

Technological advances can also facilitate the ability for newly trained clinicians to get feedback and supervision from experienced specialists in the field. BI Capture is one such program that allows the clinician to record an event in the session with just a click of a remote. Digital buffering allows the visual and auditory recording of 15 min prior to the time the system is activated. Clinicians can annotate events that are recorded on their computers and then send them to specialists for feedback. This tool is ideal for a newly trained clinician conducting an imaginal exposure exercise who finds the patient suddenly distraught. Activating the system allows the recording of the events leading up to the distress and going forward. The clinician may add specific notes to the tape and send it to an expert in exposure who can offer direct feedback on the implementation of the technique. This technology may facilitate the process of supervision and feedback for training clinicians, and may promote the use of exposure-based therapies.

Discussion

Technological innovations in psychiatry, such as telemedicine, VR, and VHs, have enormous potential as tools to address logistical, as well as psychological, barriers to psychiatric care, from the treatment of patients to the education of providers. Given the multitude of barriers to care and the pervasive stigma associated with a psychiatric diagnosis, utilizing videoconferencing offers a promising and novel option to improve access to and acceptability of care, whereas VHs offer a powerful tool both for the education of the provider as well as the treatment of patients.

However, there are numerous challenges to confront before use of telemedicine and VR technology become widespread by mental health providers. These challenges include (1) resistance to change, (2) licensing and jurisdiction issues, and (3) reimbursement by insurance plans. Perhaps the most formidable challenge is overcoming the psychological barriers to the use of VR and distance technology among providers. Advances in the use of telemedicine equipment as a tool to deliver treatment has met with resistance by providers. Several studies cited above note the reluctance to using evidence-based treatments and telemedicine based on myths and fear—not on any hard evidence pointing to their detrimental nature. Additionally, licensing of health care providers currently is a state-based function. Education of our state and federal legislators about the use of telemedicine by our professional guilds is a crucial next step in solving jurisdictional issues, so that the needs of patients in remote areas can be met. Finally, ensuring that services provided via telemedicine are reimbursed by all insurance plans is crucial; it will likely require legislative intervention as well.

The legal and policy issues concerning licensing jurisdiction and reimbursement are certainly significant, but solvable, issues. The most daunting challenge to creating the momentum for change will be in motivating providers to examine their prejudices regarding the use of technology in psychiatric care.

Conflicts of interest

The authors declare no conflicts of interest.

References

1. Caspar, F. 2004. Technological developments and applications in clinical psychology and psychotherapy: introduction. *J. Clin. Psychol.* **60:** 221–238.
2. Hoge, C.W. *et al.* 2004. Combat duty in Iraq and Afghanistan, mental health problems, and barriers to care. *N. Engl. J. Med.* **351:** 13–22.
3. Druss, B.G. & R.A. Rosenheck. 1997. Use of medical services by veterans with mental disorders. *Psychosomatics* **38:** 451–458.
4. Burnam, M.A. *et al.* 2008. Systems of care: challenges and opportunities to improve access to high quality care. In *Invisible Wounds of War*. T. Tanielian & L.H. Jaycox, Eds.: 245–428. RAND Corporation. Santa Monica, CA.
5. Greene-Shortridge, T.M., T.W. Britt & C.A. Castro. 2007. The stigma of mental health problems in the military. *Mil. Med.* **172:** 157–161.
6. Langston, V., M. Gould & N. Greenberg. 2007. Culture: what is its effect on stress in the military? *Mil. Med.* **172:** 931–935.
7. Cawkill, P. 2004. A study into commanders' understanding of, and attitudes to, stress and stress-related problems. *J. R. Army Med. Corps* **150:** 91–96.
8. Warner, C.H., G.N. Appenzeller, K. Mullen, *et al.* 2008. Soldier attitudes toward mental health screening and seeking care upon return from combat. *Mil. Med.* **173:** 563–569.
9. Burnam, M.A., L.S. Meredith, T. Tanielian & L.H. Jaycox. 2009. Mental health care for Iraq and Afghanistan war veterans. *Health Aff. (Millwood)* **28:** 771–782.
10. Stecker, T., J.C. Fortney, F. Hamilton & I. Ajzen. 2007. An assessment of beliefs about mental health care among veterans who served in Iraq. *Psychiatr. Serv.* **58:** 1358–1361.
11. Pietrzak, R.H., D.C. Johnson, M.B. Goldstein, *et al.* 2009. Perceived stigma and barriers to mental health care utilization among OEF-OIF veterans. *Psychiatr. Serv.* **60:** 1118–1122.
12. Foa, E.B., R.T. Davidson & A. Frances. 1999. The Expert Consensus Guideline Series: treatment of posttraumatic stress disorder. *Am. J. Clin. Psychiatry* **60:** 5–76.
13. Institute of Medicine (IOM). 2008. *Treatment of Posttraumatic Stress Disorder: An Assessment of the Evidence*. The National Academies Press. Washington, DC.
14. Bradley, R., J. Greene, E. Russ, *et al.* 2005. A multidimensional meta-analysis of psychotherapy for PTSD. [Erratum appears in Am. J. Psychiatry 2005; 162:832.] *Am. J. Psychiatry* **162:** 214–227.
15. Cahill, S.P. *et al.* 2006. Dissemination of exposure therapy in the treatment of posttraumatic stress disorder. *J. Trauma. Stress* **19:** 597–610.
16. Beckert, C.B., C. Zayfert & E. Anderson. 2004. A survey of psychologists' attitudes towards and utilization of exposure therapy for PTSD. *Behav. Res. Ther.* **42:** 277–292.

17. Tuerk, P.W. *et al.* 2010. A pilot study of prolonged exposure therapy for posttraumatic stress disorder delivered via telehealth technology. *J. Trauma. Stress* **23:** 116–123.

18. Shore, J.H. & S.M. Manson. 2004. Telepsychiatric care of American Indian veterans with post-traumatic stress disorder: bridging gaps in geography, organizations, and culture. *Telemed. J. E Health* **10:** 64–69.

19. Germain, V., A. Marchand, S. Bouchard, *et al.* 2009. Effectiveness of cognitive behavioural therapy administered by videoconference for posttraumatic stress disorder. *Cogn. Behav. Ther.* **38:** 42–53.

20. Deitsch, S.E., B.C. Frueh & A.B. Santos. 2000. Telepsychiatry for post-traumatic stress disorder. *J. Telemed. Telecare* **6:** 184–186.

21. Morland, L.A., K. Pierce & M.Y. Wong. 2004. Telemedicine and coping skills groups for Pacific Island veterans with post-traumatic stress disorder: a pilot study. *J. Telemed. Telecare* **10:** 286–289.

22. Frueh, B.C. *et al.* 2007. A randomized trial of telepsychiatry for post-traumatic stress disorder. *J. Telemed. Telecare* **13:** 142–147.

23. Morland, L.A. *et al.* 2010. Telemedicine for anger management therapy in a rural population of combat veterans with posttraumatic stress disorder: a randomized noninferiority trial. *J. Clin. Psychiatry* **71:** 855–863.

24. O'Reilly, R. *et al.* 2007. Is telepsychiatry equivalent to face-to-face psychiatry? Results from a randomized controlled equivalence trial. *Psychiatr. Serv.* **58:** 836–843.

25. Williams, J.B., A. Ellis, A. Middleton & K.A. Kobak. 2007. Primary care patients in psychiatric clinical trials: a pilot study using videoconferencing. *Ann. Gen. Psychiatry* **6:** 6 pp.

26. Dobscha, S.K., K. Corson, J. Solodky & M.S. Gerrity. 2005. Use of videoconferencing for depression research: enrollment, retention, and patient satisfaction. *Telemed. J. E Health* **11:** 84–89.

27. Shepherd, L. *et al.* 2006. The utility of videoconferencing to provide innovative delivery of psychological treatment for rural cancer patients: results of a pilot study. *J. Pain Symptom Manage.* **32:** 453–461.

28. Ruskin, P.E. *et al.* 2004. Treatment outcomes in depression: comparison of remote treatment through telepsychiatry to in-person treatment. *Am. J. Psychiatry* **161:** 1471–1476.

29. Fortney, J.C. *et al.* 2007. A randomized trial of telemedicine-based collaborative care for depression. *J. Gen. Intern. Med.* **22:** 1086–1093.

30. Garcia-Lizana, F. & I. Munoz-Mayorga. 2010. Telemedicine for depression: a systematic review. *Perspect. Psychiatr. Care* **46:** 119–126.

31. Kaplan, M.S., N. Huguet, B.H. McFarland & J.T. Newsom. 2007. Suicide among male veterans: a prospective population-based study. [Erratum appears in *J. Epidemiol. Community Health* 2007; 61:751.] *J. Epidemiol. Community Health* **61:** 619–624.

32. Godleski, L., J.E. Nieves, A. Darkins & L. Lehmann. 2008. VA telemental health: suicide assessment. *Behav. Sci. Law* **26:** 271–286.

33. Shore, J.H., D.M. Hilty & P. Yellowlees. 2007. Emergency management guidelines for telepsychiatry. *Gen. Hosp. Psychiatry* **29:** 199–206.

34. Jong, M. 2004. Managing suicides via videoconferencing in a remote northern community in Canada. *Int. J. Circumpolar Health* **63:** 422–428.

35. King, V.L. *et al.* 2009. Assessing the effectiveness of an Internet-based videoconferencing platform for delivering intensified substance abuse counseling. *J. Subst. Abuse Treat.* **36:** 331–338.

36. Oakes, J., M.W. Battersby, R.G. Pols & P. Cromarty. 2008. Exposure therapy for problem gambling via videoconferencing: a case report. *J. Gambl. Stud.* **24:** 107–118.

37. Myers, K.M., J.M. Valentine & S.M. Melzer. 2008. Child and adolescent telepsychiatry: utilization and satisfaction. *Telemed. J. E Health* **14:** 131–137.

38. Yellowlees, P.M., D.M. Hilty, S.L. Marks, *et al.* 2008. A retrospective analysis of a child and adolescent eMental Health program. *J. Am. Acad. Child Adolesc. Psychiatry* **47:** 103–107.

39. Barretto, A., D.P. Wacker, J. Harding, *et al.* 2006. Using telemedicine to conduct behavioral assessments. *J. Appl. Behav. Anal.* **39:** 333–340.

40. Myers, K., J. Valentine, R. Morganthaler & S. Melzer. 2006. Telepsychiatry with incarcerated youth. *J. Adolesc. Health* **38:** 643–648.

41. Savin, D., M.T. Garry, P. Zuccaro & D. Novins. 2006. Telepsychiatry for treating rural American Indian youth. *J. Am. Acad. Child Adolesc. Psychiatry* **45:** 484–488.

42. Witmans, M.B. *et al.* 2008. Delivery of pediatric sleep services via telehealth: the Alberta experience and lessons learned. *Behav. Sleep Med.* **6:** 207–219.

43. Himle, M.B., E. Olufs, J. Himle, *et al.* 2010. Behavior therapy for tics via videoconference delivery: an initial pilot test in children. *Cogn. Behav. Pract.* **17:** 329–337.

44. Nelson, E.-L., M. Barnard & S. Cain. 2006. Feasibility of telemedicine intervention for childhood depression. *Couns. Psychother. Res.* **6:** 191–195.

45. Glueckauf, R.L. *et al.* 2002. Videoconferencing-based family counseling for rural teenagers with epilepsy: phase 1 findings. *Rehabil. Psychol.* **47:** 49–72.

46. Wade, S.L., N.C. Walz, J.C. Carey & K.M. Williams. 2008. Preliminary efficacy of a Web-based family problem-solving treatment program for adolescents with traumatic brain injury. *J. Head Trauma Rehabil.* **23:** 369–377.

47. Wade, S.L., N.C. Walz, J.C. Carey & K.M. Williams. 2009. Brief report: description of feasibility and satisfaction findings from an innovative online family problem-solving intervention for adolescents following traumatic brain injury. *J. Pediatr. Psychol.* **34:** 517–522.

48. Gilkey, S.N.L., J. Carey & S.L. Wade. 2009. Families in crisis: considerations for the use of web-based treatment models in family therapy. *Fam. Soc. J. Contemp. Soc. Serv.* **90:** 37–45.

49. Steffen, A.M. 2000. Anger management for dementia caregivers: a preliminary study using video and telephone interventions. *Behav. Ther.* **31:** 281–299.

50. Sander, A.M., A.N. Clark, T.B. Atchison & M. Rueda. 2009. A web-based videoconferencing approach to training caregivers in rural areas to compensate for problems related to traumatic brain injury. *J. Head Trauma Rehabil.* **24:** 248–261.

51. Taylor, D.M. *et al.* 2009. Exploring the feasibility of videoconference delivery of a self-management program to rural participants with stroke. *Telemed. J. E Health* **15:** 646–654.

52. Rotondi, A.J. *et al.* 2005. A clinical trial to test the feasibility of a telehealth psychoeducational intervention for persons with schizophrenia and their families: intervention and 3-month findings. *Rehabil. Psychol.* **50:** 325–336.

53. Wade, S.L., J. Carey & C.R. Wolfe. 2006. An online family intervention to reduce parental distress following pediatric brain injury. *J. Consult. Clin. Psychol.* **74:** 445–454.

54. Lutz, B.J., N.R. Chumbler, T. Lyles, *et al.* 2009. Testing a home-telehealth programme for US veterans recovering from stroke and their family caregivers. *Disabil. Rehabil.* **31:** 402–409.

55. Elliott, T.R., D. Brossart, J.W. Berry & P.R. Fine. 2008. Problem-solving training via videoconferencing for family caregivers of persons with spinal cord injuries: a randomized controlled trial. *Behav. Res. Ther.* **46:** 1220–1229.

56. Wray, B.T. & C.S. Rees. 2003. Is there a role for videoconferencing in cognitive behavioral therapy? In *Australian Association for Cognitive and Behaviour Therapy State Conference.* Perth, Western Australia, Australia.

57. Rees, C.S. & S. Stone. 2005. Therapeutic alliance in face-to-face versus videoconferenced psychotherapy. *Prof. Psychol. Res. Pract.* **36:** 649–653.

58. Frueh, B.C. *et al.* 2007. Therapist adherence and competence with manualized cognitive-behavioral therapy for PTSD delivered via videoconferencing technology. *Behav. Modif.* **31:** 856–866.

59. Courtois, C.A. & S.N. Gold. 2009. The need for inclusion of psychological trauma in the professional curriculum: a call to action. *Psychol. Trauma Theory Res. Pract. Policy* **1:** 3–23.

60. Department of Defense Task Force on Mental Health. 2007. An achievable vision: report of the Department of Defense Task Force on Mental Health June 2007. http://www.health.mil/dhb/mhtf/MHTF-Report-Final.pdf (accessed April 14, 2010).

61. Difede, J., J. Cukor, N. Jayasinghe & H. Hoffman. 2006. Developing a virtual reality treatment protocol for post-traumatic stress disorder following the World Trade Center attack. In *Novel Approaches to the Diagnosis and Treatment of PTSD.* M.J. Ray, Ed.: 219–234. IOS Press. Amsterdam, the Netherlands.

62. Rizzo, A.A., T. Parsons, J.G. Buckwalter, B. Lange & P. Kenny. 2010. A new generation of intelligent virtual patients in clinical training. *Am. Behav. Sci.* In press.

63. Beutler, L.E. & T.M. Harwood. 2004. Virtual reality in psychotherapy training. *J. Clin. Psychol.* **60:** 317–330.

Ann. N.Y. Acad. Sci. ISSN 0077-8923

ANNALS OF THE NEW YORK ACADEMY OF SCIENCES
Issue: *Psychiatric and Neurologic Aspects of War*

Improvement in cerebral function with treatment of posttraumatic stress disorder[a]

Michael J. Roy,[1] Jennifer Francis,[1] Joshua Friedlander,[1] Lisa Banks-Williams,[1] Raymond G. Lande,[1] Patricia Taylor,[1] James Blair,[2] Jennifer McLellan,[2] Wendy Law,[1] Vanita Tarpley,[1] Ivy Patt,[1] Henry Yu,[2] Alan Mallinger,[2] Joann Difede,[3] Albert Rizzo,[4] and Barbara Rothbaum[5]

[1]Uniformed Services University, Bethesda, Maryland, and Walter Reed Army Medical Center, Washington, DC. [2]National Institute of Mental Health, National Institutes of Health, Bethesda, Maryland. [3]Weill Medical College of Cornell University, New York, New York. [4]Institute for Creative Technologies, University of Southern California, Los Angeles, California. [5]Emory University School of Medicine, Atlanta, Georgia

Address for correspondence: Michael J. Roy, M.D. M.P.H., Department of Medicine, Room A3062, Uniformed Services University of the Health Sciences, 4301 Jones Bridge Road, Bethesda, Maryland 20814. mroy@usuhs.mil

Posttraumatic stress disorder (PTSD) and mild traumatic brain injury (mTBI) are signature illnesses of the Iraq and Afghanistan wars, but current diagnostic and therapeutic measures for these conditions are suboptimal. In our study, functional magnetic resonance imaging (fMRI) is used to try to differentiate military service members with: PTSD and mTBI, PTSD alone, mTBI alone, and neither PTSD nor mTBI. Those with PTSD are then randomized to virtual reality exposure therapy or imaginal exposure. fMRI is repeated after treatment and along with the Clinician-Administered PTSD Scale (CAPS) and Clinical Global Impression (CGI) scores to compare with baseline. Twenty subjects have completed baseline fMRI scans, including four controls and one mTBI only; of 15 treated for PTSD, eight completed posttreatment scans. Most subjects have been male (93%) and Caucasian (83%), with a mean age of 34. Significant improvements are evident on fMRI scans, and corroborated by CGI scores, but CAPS scores improvements are modest. In conclusion, CGI scores and fMRI scans indicate significant improvement in PTSD in both treatment arms, though CAPS score improvements are less robust.

Keywords: posttraumatic stress disorder; traumatic brain injury; combat stress; functional magnetic resonance imaging; virtual reality; exposure therapy

Introduction

Many wars are characterized by a signature illness, such as "soldier's heart" after the American Civil War, or shell shock and mustard gas injuries after World War I. Vietnam brought posttraumatic stress disorder (PTSD) to our lexicon, and Desert Storm heralded "Gulf War syndrome." War also spurs innovative responses that galvanize medical advances

that benefit humanity at large. For example, the American Revolution spawned litters for carrying wounded soldiers, Napoleon's forces assigned specific litter-bearing teams, and the American Civil War introduced horse-drawn "ambulances." The wars in Iraq and Afghanistan have been characterized by widespread use of improvised explosive devices and other unconventional warfare methods that have led to high rates of PTSD and traumatic brain injury (TBI). This provides an opportunity to improve the diagnosis and treatment of PTSD and TBI.

PTSD has been reported in 10–20% of veterans after recent wars,[1–3] but reliance on self-report, in addition to issues, such as stigma, raises concerns

---

[a]The opinions expressed herein are those of the authors and do not necessarily reflect the official policy or opinions of the Department of the Army or Department of Defense.

doi: 10.1111/j.1749-6632.2010.05689.x

of both underreporting, and overendorsement. The 17-page Clinician-Administered PTSD Scale (CAPS) is the best-validated diagnostic instrument, but requires an hour-long administration by a trained professional,[4,5] and remains dependent on the unsubstantiated report of the individual patient. Since PTSD is associated with substantially greater use of health care resources and worse physical and mental health and overall functional status,[6–9] an objective diagnostic tool, such as functional magnetic resonance imaging (fMRI), could reduce stigma, facilitate targeted treatment, and enable appropriate compensation.

Diagnosis of moderate to severe TBI, with prolonged loss of consciousness or obvious physical trauma, is straightforward, but mild TBI (mTBI) is even more difficult to accurately diagnose than PTSD. Standardized diagnostic criteria for mTBI in the absence of loss of consciousness are not universally accepted. Efforts to incorporate immediate reactions, such as a dazed or confused sensation, are both subject to recall bias and difficult to establish a threshold of significance for, since surprise and confusion are almost universal with an unanticipated explosion. Subsequent symptoms, such as memory or concentration problems, irritability, sleep difficulties, and headaches are nonspecific, and overlap features of depression and PTSD.[10] Since mTBI is so poorly defined, we use "blast exposure" as a surrogate for initially classifying study participants with mTBI, while acknowledging this term retains ambiguity.

There are several variants of fMRI; we employ the most common and best evidenced method, blood oxygen level dependent (BOLD) fMRI, which has potential to objectively measures oxygenation, a manifestation of blood flow, to specific areas of the brain. T2-weighted MRI images are sensitive to oxygenation levels, facilitating assay of changes in neuronal oxygenation induced by sensory stimuli. Patients with PTSD (including combat veterans) exposed to various stimuli have been shown to have increased activation in the amygdala and decreased activation in the anterior cingulate gyrus as compared to trauma-exposed controls.[11–13] We use the Affective Stroop test, which requires subjects to make a combination of numeric and photographic distinctions; this has proven effective in distinguishing individuals with PTSD from trauma-exposed controls,[14,15] but the potential confounding effect

of mTBI has not been assessed with this or other methods.

Improved identification of PTSD and TBI is key, but better treatment is also essential. A recent Institute of Medicine report concluded that cognitive behavioral therapy with exposure therapy is the only therapy for PTSD with sufficient evidence to recommend it.[16] Imaginal exposure is the most commonly used exposure method, but many patients find it prohibitively difficult to repeatedly recount their traumatic experience in progressively greater detail. Virtual reality (VR) is a promising alternative that may effectively engage more patients in exposure therapy. Previous studies of VR exposure therapy (VRET) for PTSD have shown some evidence of benefit, including an open trial in Vietnam veterans[17] and a waitlist-controlled study of 9/11 World Trade Center workers.[18] However, our study represents the first randomized-controlled trial comparing VRET directly with Prolonged Exposure (PE), the best-evidenced form of imaginal exposure.

Methods

Baseline assessment
After obtaining informed consent, participants complete a medical history and physical examination and these self-administered questionnaires: the Defense and Veterans Brain Injury Center Brief Questionnaire for TBI,[19] PTSD Checklist-Military Version (PCL-M), Beck Depression Inventory-II (BDI),[20–24] Beck Anxiety Inventory (BAI),[25] CAGE,[26] AUDIT-C,[27] the SF-36,[28] and WHODAS-II.[29,30] A mental health professional, blinded to the treatment assignment of the subject, then administers the CAPS[4,5] and Structured Clinical Interview for DSM-IV (SCID).[31]

Imaging phase
The first phase of the study targets four groups of 22 military service members (SMs) who have been deployed to Iraq or Afghanistan (total of 88) each:

1. blast-exposed SMs with PTSD;
2. blast-exposed SMs without PTSD;
3. SMs with PTSD but without blast exposure; and
4. SMs without PTSD or blast exposure.

fMRI is performed on all participants, using the Affective Stroop, which includes three paradigms. The first displays pictures only, with no response required. The second includes number sequences only, with the participant required to identify the greater sequence with a computer mouse. The third features both pictures and numbers and requires a response. The fMRI scan results are then compared between the four groups, as well as before and after treatment for those treated for PTSD. Analysis of covariance models are used to test main effects and interactions between presence and absence of both PTSD and blast exposure on performance scores, reaction time, and physiologic parameters (skin conductance response). The fMRI time series data is analyzed voxel-by-voxel for changes in BOLD signal in response to different components of the tasks with multiple regression using Analysis of Functional NeuroImages software.[32] Within-run linear changes and run-to-run variation in the signal mean are controlled for within the regression model. For each individual and for each of the two experimental sessions, the statistical maps for the overall regression analysis are thresholded ($Z > 4.0$), aligned, and combined to identify the significant voxels across the two sessions. The target regions-of-interest (ROIs) (amygdala, hippocampus, and anterior cingulate cortex) are defined on high resolution anatomical MRI scans for each subject. The thresholded statistical map is overlaid with the ROI map to identify the contiguous voxels showing a significant experimental effect within each ROI. From each experimental session, the BOLD response averaged over the significant voxels within each ROI is obtained. These region time series data are analyzed using multiple regression with the same statistical model used for the whole brain analysis, with Statview software. Multiple regression analyses provide estimates of the effect size for each task component. These effect estimates are compared using analysis of variance (ANOVA) models to identify significant differences in response magnitude associated with task components, drug effects and group effects.

In addition, a voxel-wise analysis explores activations outside of the ROI using SPM 99 (Statistical Parametric Mapping; http://www.fil.ion.ucl.ac.uk/spm/). For voxel-wise analyses on normalized whole brain data, we then control false positive rates per map at $\alpha = 0.05$, using random-effects models.[33–35] Hypotheses regarding task-associated changes in the BOLD signal are initially tested by analyzing task-related hemodynamic responses in the ROIs, with corrections to control for inflation of α (Type I) error.

Treatment phase

Participants with PTSD are randomized to either VRET or PE in 12 or more 90-min sessions over ≥6 weeks. PE has been described;[36] we use a study manual adapted from Foa *et al.* at the University of Pennsylvania. For VRET, the study manual was adapted from Difede's Virtual World Trade Center study, which was in turn patterned after Rothbaum's Virtual Vietnam study. The study therapists are two Ph.D. psychologists, an advanced practice research nurse with specialization in psychiatry, and an art therapist/licensed professional counselor. All received live, detailed training for PE by a Ph.D. psychologist who worked with Foa for years, and for VRET by psychologists from the Virtual Vietnam and Virtual World Trade Center studies. Both the PE and VRET arms use the first three sessions to understand the participants' histories and symptoms, and to introduce cognitive behavioral techniques including psychoeducational elements and relaxation techniques as well as some imaginal and *in vivo* exposure elements. However, those receiving VRET spend up to half of each session in the virtual environment thereafter, whereas the PE arm spends comparable time engaged in imaginal exposure. For VRET, the therapist typically starts with stimuli disparate from the trauma of that individual, and gradually progresses to stimuli more closely mimicking the trauma. For example, for an individual who was hit by a rocket-propelled grenade while riding in a HMMV, VRET might begin on foot in an urban marketplace, and once the therapist saw reductions in both self-reported discomfort and physiologic measures, such as blood pressure and heart rate, would progress to a scenario featuring incoming fire in a HMMV. The Virtual Iraq environment was developed by the Institute of Creative Technologies at the University of Southern California, and has been described.[37] The therapist employs three computers simultaneously: one displays what the participant sees, one facilitates introduction of sensory stimuli, and one monitors physiologic responses. A vibration platform provides tactile stimuli, such as the feel of an explosion or moving vehicle. A smell machine adds pertinent smells, such as chordite, Middle Eastern spices, and burning trash. The subject controls the speed and direction of the HMMV with a game-type hand controller, and uses a controller mounted on an authentic rubberized M-16 rifle replica in ambulatory environments. The 45 min of each 90 min session spent outside of the virtual environment includes both preparations for the virtual element as well as processing the content afterward.

After completion of treatment fMRI is repeated to compare with the baseline scan. Clinician-administered instruments (CAPS, SCID) are repeated at the end of treatment as well as 12 weeks later, while self-administered questionnaires (PCL-M, BDI, BAI, CAGE, AUDIT-C, SF-36, and WHODAS-II) are completed at 2-week intervals during treatment, and 4-week intervals throughout follow-up. The primary desired outcomes are a 30% reduction in the CAPS score, and a significant improvement in fMRI patterns, at the end of treatment compared with baseline. Secondary measures include a 30% reduction in the CAPS at the end of a 12-week follow-up period, as well as improvements in the PCL-M, a 17-item self-administered PTSD scale included to enable more frequent measurement of symptoms, as well as improvements in scores on the BDI, BAI, CAGE, AUDIT-C, SCID, SF-36, and WHODAS-II, to assess comorbid disorders and overall functional status. The individual therapist for each participant assigned a Clinical Global Impression (CGI) severity score (range 1–7) at the first session and again at the conclusion of treatment, along with a global improvement score (range 1–7) at the end of treatment.[38]

Inclusion and exclusion criteria

Participants must have been deployed to Iraq or Afghanistan, provide written informed consent, and be in good physical health. In addition, for specific subcategories:

1. those with PTSD must have a CAPS score ≥40;
2. blast exposure (mTBI) requires having been close enough to an explosion to have felt the impact: as little as the pressure wave, up to direct impact with bodily injury and/or transient (<2 min) loss of consciousness; and
3. non-PTSD, nonblast exposed controls must have been deployed to Iraq or Afghanistan for at least 3 months, must never have been treated for PTSD, and must have a PCL-M score less than 35. Those without blast injury must never have had a concussion or trauma-related loss

of consciousness, including in a motor vehicle accident or in sports or recreational activities.

Individuals are excluded for dementia or an inability to read or understand written and oral questions; a clinically significant or unstable medical disorder (e.g., unstable angina, uncontrolled diabetes mellitus, uncontrolled hypertension, and symptomatic liver disease); meeting DSM-IV criteria for alcohol or substance abuse or dependence within the past month; currently at high risk for homicide or suicide; or a current or past history of schizophrenia, schizoaffective disorder, or bipolar disorder. Participation in the imaging phase is also prohibited for those with residual shrapnel fragments from a blast injury, or any metallic devices within the body that would pose health risks with the use of MRI. Finally, a history of claustrophobia or inability to tolerate a prior MRI without sedation is exclusionary, as sedating medicine could interfere with fMRI interpretation.

Results

To date, a total of 45 SMs have consented to participate in the study, though 10 withdrew from the study of their own volition prior to performing the baseline fMRI scan, and six failed to meet eligibility criteria, resulting in 29 active study participants to date. This number includes 15 with both PTSD and TBI, nine with PTSD only, one with TBI only, and four controls. Of those with PTSD, eight also completed a posttreatment scan (five with both PTSD and TBI, three with PTSD only), and one is still in treatment; eight (five PTSD and TBI, three PTSD only) of those who completed the baseline scan withdrew prior to finishing treatment and therefore did not complete a second scan. Finally, another six subjects (five with PTSD and TBI, one with PTSD only) could not be scanned owing to embedded shrapnel or surgical hardware, so they were referred directly to the treatment phase and completed treatment, and another in this category is still in treatment.

Of the 29 active participants, only three have been female. Three have been African-American, two Hispanic, one Asian, and 20 Caucasian. The age range is 24–59, with a mean of 34. Table 1 compares demographic factors between those completing PE and VRET, as well as withdrawals, with controls and TBI alone also lumped together because of their small numbers.

Table 1. Demographics

Variable	Controls and TBI only	Withdrawals	PE completers	VR completers
Mean age	37.2	33.3	34.1	34.5
% Male	80	94	100	88
% Caucasian	60	76	100	63

Fifteen have completed treatment thus far, seven with VRET and eight with PE. One in the VRET arm achieved the targeted 30% decrease in CAPS score at the end of treatment, and one in the PE arm did by the end of the 12-week follow-up period. The numbers to have completed the study thus far are not sufficient to compare the efficacy of VRET versus PE, but pooled data combining both arms together is provided in Table 2. The great majority of subjects reported important behavioral changes to their study therapists, such as using the subway and attending restaurants, sporting events, and movie theaters. This is corroborated by the CGI severity scores shown in Table 2, with improvement from an average of moderately ill (4.1) to mildly ill (3.25). The CGI global improvement score is consistent with these findings as well, with a mean of 2.6 reflecting that subjects were seen as nearly evenly split between the mildly improved and much improved categories. Six participants withdrew prior to completing treatment.

Figure 1 demonstrates pooled fMRI data for the first eight study participants to complete either VRET and PE as well as pre- and posttreatment scans. The figure shows that prior to treatment there were substantial increases in oxygenation, representing increased blood flow, in the amygdala and

Table 2. Results on PTSD and depression scales (mean scores for 15 subjects completing treatment)

	PE arm		
Participant #	Pretreatment score	Posttreatment score	12-week f/u score
CAPS	81.8	74.1	69.5
PCL-M	62.7	51.2	51.4
BDI	27.2	23.7	22.3
CGI	4.1	3.25	–

the subcallosal gyrus in response to stimuli, along with a more moderate increase in the lateral prefrontal cortex and a marked decrease in the anterior cingulate cortex of the frontal lobe. Treatment of PTSD resulted in dramatic shifts in oxygenation in response to stimuli within the amygdala, subcallosal gyrus and lateral prefrontal cortex, along with lessening of the decrease that had been seen prior to treatment in the anterior cingulate cortex. Figure 2 distinguishes the relative impact of negative versus neutral stimuli on the amygdala, a distinction echoed in the inferior frontal gyrus. This figure demonstrates that before treatment, negative, but not neutral, stimuli, resulted in dramatic increases in bloodflow to the amygdala; treatment of PTSD dramatically reduced the amygdala response to negative stimuli while having relatively little impact upon the response to neutral stimuli.

Discussion

This paper provides compelling evidence of the utility of fMRI to document response to treatment in PTSD. The analysis of the fMRI data takes the entire brain into account, and employs ANOVA to assess voxel-wise repeated measures comparisons, with beta weights of 12 regressors of interest as the dependent measures; with this approach, an activation level of 0.2 in a given area of the brain represents a quite significant response to a stimulus. As shown in Figure 1, our SMs with PTSD had quite significant responses in multiple key areas of the brain; moreover, treatment was associated with marked improved these areas. The increases in bloodflow to the amygdala and lateral prefrontal cortex, as well as the decrease in bloodflow to the anterior cingulate cortex, have also been reported by other researchers studying PTSD. It has been hypothesized that the areas in which increases are seen may be associated with symptoms of hypervigilance and arousal, whereas the inhibition in the anterior cingulate

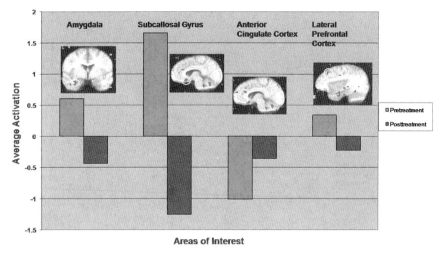

Figure 1. fMRI before versus after treatment; activation across areas of interest. (In color in *Annals* online.)

gyrus may be a manifestation of the numbing and withdrawal characteristics of PTSD. Subcallosal gyrus responses to stimulation have been previously associated with depressive symptoms, so the pattern seen for this region in Figure 1 may be a manifestation of the BDI scores we report in this population. The fact that treatment correlates with a return to normalcy in each brain area of interest is promising evidence of treatment efficacy.

The results we report here position fMRI as a particularly valuable tool, with potential as both an objective diagnostic instrument upon presentation with PTSD, and to document response to therapy. Current instruments that rely on the validity of individual recall, whether self-administered (e.g., PCL-M) or clinician-administered (e.g., CAPS), are dependent upon the memory and honesty of the respondent. Among military SMs, some may be reluctant to acknowledge symptoms they are feeling for fear that such admission might adversely affect their chances for promotion or select duty assignments. In fact, some participants who remain on active duty withdrew from the study because they found it too difficult to fully engage in exposure therapy while maintaining a busy work schedule. Conversely, others who were already far along in the disability assessment process and highly unlikely to return to active duty might, either consciously or subconsciously, decline to acknowledge improvement for fear that it would reduce their level of disability compensation. It is also important to note that most study participants have relatively high

scores on both the CAPS and PCL, and most have been on multiple psychotropic medications upon referral, though with little apparent response to the pharmacotherapeutics. The population we have identified at a tertiary medical center (Walter Reed) may represent relatively severe, treatment-resistant PTSD. Perhaps it is a manifestation of the relatively horrific or PEs that SMs are subject to, but it is plausible that this might be the result of mTBI, something that our study design should ultimately give us the ability to address.

While it is important to remember that these results are preliminary and need replication with larger numbers and other populations to try to delineate sensitivity and specificity, we believe there is reason to be optimistic about the use of fMRI in documenting both the initial diagnosis of PTSD, and evidence of response to therapy. Improvements on fMRI are consistent with improvements documented by our study therapists on the CGI. The modest improvement in PTSD symptoms documented on the CAPS and PCL-M thus far is undeniably disappointing, but it should be noted that other investigators have also reported lower response rates for combat veterans than for civilians with PTSD. Most relevant to our report is the fact that Rothbaum and Hodges *et al.* found modest efficacy with VRET for Vietnam War veterans,[17] whereas Difede *et al.* demonstrated much more robust improvements in World Trade Center workers suffering from PTSD who were treated with VRET compared to waitlist controls.[18]

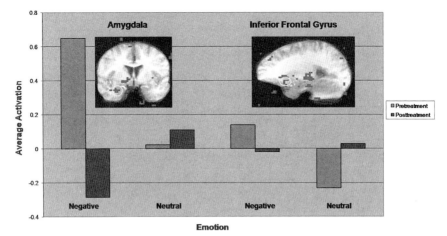

Figure 2. Amygdala activation with emotional stimuli, pre- and posttreatment. (In color in *Annals* online.)

Limitations to the results described here include that this is a preliminary report with relatively small numbers. Although the numbers are already sufficient to show the value of fMRI, they do not yet allow us to compare PTSD and TBI, or VRET and PE. To date, garnering participation of those without PTSD has been more difficult than identification of those with PTSD, likely in part because treatment of PTSD provides significant incentive for those who have it to participate, but there is not a comparable incentive for controls or those with TBI alone. The correlation of fMRI findings within particular brain regions with specific PTSD symptoms is not much more than conjecture at this point, but studies may eventually confirm such a relationship. Hopefully, we will ultimately find that fMRI can clearly discriminate between TBI, PTSD, and the combination, making it an attractive test for any with symptoms in this realm.

While the coupling of imaging and therapy together in a single study makes the design a bit more cumbersome, but we already have compelling evidence that it is worthwhile. Conduct of fMRI both before and after treatment enables us to determine what changes occur with response to therapy, which may provide a tremendously valuable method for overcoming the limitations of self-report. It is not inconceivable that fMRI may even yield patterns that enable prediction of whom is more likely to respond to one form of treatment than another. fMRI warrants significant additional study as an instrument for the diagnosis and monitoring of PTSD and related conditions.

Conflicts of interest

The authors declare no conflicts of interest.

References

1. Stein, M.B., J.R. Walker, A.L. Hazen & D.R. Forde. 1997. Full and partial posttraumatic stress disorder: findings from a community survey. *Am. J. Psychiatry* **154:** 1120–1126.
2. Roy, M.J., P.A. Koslowe, K. Kroenke & C. Magruder. 1998. Signs, symptoms, and ill-defined conditions in Persian Gulf War Veterans: findings from the comprehensive clinical evaluation program. *Psychosom. Med.* **60:** 663–668.
3. Hoge, C.W., C.A. Castro, S.C. Messer, *et al.* 2004. Combat duty in Iraq and Afghanistan, mental health problems, and barriers to care. *N. Engl. J. Med.* **351:** 13–22.
4. Blake, D.D., F.W. Weathers, L.M. Nagy, *et al.* 1995. The development of a clinician-administered PTSD scale. *J. Trauma. Stress* **8:** 75–90.
5. Weathers, F.W., T.M. Keane & J.R. Davidson. 2001. Clinician-administered PTSD scale: a review of the first ten years. *Depress. Anxiety* **13:** 132–156.
6. Ullman, S.E. & J.M. Siegel. 1996. Traumatic events and physical health in a community sample. *J. Trauma. Stress* **9:** 703–720.
7. Kessler, R.C. 2000. Posttraumatic stress disorder: the burden to the individual and to society. *J. Clin. Psychiatry* **61**(Suppl. 5): 4–14.
8. Wagner, A.W., J. Wolfe, A. Rotnitsky, *et al.* 2000. An investigation of the impact of posttraumatic stress disorder on physical health. *J. Trauma. Stress* **13:** 41–55.
9. Walker, E.A., W. Katon, J. Russo, *et al.* 2003. Health care costs associated with posttraumatic stress disorder symptoms among women. *Arch. Gen. Psychiatry* **60:** 369–374.
10. Hoge, C.W., D. McGurk, J.L. Thomas, *et al.* 2008. Mild traumatic brain injury in U.S. soldiers returning from Iraq. *N. Engl. J. Med.* **358:** 453–463.
11. Thomas, K.M., W.C. Drevets, R.E. Dahl, *et al.* 2001. Amygdala response to fearful faces in anxious and depressed children. *Arch. Gen. Psychiatry* **58:** 1057–1063.

12. Shin, L.M., P.J. Whalen, R.K. Pitman, *et al.* 2001. An fMRI study of anterior cingulate function in posttraumatic stress disorder. *Biol. Psychiatry* **50:** 932–942.

13. Shin, L.M., C.I. Wright, P.A. Cannistraro, *et al.* 2005. A functional magnetic resonance imaging study of amygdale and medial prefrontal cortex responses to overtly presented fearful faces in posttraumatic stress disorder. *Arch. Gen. Psychiatry* **62:** 273–281.

14. Blair, R.J.R., J.S. Morris, C.D. Frith, *et al.* 1999. Dissociable neural responses to facial expressions of sadness and anger. *Brain* **122:** 883–893.

15. Nakic, M., B.W. Smith, S. Busis, *et al.* 2006. The impact of affect and frequency on lexical decision: the role of the amygdala and inferior frontal cortex. *Neuroimage* **31:** 1752–1761.

16. Berg, A.O., N. Breslau, M.D. Lezak, *et al.* 2008. *Treatment of Posttraumatic Stress Disorder: An Assessment of the Evidence.* National Academies Press. Washington, DC.

17. Rothbaum, B.O., L.F. Hodges, D. Ready, *et al.* 2001. Virtual reality & exposure therapy for Vietnam veterans with posttraumatic stress disorder. *J. Clin. Psychiatry* **62:** 617–622.

18. Difede, J., N. Cukor, I. Jayasinghe, *et al.* 2007. Virtual reality exposure therapy for the treatment of posttraumatic stress disorder following September 11, 2001. *J. Clin. Psychiatry* **68:** 1639–1647.

19. Schwab, K.A., G. Baker, B. Ivins, *et al.* 2006. The Brief Traumatic Brain Injury Screen (BTBIS): investigating the validity of a self-report instrument for detecting traumatic brain injury (TBI) in troops returning from deployment in Afghanistan and Iraq. *Neurology* **66**(5, Suppl. 2): A235.

20. Cole, J.C., I. Grossman, C. Prilliman & E. Hunsaker. 2003. Multimethod validation of the Beck Depression Inventory-II and Grossman-Cole Depression Inventory with an inpatient sample. *Psychol. Rep.* **93:** 1115–1129.

21. Dutton, G.R., K.B. Grothe, G.N. Jones, *et al.* 2004. Use of the Beck Depression Inventory-II with African American primary care patients. *Gen. Hosp. Psychiatry* **26:** 437–442.

22. Dozois, D.J.A. & R. Covin. 2004. The Beck Depression Inventory-II (BDI-II), Beck Hopelessness Scale (BHS), and Beck Scale for Suicide Ideation (BSS). In *Comprehensive Handbook of Psychological Assessment, Vol. 2: Personality Assessment.* M.J. Hilsenroth & D.L. Segal, Eds.: 50–69. Wiley & Sons. Hoboken, NJ.

23. Longwell, B.T. & P. Truax. 2005. The differential effects of weekly, monthly, and bimonthly administrations of the Beck Depression Inventory-II: psychometric properties and clinical implications. *Behav. Ther.* **36:** 265–275.

24. Contreras, S., S. Fernandez, V.L. Malcarne, *et al.* 2004. Reliability and validity of the Beck depression and anxiety inventories in Caucasian Americans and Latinos. *Hisp. J. Behav. Sci.* **26:** 446–462.

25. Derogatis, L.R. & W.J. Culpepper. 2004. Beck Anxiety Inventory. In *The Use of Psychological Testing for Treatment Planning and Outcomes Assessment, Vol. 3: Instruments for Adults.* 3rd ed. M.E. Maruish, Ed.: 59–100. Lawrence Erlbaum Associates. Mahwah, NJ.

26. King, M. 1986. At risk drinking among general practice attenders: validation of the CAGE questionnaire. *Psychol. Med.* **16:** 213–217.

27. Bradley, K.A., A.F. DeBenedetti, R.J. Volk, *et al.* 2007. AUDIT-C as a brief screen for alcohol misuse in primary care. *Alcohol. Clin. Exp. Res.* **31:** 1208–1217.

28. Ware, J.E. & C.D. Sherbourne. 1992. The MOS 36-item Short-Form Health Survey (SF-36). *Med. Care* **30:** 473–483.

29. Van Tubergen, A., R. Landewe, L. Heuft-Dorenbosch, *et al.* 2003. Assessment of disability with the World Health Organisation Diasability Assessment Schedule II in patients with ankylosing spondylitis. *Ann. Rheum. Dis.* **62:** 140–145.

30. Chisolm, T.H., H.B. Abrams, R. McArdle, *et al.* 2005. The WHO-DAS II: psychometric properties in the measurement of functional health status in adults with acquired hearing loss. *Trends Amplif.* **9:** 111–126.

31. Spitzer, R.L., J.B. Williams, M. Gibbon & M.B. First. 1992. The structured Clinical Interview for DSM-III-R (SCID). I: history, rationale, and description. *Arch. Gen. Psychiatry* **49:** 624–629.

32. Cox, R.W. 1996. AFNI: software for analysis and visualization of functional magnetic resonance neuroimages. *Comput. Biomed. Res.* **29:** 162–173.

33. Pine, D.S., J. Grun, E.A. Maguire, *et al.* 2010. Neurodevelopmental aspects of virtual reality navigation: an fMRI study. *Neuroimage* In press.

34. Zarahn, E. 2000. Testing for neural responses during temporal components of trials with BOLD fMRI. *Neuroimage* **11:** 783–796.

35. Zarahn, E., G. Aguirre & M. D'Esposito. 2000. Replication and further studies of neural mechanisms of spatial mnemonic processing in humans. *Brain Res. Cogn. Brain Res.* **9:** 1–17.

36. Foa, E.B., B.O. Rothbaum, D.S. Riggs & T.B. Murdock. 1991. Treatment of posttraumatic stress disorder in rape victims: a comparison between cognitive-behavioral procedures and counseling. *J. Consult. Clin. Psychol.* **59:** 715–723.

37. Rizzo, A.A., K. Graap, K. Perlman, *et al.* 2008. Virtual Iraq: initial results from a VR exposure therapy application for combat-related PTSD. *Stud. Health Technol. Inform.* **132:** 420–425.

38. Guy, W. 1976. *ECDEU Assessment Manual for Psychopharmacology.* U.S. Department of Health, Education and Welfare. Rockville, MD.

Ann. N.Y. Acad. Sci. ISSN 0077-8923

ANNALS OF THE NEW YORK ACADEMY OF SCIENCES
Issue: *Psychiatric and Neurologic Aspects of War*

Variant brain-derived neurotrophic factor Val66Met endophenotypes: implications for posttraumatic stress disorder

Helena Frielingsdorf,[1,2] Kevin G. Bath,[1,2,3] Fatima Soliman,[1,2] JoAnn DiFede,[2] B. J. Casey,[1,2] and Francis S. Lee[2]

[1]The Sackler Institute for Developmental Psychobiology, Weill Medical College of Cornell University, New York, New York. [2]Department of Psychiatry, Weill Medical College of Cornell University, New York, New York [3]Department of Neuroscience, Brown University, Providence, Rhode Island

Address for correspondence: Helena Frielingsdorf or Francis S. Lee, Department of Psychiatry, Weill Cornell Medical College, 1300 York Avenue, Box 244, New York, New York 10065. hef2004@med.cornell.edu or fslee@med.cornell.edu

Recently, a common single nucleotide polymorphism (SNP) has been identified in the gene encoding brain-derived neurotrophic factor (BDNF). The variant BDNF$_{Met}$ has been shown to have decreased activity-dependent BDNF secretion from neurons and to lead to impairments in specific forms of learning and altered susceptibility to stress. A mouse model containing BDNF$_{Met}$ has also been linked to increased anxiety-like behavior. In a translational study, mice and human carriers of the BDNF$_{Met}$ allele were compared in their ability to extinguish a learned fear memory. Both showed slower suppression of the learned fear response. In humans, the neural correlates of this behavior were validated using fMRI. As anxiety and fear extinction lie at the core of symptoms and therapeutic approaches to posttraumatic stress disorder (PTSD), we propose that BDNF genotype and neuroimaging may be useful as biomarkers to provide guidance for more customized therapeutic directions. The aim of this paper is to review the available knowledge on the BDNF Val66Met SNP, with emphasis on anxiety- and fear-related endophenotypes and its potential implications for PTSD.

Keywords: BDNF; Val66Met; anxiety; PTSD; fear extinction

Introduction

Brain-derived neurotrophic factor (BDNF), a member of the neurotrophin family of polypeptide growth factors, is widely expressed in the developing and adult mammalian brain and has been identified as a key regulator of neuronal development within the central nervous system.[1,2] In recent years, BDNF has been implicated in the development and treatment of a number of psychiatric disorders, including depression, anxiety, and eating disorders. In this review, we will focus on a recently identified single nucleotide polymorphism (SNP) that has been identified in the gene encoding BDNF. We specifically examine its role in the development of emotional and cognitive disorders. We will then expand upon this wealth of recent work to provide an argu-

ment for the potential role for this BDNF variant in additional forms of psychiatric disorders with their roots in emotional dysregulation, specifically posttraumatic stress disorder (PTSD).

BDNF is synthesized as a precursor protein (proBDNF) that is proteolytically cleaved to generate mature BDNF.[3] Throughout life, BDNF influences the proliferation, differentiation, morphology, and functional activity of neuronal cells. BDNF action is dictated by its binding to either of two functionally different classes of cell surface receptors, the TrkB receptor tyrosine kinase or the p75 neurotrophin receptor (p75^{NTR}), a member of the tumor necrosis factor receptor super family.[1] ProBDNF is preferentially bound by p75^{NTR}, whereas mature BDNF preferentially binds to the TrkB receptor.[4,5] BDNF binding to the TrkB receptor

doi: 10.1111/j.1749-6632.2010.05722.x

produces neurotrophic responses through rapid activation of the PI-3 kinase, Ras/MAPK, and PLC-γ pathways, thus influencing transcriptional events affecting the cell-cycle, neurite outgrowth, and synaptic plasticity.[6–9] ProBDNF binding to the p75[NTR] gives rise to an increase in JNK (c-Jun N-terminal kinase) and NF-κB (nuclear factor κB), which triggers apoptosis, axonal retraction, or the pruning of dendritic spines.[10]

As mentioned, an SNP in the gene encoding BDNF has recently been identified. This SNP results in an amino acid change from a valine (Val) to a methionine (Met) at position 66 (Val66Met) in the prodomain of BDNF ($BDNF_{Met}$). Thus far, this SNP in the BDNF gene has only been found in humans. The frequency of the $BDNF_{Met}$ allele is relatively common and is ethnically stratified. Approximately, 50% of Asians, 30% of Caucasians, and 4% of African Americans carry at least one $BDNF_{Met}$ allele.[11,12] In Asian and Caucasian populations, the incidence of homozygous $BDNF_{Met}$ allele carriers is around 20% and 4%, respectively.[13]

Impact of BDNF Val66Met on BDNF availability

The molecular and cellular effects of BDNF Val66Met have been studied using a number of model systems, including cell culture and animals models. The initial work was carried out in *in vitro* cell culture systems. Transfection of $BDNF_{Met}$ into neurons does not alter total levels of BDNF.[14,15] This was shown in neuronal cultures from mice in which $BDNF_{Met}$ was genetically knocked into the endogenous BDNF locus. Specifically, $BDNF_{Met}$ was less efficiently trafficked to neuronal processes and 20–30% less BDNF was released under depolarizing conditions in cells from hetero- and homozygous $BDNF_{Met}$ carriers, respectively.[14] A number of groups hypothesized that $BDNF_{Met}$ could lead to less efficient sorting of BDNF into secretory granules. Subsequently, it was demonstrated that $BDNF_{Met}$ bound less efficiently to the protein sortilin, a molecule implicated both in the trafficking of BDNF in the biosynthetic pathway and as a coreceptor with p75[NTR] that binds proBDNF.[5,16]

Impact of BDNF Val66Met on neuronal survival and morphology

As mentioned previously, BDNF plays a significant role in the development of neuronal cells. To study the potential role of BDNF Val66Met on neuronal development, we and another lab developed lines of mice in which the BDNF Val66Met allele was genetically knocked into mice in a targeted fashion. In our lab, the endogenous mouse BDNF gene was replaced with a modified version of the mouse BDNF gene containing the Val66Met SNP.[14] In a second lab, Cao and colleagues developed a mouse in which the human version of the BDNF gene containing the Val66Met SNP was genetically knocked into the mouse genome.[17] To study the impact of BDNF Val66Met on neuronal birth, we carried out a series of studies in which we tracked rates of proliferation of new cells within the subventricular zone and their eventual migration and survival within the olfactory bulb (OB) in wild-type and $BDNF_{Met}$ homozygous mice. Interestingly, we found that $BDNF_{Met}$ led to a significant reduction in the survival of newly born cells in the OB, suggesting that altered BDNF availability as a result of the Val66Met SNP could lead to a reduction in the birth of new cells in the adult brain.[18] In a separate series of studies, Cao and colleagues demonstrated that, during development, $BDNF_{Met}$ alters the ability of axons to survive within the developing olfactory system, indicative of potentially significant effects on axonal development throughout the brain.[17] Finally, using Golgi impregnation, we have demonstrated that the complexity of dendritic arbors of neurons in the hippocampus is significantly less elaborate in $BDNF_{Met}$ homozygous mice compared to wild-type mice.[14] This reduction in dendritic complexity mirrors that of mice that have been exposed to chronic stress regimens.[19] In these same $BDNF_{Met}$ mice, we found that in the hippocampus, a BDNF rich region, there was a significant reduction in volume. These data replicated findings from human imaging studies in which $BDNF_{Met}$ carriers were found to have reduced hippocampal volume compared to age- and sex-matched controls.

BDNF Val66Met leads to altered neuronal function

BDNF has been implicated in the electrical plasticity of neurons, specifically in the processes of long-term potentiation (LTP) and long-term depression (LTD). In a recent series of experiments, we examined whether and how the BDNF Val66Met polymorphism affects hippocampal neurotransmission and synaptic plasticity using mice homozygous for the $BDNF_{Met}$ allele. We found that both young and adult BDNF$_{Met}$ homozygous mice exhibited a decrease in TBS (theta-burst stimulation)-induced LTP at the CA3-CA1 synapses. We also observed a decrease in N-methyl-D-aspartate (NMDA) receptor-dependent LTD in these mice. These data suggest that in human BDNF$_{Met}$ carriers, electrophysiological processes associated with memory function could be disrupted as a result of the BDNF Val66Met SNP.[20]

BDNF Val66Met is associated with altered hippocampal memory function

BDNF$_{Met}$ has been associated with alterations in hippocampal plasticity and morphology. In a study of human schizophrenic patients and age-matched controls, Egan and colleagues demonstrated that BDNF$_{Met}$ allele carriers have impairments in an episodic memory task.[15] Subsequently, these findings were in part replicated by Dempster *et al.*[21] using a healthy control group. This same task, when tested using functional magnetic resonance imaging (fMRI), demonstrated that BDNF$_{Met}$ homozygous individuals had reduced hippocampal activation compared with controls and had a gene-dose-dependent reduction in *n*-acetyl aspartate, an intracellular marker of neuronal activity, indicating potential hippocampal dysregulation. These findings were later confirmed in another fMRI study by the same group.[22] They found again that BDNF$_{Met}$ carriers showed a relative decrease in hippocampal activation during encoding and retrieval of a declarative memory task. The BDNF$_{Met}$ allele carriers also made more errors on a retrieval memory task. A separate group in Australia found a similar decrease in hippocampal gray matter in BDNF$_{Met}$ carriers and also found that BDNF$_{Met}$ homozygous individuals make more errors on a verbal recall task.[23] Finally, in a fMRI study, Sambataro and colleagues found that BDNF$_{Met}$ allele carriers show a steeper decline in age-related hippocampal activation during a declarative memory task.[24]

To get a clearer picture of the potential effects of the BDNF$_{Met}$ allele on memory function, we used our knockin BDNF Val66Met mouse model. This manipulation allows us to assay memory function on genetically homogenous background as well as control many of the potential environmental factors that may impact gene function and neural development. Using a contextual fear-conditioning task, we tested mice on their ability to recall and generate a fear response to a context in which they previously received a series of three footshocks. This task has previously been shown to rely on the hippocampus. We found that contextual fear memory was significantly impaired in BDNF$_{Met}$ homozygous mice. These data provide additional convergent evidence for a role for BDNF Val66Met and alterations in hippocampal memory function.[14]

BDNF Val66Met and affective disorders

Human studies attempting to link the Val66Met SNP with affective/anxiety disorders have resulted in mixed results. A 2008 meta-analysis focusing on the Val66Met polymorphism and anxiety-related traits reported no significant association between the SNP and anxiety disorder or with harm avoidance, a trait that is thought to be closely associated with anxiety and depression.[25] They found that healthy BDNF$_{Met}$ carrying subjects had significantly lower neuroticism scores than noncarriers. However, in these studies the sample and effect sizes were small. Another recent meta-analysis found no overall association between carrying the BDNF$_{Met}$ allele and diagnosis with major depressive disorder (MDD),[26] an effect that remained when stratified for ethnicity (Caucasian or Asian). Interestingly, when gender was taken into account, male homozygous carriers of the BDNF$_{Met}$ allele were significantly more likely to be diagnosed with MDD than noncarriers. These results are consistent with another recent study in which BDNF$_{Met}$ homozygous subjects exhibited significantly increased anxiety-related traits (e.g., harm avoidance, fear of uncertainty, and anticipatory worry) compared with noncarriers.[27]

Other studies have begun to investigate the response to stress in BDNF$_{Met}$ allele carriers. In one such study, an interaction between early life stress and Val66Met status was found for measures of anxiety and depression.[23] Individuals carrying the BDNF$_{Met}$ allele who had been exposed to early life stress were found to have reduced hippocampal volume compared to noncarriers. The size of the hippocampi of these subjects was correlated with reduced lateral prefrontal cortex (PFC) volume and higher depression scores. The interaction between BDNF genotype and early life stress also indirectly predicted higher scores on neuroticism and anxiety, albeit with modest effect sizes. In a separate study of healthy twins with either high or low familial risk for affective disorder, an interaction was found between risk level and stress response. Individuals in the high-risk group and carrying the BDNF$_{Met}$ allele were found to have higher levels of evening cortisol, suggesting that familial risk of affective disorders in combination with carrying the BDNF$_{Met}$ allele may impact stress responsiveness.[28] This finding is consistent with another recent study of subjects admitted with major depression in which BDNF$_{Met}$ homozygous individuals were found to have a greater hypothalamus-pituitary-adrenal response to dexamethasone challenge compared with BDNF$_{Met}$ heterozygotes and noncarriers.[29]

Because of its relative scarcity in the population, most human studies have difficulties reaching statistical power for groups of BDNF$_{Met}$ homozygous subjects. In the mouse model, this problem can be avoided. In the studies by Chen *et al.*[14] only homozygous BDNF$^{Met/Met}$ mice showed significantly increased anxiety-related behavior. The reported behaviors included less spontaneous exploratory behavior of the center of the open field and less time and fewer entries into the open arms of the elevated plus maze compared with littermate control BDNF$^{Val/Val}$ mice. Furthermore, the BDNF$^{Met/Met}$ mice had greater latency to consume sweetened milk in the novelty-induced hypophagia task, a test that is regarded especially sensitive to chronic antidepressant-induced modulation of anxiety-like behavior.[30] Interestingly, the BDNF$^{Met/Met}$ mice did not respond with decreased anxiety-like behavior to chronic (21 days) treatment with the selective serotonin reuptake inhibitor (SSRI) fluoxetine. In the experiments performed by Chen *et al.*,[14] only male BDNF$_{Met}$ mice were used; however, the finding of increased anxiety-related behavior in the open field task has also been replicated in female BDNF$^{Met/Met}$ mice.[31]

BDNF Val66Met and fear-related behavior

Models of fear memory assess the response to fearful or neutral stimuli. The most commonly used fear conditioning, Pavlovian classical conditioning, consists of a form of learning in which a neutral stimulus and/or context is associated with an aversive one, resulting in a fear response to the originally neutral stimulus/context. The term fear extinction is used to describe the process of gradual attenuation of a fear response to that stimulus after it is no longer associated with danger.

As already mentioned, Chen *et al.*[14] showed that contextual fear memory (i.e., fear response to the environment, where the aversive stimulus was delivered) was attenuated in homozygous BDNF$^{Met/Met}$ mice. However, in that same study, they noted no difference between genotypes for cued-dependent fear memory.[14]

The first association between the Val66Met polymorphism and ability to extinguish fearful memories in the Val66Met transgenic mouse model was described by Yu *et al.*,[32] using a conditioned taste aversion task, in which mice were conditioned to associate sucrose water with LiCl-induced nausea. The authors reported no effect of genotype on the acquisition or retention of the aversive memory. However, mice homozygous for the BDNF$_{Met}$ allele showed a marked decrease in the rate of extinction for this learned aversion. The slower extinction in BDNF$_{Met}$ homozygous mice was accompanied with lower levels of c-Fos expression in the ventromedial PFC (vmPFC), an area implicated in the extinction of aversive memories.[33–35] In addition, compared to wild-type, littermate controls, naïve BDNF$_{Met}$ homozygous mice had diminished dendritic arborization as well as a 17% volume reduction of the vmPFC. Finally, the authors found that the impairment in fear extinction could be rescued by a single injection of the partial NMDA-receptor agonist D-cycloserine (DCS) during extinction training. In a cohort of healthy human subjects, Hajcak *et al.*[36] studied the relationship between the BDNF$_{Met}$ allele and generalization of fear conditioned startle using a paradigm similar to that originally developed by Lissek *et al.*[37] In this study, a paradigm where the danger and safety cues consisted of rectangles of different sizes and the aversive stimulus, a mild shock to the triceps was always paired with the middle-sized rectangle. It was found that BDNF$_{Met}$ allele carriers showed a specific deficit in the startle response to the medium-sized rectangle (danger cue) but not to the rectangle most similar in size. However, the sample size was small (44 noncarriers, and 10 BDNF$_{Met}$ heterozyotes and three BDNF$_{Met}$ homozygous carriers grouped together). In another study investigating fear potentiated startle, where a picture was paired with a mild shock to the ankle, the authors reported that BDNF$_{Met}$ allele carriers showed a reduced startle response to the aversive stimulus in late acquisition and early extinction blocks, but no effect on skin conductance. Again, the sample size was small

(39 noncarriers, and seven BDNF$_{Met}$ heterozygotes and two BDNF$_{Met}$ homozygotes).

In a recent translational study, we found that human BDNF$_{Met}$ allele carriers have intact fear conditioning but impairments in the extinction of a learned fear response, as measured by skin conductance.[38] This finding was replicated in a parallel study conducted in BDNF Val66Met knockin mice. In mice that were conditioned to anticipate a mild footshock following a tone, BDNF$_{Met}$ mice failed to suppress the learned fear response over the course of 30 extinction trials. This impairment was dose-dependent, such that mice homozygous for BDNF$_{Met}$ were significantly slower than heterozygous mice. The parallel human experiments involved 36 healthy young adults (noncarriers) and 36 BDNF$_{Met}$ allele carriers (31 heterozygotes and five BDNF homozygotes). While undergoing fMRI, participants were fear conditioned by presentation of two different colored squares, one of which was paired with an aversive sound. Once an association was formed, extinction was carried out by multiple presentations of both squares in the absence of the aversive sound. The BDNF$_{Met}$ human subjects were found to have decreased activation of the vmPFC compared with noncarriers, a finding consistent with a failure to effectively engage circuitry implicated in fear extinction. This was consistent with findings in BDNF$_{Met}$ mice, in which lower levels of c-Fos were found in the vmPFC of BDNF$_{Met}$ mice following extinction training.

Discussion: relevance for PTSD

PTSD is a condition characterized by increased anxiety as well as a reduced ability to extinguish fearful memories after exposure to one or more traumatic events. There is also a significant comorbidity with MDD. To date, only one publication provides data on a possible link between Val66Met status and PTSD. In that study, no overrepresentation of BDNF$_{Met}$ allele carriers was seen in a cohort of 96 war veterans diagnosed with PTSD.[39] However, this result was inconclusive because of low statistical power, and further studies are warranted. In the largest study focusing on the acquisition of fear-related behavior, neither humans nor mice carrying the BDNF$_{Met}$ allele showed any difference in the ability to learn to generate a conditioned fear response to a cue.[38] BDNF$_{Met}$ mice had decreased expression of

a contextual fear memory,[14] which in theory could partially be a protective factor for the development of PTSD symptoms. However, that protective effect would likely be overshadowed by the impaired or slowed ability to extinguish fearful memories.

We concluded, based on the currently available literature, that the variant BDNF Val66Met polymorphism does not consistently confer an increased overall risk for affective- or anxiety-related disorders or traits. The only correlation found in a large meta-analysis suggested that males homozygous for the BDNF$_{Met}$ allele have an increased risk of developing MDD.[26]

Although most of the human studies to date have not found a conclusive relationship between a single BDNF$_{Met}$ allele and anxiety-related traits, it is still unclear whether the same is true for homozygous BDNF$_{Met}$ allele carriers. This is in part due to low statistical power given the low percentage of homozygous individuals in the population. By contrast, the mouse model clearly indicates there is a dose–response relationship between the number of alleles and anxiety-related behavior.[14] Hence, the mouse model provides robust evidence for an anxiety-like endophenotype that has been replicated in both male and female homozygous mice. In support of these findings, a recent study on healthy volunteers with a large number of homozygotes found that only homozygote carriers of the BDNF$_{Met}$ allele scored significantly higher on measures of anxiety compared to noncarriers. This effect replicated across both sexes.[27]

Both human and rodent BDNF$_{Met}$ allele carriers, after being exposed to an aversive event, are slower to show an attenuated response to a cue that has previously been associated with that aversive event, even after that cue no longer represents danger, that is, impaired fear extinction.[32,38] The study by Soliman *et al.*[38] found a significant impairment in fear extinction in heterozygous BDNF$^{Val/Met}$ individuals. In addition to the behavioral findings, Soliman *et al.*[38] also show that BDNF$_{Met}$ allele carriers recruit the amygdala and vmPFC differently than noncarriers. This is a similar pattern of increased amygdala activation and decreased medial PFC (mPFC) activation to what has been observed in fMRI studies of PTSD patients.[40,41] In addition, the relative extent of decrease in amygdala activation during fear extinction has been correlated with the degree of extinction success in healthy volunteers.[35]

Extinction of fearful memories is thought to be brought on by the formation of a new memory, one that associates the stimulus previously paired with a fearful event with one that signals safety. This is in contrast to the notion that fear extinction is in fact an erasure of the original memory. Recent findings suggest that BDNF availability in the infralimbic mPFC from hippocampal projections is critical for the formation of such new memories.[42] It is therefore conceivable that the reduced activity-dependent secretion of BDNF associated with the BDNF$_{Met}$ allele leads to decreased synaptic plasticity in the mPFC and thereby deficiency in the formation of the new memory required for fear extinction.

There is a significant need for new therapeutic directions for many psychiatric disorders. In addition to new therapies, a lot would be gained if the use of currently available pharmacological and psychotherapeutic therapies could be more effectively used. In the case of PTSD, a recent meta-analysis showed that, on average, 80% of PTSD patients improved by 70% using different therapeutic approaches.[43] With today's diagnostic tools, it is very difficult to predict who will benefit the most from a particular therapy. Furthermore, many patients go through a painful "trial and error" phase before the most effective therapeutic combination for that particular individual is established. Hence, biomarkers that predict treatment response would be very beneficial.

In the mouse model, adult BDNF$_{Met}$ mice show blunted alteration in anxiety-like behaviors after chronic SSRI treatment,[14] the most commonly used pharmacological treatment for PTSD. The recent study by Soliman *et al.*[38] also validates that both humans and mice carrying the Met allele are worse at, or at least take longer, to extinguish fearful memories. This finding implies that they may not respond as readily to exposure therapy, which is one of the best documented and most widely used psychotherapeutic approaches for PTSD.[44] The fact that exposure therapy relies on intact ability to extinguish fearful memories suggests that it could be informative to genotype PTSD patients with regard to BDNF Val66Met in order to be able to offer modified or alternative treatment strategies.

Therapies aimed at normalizing BDNF function could be divided into at least two different categories: (i) therapies aimed at normalizing BDNF secretion during development in order to rescue structural changes caused by BDNF Val66Met and (ii) therapies aimed at normalizing BDNF secretion in adult life in order to ensure intact moment to moment BDNF-dependent synaptic plasticity and related functions. Drug discovery strategies to increase BDNF release from synapses or to prolong the half-life of secreted BDNF may improve therapeutic responses for humans with this common BDNF polymorphism.

Alternatively, therapies that do not involve BDNF signaling could be used to circumvent the deficit in BDNF signaling as well as the decreased response seen after SSRI treatment. As BDNF Val66Met status is suggested to be associated with an impaired ability to extinguish fearful memories, therapies aimed at enhancing fear extinction could be extremely useful. DCS, a partial NMDA receptor agonist, has emerged as one of the most promising pharmacological therapies aimed at enhancing fear extinction, that is, the efficacy of exposure therapy.[45,46] Several studies report beneficial effects of DCS administered before early sessions of exposure therapy for patients diagnosed with acrophobia and social phobia.[46,47] Clinical studies evaluating the effects of DCS in enhancing exposure therapy for PTSD are currently under way. As NMDA receptors are necessary for BDNF-induced fear extinction,[42] it is plausible that NMDA receptor modulation could be an efficient means of bypassing the deficit in fear extinction supposedly caused by disrupted BDNF secretion in BDNF$_{Met}$ allele carriers. In the mouse model, Yu *et al.*[32] demonstrated that one dose of DCS at a critical time during fear extinction can rescue the impairment associated with the Val66Met status. Future studies are needed to confirm whether exposure therapy combined with NMDA receptor modulators could be of similar value for PTSD patients carrying the BDNF$_{Met}$ allele.

Propranolol, a nonselective β-blocker, has also been proposed to attenuate subsequent fear response when administered directly after retrieval of a previously experienced traumatic event.[48] However, preliminary results from clinical trials using propranolol in the immediate aftermath of a traumatic event to prevent development of PTSD have failed to show a significant effect of the treatment.[49,50]

Recent findings from both rodent and human studies also suggest that fear memories can be disrupted without the use of any drugs by performing fear extinction during reconsolidation within a limited time window after reexposure to a cue that predicts the aversive event,[51,52] an approach that may be beneficial in $BDNF_{Met}$ allele carriers.

In conclusion, several new therapies are emerging that may be used alone or in concert for PTSD patients who do not successfully respond to SSRI and conventional exposure therapy alone. Further studies are needed to clarify whether Val66Met genotype confers an increased risk for the development of affective disorders, including PTSD. Independent of that, recent studies suggest that BDNF genotype based therapy could be applicable for PTSD as well as other affective- and anxiety-related disorders. The study by Soliman *et al.*[38] also implicates that, aside from genotype, behavioral tests of extinction capacity and neuroimaging could also serve as biomarkers to direct more personalized psychiatric treatment. Future studies on patient cohorts will elucidate whether these biomarkers prove to be useful in a clinical setting.

Acknowledgments

We acknowledge support from the Swedish Brain Foundation (H.F.), the Gylling family (H.F.), NIH Grants MH079513 (B.J.C., F.S.L.), MH060478 (B.J.C.), NS052819 (F.S.L.), GM07739 (F.S.), and United Negro College Fund–Merck Graduate Science Research Dissertation Fellowship (F.S.), Burroughs Wellcome Foundation (F.S.L.), and the International Mental Health Research Organization (F.S.L).

Conflicts of interest

The authors declare no conflicts of interest.

References

1. Chao, M.V. 2003. Neurotrophins and their receptors: a convergence point for many signalling pathways. *Nat. Rev. Neurosci.* **4:** 299–309.

2. Huang, E.J. & L.F. Reichardt. 2001. Neurotrophins: roles in neuronal development and function. *Annu. Rev. Neurosci.* **24:** 677–736.

3. Greenberg, M.E. *et al.* 2009. New insights in the biology of BDNF synthesis and release: implications in CNS function. *J. Neurosci.* **29:** 12764–12767.

4. Lee, R. *et al.* 2001. Regulation of cell survival by secreted proneurotrophins. *Science* **294:** 1945–1948.

5. Teng, H.K. *et al.* 2005. ProBDNF induces neuronal apoptosis via activation of a receptor complex of p75NTR and sortilin. *J. Neurosci.* **25:** 5455–5463.

6. Chao, M.V., R. Rajagopal & F.S. Lee. 2006. Neurotrophin signalling in health and disease. *Clin. Sci. (Lond.)* **110:** 167–173.

7. Cowley, S. *et al.* 1994. Activation of MAP kinase kinase is necessary and sufficient for PC12 differentiation and for transformation of NIH 3T3 cells. *Cell* **77:** 841–852.

8. Mazzucchelli, C. *et al.* 2002. Knockout of ERK1 MAP kinase enhances synaptic plasticity in the striatum and facilitates striatal-mediated learning and memory. *Neuron* **34:** 807–820.

9. Rosenblum, K. *et al.* 2002. The role of extracellular regulated kinases I/II in late-phase long-term potentiation. *J. Neurosci.* **22:** 5432–5441.

10. Roux, P.P. & P.A. Barker. 2002. Neurotrophin signaling through the p75 neurotrophin receptor. *Prog. Neurobiol.* **67:** 203–233.

11. Shimizu, E., K. Hashimoto & M. Iyo. 2004. Ethnic difference of the BDNF 196G/A (val66met) polymorphism frequencies: the possibility to explain ethnic mental traits. *Am. J. Med. Genet. B. Neuropsychiatr. Genet.* **126B:** 122–123.

12. Pivac, N. *et al.* 2009. Ethnic differences in brain-derived neurotrophic factor Val66Met polymorphism in Croatian and Korean healthy participants. *Croat. Med. J.* **50:** 43–48.

13. Petryshen, T.L. *et al.* 2009. Population genetic study of the brain-derived neurotrophic factor (BDNF) gene. *Mol. Psychiatry* Mar 3 [Epub ahead of print].

14. Chen, Z.Y. *et al.* 2006. Genetic variant BDNF (Val66Met) polymorphism alters anxiety-related behavior. *Science* **314:** 140–143.

15. Egan, M.F. *et al.* 2003. The BDNF val66met polymorphism affects activity-dependent secretion of BDNF and human memory and hippocampal function. *Cell* **112:** 257–269.

16. Chen, Z.Y. *et al.* 2005. Sortilin controls intracellular sorting of brain-derived neurotrophic factor to the regulated secretory pathway. *J. Neurosci.* **25:** 6156–6166.

17. Cao, L. *et al.* 2007. Genetic modulation of BDNF signaling affects the outcome of axonal competition in vivo. *Curr. Biol.* **17:** 911–921.

18. Bath, K.G. *et al.* 2008. Variant brain-derived neurotrophic factor (Val66Met) alters adult olfactory bulb neurogenesis and spontaneous olfactory discrimination. *J. Neurosci.* **28:** 2383–2393.

19. Magarinos, A.M. *et al.* 2010. Effect of brain-derived neurotrophic factor haploinsufficiency on stress-induced remodeling of hippocampal neurons. *Hippocampus* Jan 21 [Epub ahead of print].

20. Ninan, I. *et al.* 2010. The BDNF Val66Met polymorphism impairs NMDA receptor-dependent synaptic plasticity in the hippocampus. *J. Neurosci.* **30:** 8866–8870.

21. Dempster, E. *et al.* 2005. Association between BDNF val66 met genotype and episodic memory. *Am. J. Med. Genet. B Neuropsychiatr. Genet.* **134B:** 73–75.

22. Hariri, A.R. *et al.* 2003. Brain-derived neurotrophic factor val66met polymorphism affects human memory-related hippocampal activity and predicts memory performance. *J. Neurosci.* **23:** 6690–6694.

23. Gatt, J. M. *et al.* 2009. Interactions between BDNF Val66Met polymorphism and early life stress predict brain and arousal

pathways to syndromal depression and anxiety. *Mol. Psychiatry* **14:** 681–695.

24. Sambataro, F. *et al.* 2010. BNDF modulates normal human hippocampal ageing. *Mol. Psychiatry* **15:** 116–118.

25. Frustaci, A. *et al.* 2008. Meta-analysis of the brain-derived neurotrophic factor gene (BDNF) Val66Met polymorphism in anxiety disorders and anxiety-related personality traits. *Neuropsychobiology* **58:** 163–170.

26. Verhagen, M. *et al.* 2010. Meta-analysis of the BDNF Val66Met polymorphism in major depressive disorder: effects of gender and ethnicity. *Mol. Psychiatry* **15:** 260–271.

27. Montag, C. *et al.* 2010. The BDNF Val66Met polymorphism and anxiety: support for animal knock-in-studies from a genetic association study in humans. *Psychiatry Res* Jul 16 [Epub ahead of print].

28. Vinberg, M. *et al.* 2009. The BDNF Val66Met polymorphism: relation to familiar risk of affective disorder, BDNF levels and salivary cortisol. *Psychoneuroendocrinology* **34:** 1380–1389.

29. Schule, C. *et al.* 2006. Brain-derived neurotrophic factor Val66Met polymorphism and dexamethasone/CRH test results in depressed patients. *Psychoneuroendocrinology* **31:** 1019–1025.

30. Dulawa, S.C. & R. Hen. 2005. Recent advances in animal models of chronic antidepressant effects: the novelty-induced hypophagia test. *Neurosci Biobehav Rev.* **29:** 771–783.

31. Spencer, J.L. *et al.* 2010. BDNF variant Val66Met interacts with estrous cycle in the control of hippocampal function. *Proc. Natl. Acad. Sci. USA* **107:** 4395–4400.

32. Yu, H. *et al.* 2009. Variant BDNF Val66Met polymorphism affects extinction of conditioned aversive memory. *J. Neurosci.* **29:** 4056–4064.

33. Milad, M.R. & G.J. Quirk. 2002. Neurons in medial prefrontal cortex signal memory for fear extinction. *Nature* **420:** 70–74.

34. Milad, M.R. *et al.* 2007. Recall of fear extinction in humans activates the ventromedial prefrontal cortex and hippocampus in concert. *Biol. Psychiatry* **62:** 446–454.

35. Phelps, E.A. *et al.* 2004. Extinction learning in humans: role of the amygdala and vmPFC. *Neuron* **43:** 897–905.

36. Hajcak, G. *et al.* 2009. Genetic variation in brain-derived neurotrophic factor and human fear conditioning. *Genes Brain Behav.* **8:** 80–85.

37. Lissek, S. *et al.* 2008. Generalization of conditioned fear-potentiated startle in humans: experimental validation and clinical relevance. *Behav. Res. Ther.* **46:** 678–687.

38. Soliman, F. *et al.* 2010. A genetic variant BDNF polymorphism alters extinction learning in both mouse and human. *Science* **327:** 863–866.

39. Zhang, H. *et al.* 2006. Brain derived neurotrophic factor (BDNF) gene variants and Alzheimer's disease, affective disorders, posttraumatic stress disorder, schizophrenia, and substance dependence. *Am. J. Med. Genet. B Neuropsychiatr. Genet.* **141B:** 387–393.

40. Williams, L.M. *et al.* 2006. Trauma modulates amygdala and medial prefrontal responses to consciously attended fear. *Neuroimage* **29:** 347–357.

41. Protopopescu, X. *et al.* 2005. Differential time courses and specificity of amygdala activity in posttraumatic stress disorder subjects and normal control subjects. *Biol. Psychiatry* **57:** 464–473.

42. Peters, J. *et al.* 2010. Induction of fear extinction with hippocampal-infralimbic BDNF. *Science* **328:** 1288–1290.

43. Bradley, R. *et al.* 2005. A multidimensional meta-analysis of psychotherapy for PTSD. *Am. J. Psychiatry* **162:** 214–227.

44. Butler, A.C. *et al.* 2006. The empirical status of cognitive-behavioral therapy: a review of meta-analyses. *Clin. Psychol. Rev.* **26:** 17–31.

45. Ledgerwood, L., R. Richardson & J. Cranney. 2003. Effects of D-cycloserine on extinction of conditioned freezing. *Behav. Neurosci.* **117:** 341–349.

46. Ressler, K.J. *et al.* 2004. Cognitive enhancers as adjuncts to psychotherapy: use of D-cycloserine in phobic individuals to facilitate extinction of fear. *Arch. Gen. Psychiatry* **61:** 1136–1144.

47. Hofmann, S.G. *et al.* 2006. Augmentation of exposure therapy with D-cycloserine for social anxiety disorder. *Arch. Gen. Psychiatry* **63:** 298–304.

48. Brunet, A. *et al.* 2008. Effect of post-retrieval propranolol on psychophysiologic responding during subsequent script-driven traumatic imagery in post-traumatic stress disorder. *J. Psychiatr. Res.* **42:** 503–506.

49. McGhee, L.L. *et al.* 2009. The effect of propranolol on post-traumatic stress disorder in burned service members. *J. Burn Care Res.* **30:** 92–97.

50. Nugent, N.R. *et al.* 2010. The efficacy of early propranolol administration at reducing PTSD symptoms in pediatric injury patients: a pilot study. *J. Trauma Stress* **23:** 282–287.

51. Schiller, D. *et al.* 2010. Preventing the return of fear in humans using reconsolidation update mechanisms. *Nature* **463:** 49–53.

52. Monfils, M.H. *et al.* 2009. Extinction-reconsolidation boundaries: key to persistent attenuation of fear memories. *Science* **324:** 951–955.

Ann. N.Y. Acad. Sci. ISSN 0077-8923

ANNALS OF THE NEW YORK ACADEMY OF SCIENCES

Issue: *Psychiatric and Neurologic Aspects of War*

Using biological markers to inform a clinically meaningful treatment response

Rachel Yehuda,[1,2] Linda M. Bierer,[1,2] Laura C. Pratchett,[1] and Michelle Pelcovitz[2]

[1]Department of Psychiatry, James J. Peters Veterans Affairs Medical Center, Bronx, New York. [2]Department of Psychiatry, Mount Sinai School of Medicine, New York, New York

Address for correspondence: Rachel Yehuda, Ph.D., James J. Peters VAMC, 526 OOMH, 130 W. Kingsbridge Rd., Bronx, New York. rachel.yehuda@va.gov

Combat veterans with posttraumatic stress disorder (PTSD) demonstrate less robust improvement following treatments than do civilians with PTSD. This paper discusses a theoretical model for evaluating treatment response based on the extent of change in biological markers of symptom severity or resilience between treatment initiation and termination. Such analysis permits a determination of biological change associated with the liberal criteria commonly used to determine treatment response in combat PTSD, and a comparison of this to the biological change associated with clinical response determined according to the conservative definition more appropriate to civilian PTSD. Interim data supporting the utility of this approach is presented based on preliminary analyses from our work in progress. We propose that future studies consider the unique consequences of combat trauma and develop treatments that incorporate the complex nature of the exposure and response characteristic of a veteran population.

Keywords: PTSD; treatment response; combat trauma; neuroendocrinology

Introduction

Exposure to a traumatic event can result in an enduring transformation that affects psychological, physical, and spiritual health.[1] The consequences of such exposures may include the development of posttraumatic stress disorder (PTSD). PTSD has been described as a chronic disorder because a significant number of those who develop the condition maintain symptoms for years or even decades with symptoms that can be disabling.[2] An estimated 7.7 million American adults currently have PTSD, reflecting a lifetime prevalence ranging from 7% to 14% of the population.[3] The cost of PTSD to our society is substantial. In civilians, estimates due to lost productivity are in the range of $3 billion annually.[4] Claims for psychological disability associated with PTSD in veterans accounted for over one-third of the $24 billion spent last year.[5]

The last several decades have seen the development of treatments for PTSD, though it remains unclear how to define recovery and/or resilience. An additional question concerns whether different types of trauma exposure might require different interventions and whether there should be a different expectation of recovery for combat veterans, or others, for whom the trauma exposure may have been of greater intensity and duration than a single episode trauma.

This paper will provide a theoretical model for evaluating treatment response based on the extent of change in biological markers known to be associated with symptom severity and/or resilience. The model currently informs several continuing studies at the James J. Peters Bronx Veterans Affairs Medical Center. Because the studies are ongoing, this paper does not present final results about PTSD treatment response or their biological underpinnings. Rather, the approach we describe provides a method for determining the potential clinical significance of a treatment response and for evaluating relative differences in treatment responses based on the nature of the trauma exposure or its resultant PTSD.

The paper further describes why such a conceptual model is necessary. Indeed, to date there has been very little emphasis on developing specialized

doi: 10.1111/j.1749-6632.2010.05698.x

interventions for PTSD based on trauma type. Rather, the assumption has been that treatments that have been developed specifically for civilian PTSD will naturally also be effective in combat-related PTSD. Yet, emerging data from treatment studies in combat veterans suggests that the magnitude effect in clinical response is substantially weaker in combat than in civilian PTSD. Use of the proposed biological approach allows an assessment of whether this weaker response may nonetheless result in a biologically significant change in this group.

Efficacy of PTSD treatment in civilians

Civilians with PTSD respond extremely well to cognitive behavioral psychotherapy, such as prolonged exposure (PE). Accordingly, PE has emerged as a first-line treatment for PTSD in civilians.[6–10] In women whose PTSD resulted from exposure to interpersonal violence, PE not only reduced symptoms significantly, but resulted in loss of PTSD diagnosis in 65–95% of treatment completers.[11,12] Because the field of traumatology has tended to minimize differences in PTSD clinical presentation based on trauma type and severity, it has been broadly assumed on the heels of the successful PTSD trials in civilians that combat veterans with PTSD would also respond well to PE. Indeed, when the Committee on the Treatment of Posttraumatic Stress Disorder, commissioned by the National Institute of Medicine, was asked to make recommendations to the Veterans Affairs about how to treat combat trauma, they recommended PE as a first-line treatment based on its efficacy in civilians. The suggestion came despite the committee's acknowledgment that "the scientific evidence on treatment modalities for PTSD does not reach the level of certainty that would be desired for such a common and serious condition among veterans...and that additional high quality research is essential" (p. 1).[13] The statement is particularly optimistic in light of decades of observation that combat veterans do not respond as well as civilians to any kind of treatment, even pharmacological.[14–16]

Civilian versus combat-related PTSD

Explanations for why combat veterans may not respond as well as civilians to PTSD treatments have sometimes emphasized the conflict between maintaining disability status and showing improvement.

However, this explanation overlooks the magnitude and complexity of the combat experience and implies that veterans have more control over their mental health than may be true. The prediction that combat veterans would have a similar response to treatment as civilians with PTSD does not fully consider the many associated features of PTSD in combat veterans that are related to the length and nature of their exposure. For the veteran who has served in a warzone, PTSD symptoms may co-occur with traumatic brain injury, and the resultant memory problems, and with increased substance use including nicotine use—a habit that is often begun in the context of military service and may serve to sensitize biological systems. Combat veterans with PTSD also notoriously meet criteria for several comorbid mood and anxiety disorders. Although these problems can be present in civilians with PTSD, within a combat arena there is opportunity for multiple exposures that can have synergistic or sensitizing effects.

There are several other aspects of the combat trauma itself that are likely at the nexus of understanding the attenuated response of combat veterans to classic PTSD treatments. For example, combat veterans seek and prepare for their combat experiences. That is, unlike civilian exposures, there is preparation and training for combat. Furthermore, in many cases, soldiers hope to be positively transformed by the opportunity to serve their country and engage in patriotic and heroic action; enlisting is motivated by the desire to serve, or to develop skills, even while understanding that these may take place in harms way. Indeed, one of the major differences between civilian trauma exposure and the combat experience is that the former are unequivocally horrible, whereas deployment contains some

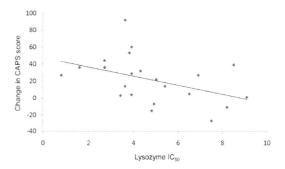

Figure 1. Moderate negative relationship between baseline GR sensitivity and change in CAPS score.

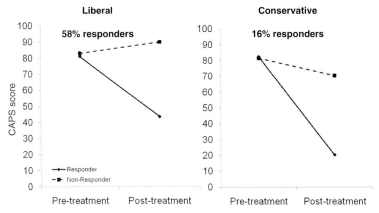

Figure 2. Definition of treatment response (liberal or conservative) produces different percentages of responders as measured by changes in CAPS score.

of the anticipated positive experiences. Often however, despite the psychological and physical preparation and training for combat, many soldiers are ill-prepared for the moral ambiguity that is experienced in combat. A blurring of the distinction between victim and perpetrator can occur as the combat soldier is sometimes placed in both roles. Despite the clearly more complex nature of combat exposure, there has not been a great effort to develop specialized approaches for combat-related PTSD.

Effect of PE in combat veterans

The few published studies examining the efficacy of PE and other cognitive behavioral therapies, such as cognitive processing therapy (CPT), in combat veterans have reported lower rates of clinical response relative to civilians.[17,18] A meta-analysis conducted several years ago demonstrated that effect sizes for PE and CPT were substantially lower for combat PTSD ($d = 0.81$) than for PTSD from civilian trauma ($d = 1.24$) or assault ($d = 1.83$).[19]

Recent studies of combat veterans have significantly adjusted the criterion for what constitutes a clinically significant response. Instead of a 50% decline in symptoms or no longer meeting the diagnostic criteria for PTSD, studies of combat veterans have used a reduction of only 10 or 12 points on the Clinician-Administered PTSD Scale for DSM-IV (CAPS) to indicate clinically meaningful response (e.g., Ref. 20). This rationale is based on an effect size of $d = 0.5$, referencing data from a 1997 study of 785 Vietnam veterans that identified a standard deviation of approximately 20 points on the CAPS.[21] However, since CAPS scores in treatment-seeking combat veterans may be as high as 80 points or more, a 10–12 point reduction may not reflect a stable or clinically substantial gain.

Most scoring approaches to the CAPS[22] require a combined frequency and intensity rating of at least three points for a symptom to be defined as occurring for diagnostic purposes (i.e., occurring at least once per month and causing distress or impairment in functioning). However, each symptom may ultimately be scored at a maximum combined frequency and intensity rating of eight points, reflecting a daily occurrence that causes severe distress and impairment. Therefore, a reduction of 10 points could reflect a change in the frequency and severity of as few as two PTSD symptoms, especially for patients who initially present with severe symptoms of the disorder, or it can reflect a modest improvement in as many as 10 symptoms. When one considers that the longitudinal trajectory of PTSD is characterized by fluctuations in severity over time it is important to know whether such a change will be sustainable. Regression to the mean, or even placebo effects (as may result from "nonspecific factors" of psychotherapies; Ref. 23) could potentially induce such a reduction, in the absence of alterations in the underlying pathophysiology of the disorder. It is therefore important to ascertain whether a decline of a 10–12 points in the CAPS score is a clinically meaningful unit for combat veterans that would be comparable to a greater reduction in civilians.

The use of biological markers

Since PTSD is associated with a unique neuroendocrine profile (e.g., Refs. 24 and 25), there is an opportunity to use biological variables in the interpretation of a clinically meaningful response. In PTSD, for example, catecholamine levels are often increased in association with symptom severity,[26] but basal cortisol levels are typically low (e.g., Refs. 27 and 28)). Several reports demonstrate an inverse relationship between PTSD severity and cortisol levels,[29,30] although sometimes cortisol levels have been linked with trauma exposure rather than symptom severity.[31,32] Furthermore, several refined measures of cortisol metabolism[33] have been developed and demonstrated in association with PTSD symptom recrudescence in longitudinal treatment studies. Measures of glucocorticoid responsiveness have also been developed for this purpose.[34] In two studies of biological alterations before and after PE in civilians,[35,36] cortisol levels were found to be altered in responders versus nonresponders at posttreatment, but not pretreatment.

Preliminary analyses suggest that at least some of the biological markers that were hypothesized to be correlates of symptom severity or recovery can be used in this manner. This is best illustrated through correlational analysis of the entire sample without regard for responder versus nonresponder status. Such analyses demonstrate, for example, that measures of glucocorticoid receptor (GR) sensitivity, as assessed by the lysozyme stimulation test in mononuclear leukocytes,[37] correlates with symptom improvement. Figure 1 shows that pretreatment lysozyme IC_{50} is moderately negatively associated with the pre- to posttreatment change in CAPS score ($r = -0.428$, $P < 0.05$). Our study (in progress) has also revealed potential markers of recovery and resilience, consistent with emerging reports. For example, dehydroepiandrosterone (DHEA), an endogenous hormone secreted by the adrenal in response to adrenocorticotrophin hormone, has been found to be higher in military trainees who performed well during extreme stress compared to those who did not.[38] In PTSD, it has been hypothesized that lower levels of DHEA may facilitate increased GR sensitivity.

Assuming the change in these biological measures reflects a clinically meaningful change, it is possible to ask whether a liberal treatment response produces a similar biological change as a more conser-

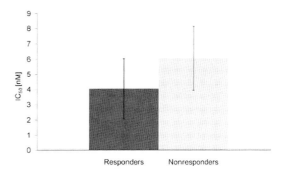

Figure 3. Baseline GR sensitivity predicts treatment response.

vative response. This involves analyzing data according to subgroups, rather than correlational analysis of the entire sample. This conceptual approach can be illustrated by pilot data from our ongoing study described below in which we hypothesized that changes associated with symptom severity and recovery would be present in responders, whereas nonresponders to treatment would show little change in these variables. Using a conservative criterion for response (50% change in CAPS score, as in civilian studies) resulted in relatively few responders.

We therefore examined the sample based on both liberal and conservative criteria of response, respectively. For the liberal criteria we used a 12 point reduction in CAPS score from pre- to posttreatment, and for the conservative criteria a 50% reduction in CAPS score from pre- to posttreatment in combination with a final CAPS score of less than 45. As of December 2009, a total of 23 participants were evaluated, all of whom had completed pre- and posttreatment biological and clinical measures, with 7 participants receiving a minimal attention condition and 16 receiving PE. The mean pretreatment CAPS score of the sample was 79.9 (standard deviation of 20.2), which is well above the score of 60 that is considered to reflect severe PTSD. On the basis of the liberal definition of response, 58% were identified as responders; on the basis of the conservative definition, only 16% were responders (Fig. 2).

In applying this scheme to the data on GR responsiveness, preliminary analyses showed that pretreatment IC_{50} predicted treatment response even when using the liberal criteria ($P = 0.039$) (Fig. 3). However, with respect to DHEA, a putative measure of resilience and recovery, the liberal criteria failed to generate a meaningful difference in biology. This is illustrated in Figure 4.

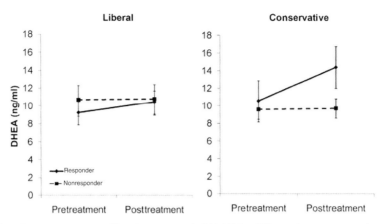

Figure 4. Definition of treatment response (liberal or conservative) highlights difference between responders and nonresponders in measures of pretreatment to posttreatment DHEA.

Although not quite reaching significance in this preliminary sample, we found that DHEA levels increased among responders (as defined conservatively) differentially from the changes observed among nonresponders ($F = 3.829$, $P = 0.064$) but that such a difference does not exist for responders versus nonresponders as liberally defined. The lack of statistical significance in the above findings should be interpreted with caution and are not being presented as definitive results from a completed study, but rather an illustration of how biological markers may ultimately be used in the service of determining a meaningful clinical response.

Conclusion

In this paper, we illustrated the use of treatment to conduct a longitudinal study examining biological correlates of PTSD. This type of study allows consideration of data in both correlational analyses and in analyses that subgroup patients dichotomously into responders and nonresponders. Within this distinction there is an opportunity to compare liberal and conservative criteria of responses. By examining persons when symptoms are high (at treatment initiation) and then again posttreatment when symptoms are lower for some, we can generate information about biological markers associated with PTSD state and/or recovery. Such information will allow determination of whether any established response criterion is biologically significant. In considering what may or may not be a significant clinical response, future studies should carefully consider the unique consequences of combat trauma and develop treat-

ments for combat-related PTSD that incorporate the complex exposure and nature of the response. Combat-related PTSD resembles civilian PTSD in some of the basic symptoms, as described by the DSM-IV, but treatment response may be related to some of the important differences between combat and civilian trauma.

Acknowledgments

This work was supported by the following funding: NIMH MH088101, DOD PT073577 and 10164894, and VA Merit Review to R.Y.

Conflicts of interest

The authors declare no conflicts of interest.

References

1. Yehuda, R. & L.M. Bierer. 2009. The relevance of epigenetics to PTSD: implications for the DSM-V. *J. Trauma Stress* **22:** 427–434.
2. American Psychiatric Association. 2000. *Diagnostic and Statistical Manual of Mental Disorders*, 4th ed. Text Revision: DSM-IV-TR. Washington, DC.
3. Kessler, R.C., W.T. Chiu, O. Demler & E.E. Walters. 2005. Prevalence, severity, and comorbidity of twelve-month DSM-IV disorders in the National Comorbidity Survey Replication (NCS-R). *Arch. Gen. Psychiatry* **62:** 617–627.
4. Kessler, R.C. 2000. Posttraumatic stress disorder: the burden to the individual and to society. *J. Clin. Psychiatry* **61**(Suppl. 5): 4–12.
5. The American Legion Benefits Center. February 2, 2010. Disability claims, homelessness top VA list. The American Legion.
6. Eisenman, D., S. Weine, B. Green, *et al.* 2006. The ISTSS/Rand guidelines on mental health training of primary healthcare providers for trauma-exposed populations in conflict-affected countries. *J. Trauma Stress* **19:** 5–17.

7. Bisson, J. & M. Andrew. 2007. Psychological treatment of post-traumatic stress disorder (PTSD). *Cochrane Database Syst. Rev.* **18**.

8. Harvey, A.G., R.A. Bryant & N. Tarrier. 2003. Cognitive behaviour therapy for posttraumatic stress disorder. *Clin. Psychol. Rev.* **23:** 501–522.

9. Foa, E.B. 2006. Psychosocial therapy for posttraumatic stress disorder. *J. Clin. Psychiatry* **67:** 40–45.

10. Rothbaum, B.O. & A.C. Schwartz. 2002. Exposure therapy for posttraumatic stress disorder. *Am. J. Psychother.* **56:** 59–75.

11. Foa, E.B., C.V. Dancu, E.A. Hembree, *et al.* 1999. A comparison of exposure therapy, stress inoculation training, and their combination for reducing posttraumatic stress disorder in female assault victims. *J. Consult. Clin. Psych.* **67:** 194–200.

12. Rothbaum, B.O., M.C. Astin & F. Marsteller. 2005. Prolonged exposure versus eye movement desensitization and reprocessing (EMDR) for PTSD rape victims. *J. Trauma Stress* **18:** 607–616.

13. Institute of Medicine's Committee on Treatment of Posttraumatic stress disorder (PTSD). 2007. Treatment of PTSD: an assessment of the evidence. Institute of Medicine of the National Academies.

14. Van Der Kolk, B.A., D. Dreyfuss, M. Michaels, *et al.* 1994. Fluoxetine in posttraumatic stress disorder. *J. Clin. Psychiatry* **55:** 517–522.

15. Zohar, J., D. Amital, C. Miodownik, *et al.* 2002. Double-blind placebo-controlled pilot study of sertraline in military veterans with posttraumatic stress disorder. *J. Clin. Psychpharmacol.* **22:** 190–195.

16. Friedman, M.J., C.R. Marmar, D.G. Baker, *et al.* 2007. Randomized, double-blind comparison of sertraline and placebo for posttraumatic stress disorder in a Department of Veterans Affairs setting. *J. Clin. Psychiatry* **68:** 711–720.

17. Monson, C.M., P.P. Schnurr, P.A. Resick, *et al.* 2006. Cognitive processing therapy for veterans with military-related posttraumatic stress disorder. *J. Consult. Clin. Psychol.* **74:** 898–907.

18. Schnurr, P.P., M.J. Friedman, C.C. Engel, *et al.* Cognitive behavioral therapy for posttraumatic stress disorder in women: a randomized controlled trial. *JAMA* **297:** 820–830.

19. Bradley, R., J. Greene, E. Russ, *et al.* 2005. A multidimensional meta-analysis of psychotherapy for PTSD [published erratum in *Am. J. Psychiatry* 2005;162:832]. *Am. J. Psychiatry* **162:** 214–227.

20. Schnurr, P.P., M.J. Friedman, C.C. Engel, *et al.* Cognitive behavioral therapy for posttraumatic stress disorder in women: a randomized controlled trial. *JAMA* **297:** 820–830.

21. Fontana, A. & R.A. Rosenheck. 1997. Effectiveness and cost of the inpatient treatment of posttraumatic stress disorder: comparison of three models of treatment. *Am. J. Psychiatry* **154:** 758–765.

22. Weathers, F.W., A.M. Ruscio & T.M. Keane. 1999. Psychometric properties of nine scoring rules for the Clinician Administered Posttraumatic Stress Disorder Scale. *Psychol. Assess.* **11:** 124–133.

23. Strupp, H.H. & S.W. Hadley 1979. Specific vs nonspecific factors in psychotherapy. A controlled study of outcome. *Arch. Gen. Psychiatry* **36:** 1125–1136.

24. Baker, D.G., S.A. West, W.E. Nicholson, *et al.* 1999. Serial CSF corticotropin-releasing hormone levels and adrenocortical activity in combat veterans with posttraumatic stress disorder [published erratum appears in *Am. J. Psychiatry* 1999: 156; 986]. *Am. J. Psychiatry* **156:** 585–588.

25. Bremner, J.D., J. Licinio, A. Darnell, *et al.* 1997. Elevated CSF corticotropin-releasing factor concentrations in posttraumatic stress disorder. *Am. J. Psychiatry* **154:** 624–629.

26. Yehuda, R. 2002. Current status of cortisol findings in posttraumatic stress disorder. *Psychiatr. Clin. North Am.* **25:** 341–368.

27. Bremner, J.D., E. Vermetten & M.E. Kelley. 2007. Cortisol, dehydroepiandrosterone, and estradiol measured over 24 hours in women with childhood sexual abuse-related posttraumatic stress disorder. *J. Nerv. Ment. Dis.* **195:** 919–927.

28. Vythilingam, M., J.M. Gill, D.A. Luckenbaugh, *et al.* 2010. Low early morning plasma cortisol in posttraumatic stress disorder is associated with co-morbid depression but not with enhanced glucocorticoid feedback inhibition. *Psychoneuroendocrinology* **35:** 442–450.

29. de Kloet, C.S., E. Bermetten, E. Geuze, *et al.* 2006. Assessment of HPA-axis function in posttraumatic stress disorder: pharmacological and non-pharmacological challenge tests, a review. *J. Psychiatr. Res.* **40:** 550–567.

30. Yehuda, R. 2002. Current status of cortisol findings in posttraumatic stress disorder. *Psychiatr. Clin. North Am.* **25:** 341–368.

31. Bremner, J.D., E. Vermetten & M.E. Kelley. 2007. Cortisol, dehydroepiandrosterone, and estradiol measured over 24 hours in women with childhood sexual abuse-related posttraumatic stress disorder. *J. Nerv. Ment. Dis.* **195:** 919–927.

32. Flory, J.D., R. Yehuda, R. Grossman, *et al.* 2009. Childhood trauma and basal cortisol in people with personality disorders. *Compr. Psychiatry* **50:** 34–37.

33. Yehuda, R. 2009. Status of glucocorticoid alterations in posttraumatic stress disorder. *Ann. N.Y. Acad. Sci.* **1179:** 56–69.

34. Yehuda, R., R.K. Yang, S.L. Guo, *et al.* 2003. Relationship between dexamethasone-inhibited lysozyme activity in peripheral mononuclear leukocytes and the cortisol and glucocorticoid receptor response to dexamethasone. *J. Psychiatr. Res.* **37:** 471–477.

35. Olff, M., G. de Vries, Y. Güzelcan, *et al.* 2007. Changes in cortisol and DHEA plasma levels after psychotherapy for PTSD. *Psychoneuroendocrinology* **32:** 619–626.

36. Yehuda, R., L.M. Bierer, C. Sarapas, *et al.* 2009. Cortisol metabolic predictors of response to psychotherapy for symptoms for PTSD in survivors of the World Trade Center attacks on September 11, 2001. *Psychoneuroendocrinology* **34:** 1304–1313.

37. Yehuda, R., R.K. Yang, S.L. Guo, *et al.* 2003. Relationship between dexamethasone-inhibited lysozyme activity in peripheral mononuclear leukocytes and the cortisol and glucocorticoid receptor response to dexamethasone. *J. Psychiatr. Res.* **37:** 471–477.

38. Morgan, C.A., 3rd, S. Southwick, G. Hazlett, *et al.* 2004. Relationships among plasma dehydroepiandrosterone sulfate and cortisol levels, symptoms of dissociation, and objective performance in humans exposed to acute stress. *Arch. Gen. Psychiatry* **61:** 819–825.

Ann. N.Y. Acad. Sci. ISSN 0077-8923

ANNALS OF THE NEW YORK ACADEMY OF SCIENCES

Issue: *Psychiatric and Neurologic Aspects of War*

Psychiatric and neurologic aspects of war: concluding comments on the ARNMD conference

David A. Silbersweig

Chairman, Department of Psychiatry, Chairman, Institute for the Neurosciences, Brigham and Women's/Faulkner Hospitals, Boston, Massachusetts

Address for correspondence: David A. Silbersweig, M.D., Brigham and Women's Hospital, Department of Psychiatry, 75 Francis Street, 2nd floor, Boston, Massachusetts 02115. dsilbersweig@partners.org

These concluding remarks address some of the main disorders that were described during the 89th Annual Conference of the Association for Research in Nervous and Mental Disease entitled "Psychiatric and Neurologic Aspects of War," held December 16, 2009 at The Rockefeller University, New York, New York. Brief remarks are also made on the roles of clinical scientists to consider some of the diagnostic, therapeutic, and societal elements that were discussed at the conference.

The 89th Annual Conference of the Association for Research in Nervous and Mental Disease entitled "Psychiatric and Neurologic Aspects of War," held December 16, 2009 at The Rockefeller University, New York, New York, has thoughtfully and rigorously dealt with issues ranging from molecular biomarkers to some of the biggest problems and biggest opportunities that face our species, historically and otherwise. On the one hand, we have conundrums and problems, such as terrorism and the potential of nuclear disaster; and on the other, we have increasing empirical knowledge and an ability to integrate it clinically and medically while also being able to think societally as to how we might address these problems. It is both a very hopeful and dangerous time.

I would like to address some of the main disorders that were described as well as to share some brief thoughts about our roles as clinical scientists and to consider some of the diagnostic, therapeutic, and societal elements that we may take from the conference. We are clearly beyond the era of brain versus mind, nature versus nurture, and individual effects versus societal/cultural effects. The increasing integration, and importantly, the increasingly mechanistic and fluid nature of our thinking, aids us as we consider how it is that we come into the world as a species, as organisms, with genetic pre-dispositions that interact with neurodevelopmental processes starting in pregnancy and lead to some hard-wired predispositions to behave a certain way and therefore prompt others to behave toward us in a certain way. This social interaction with early formative experiences—for positive or for negative—and adult as well as developmental processes, experiences, and illnesses leads to diatheses, traits, and states that can then accrue.

In this context, we consider the research of Bruce McEwen,[1] whose work from early on has thoughtfully approached the ways in which experience and the brain—including the hardware and software of the brain, the chemistry and wiring, as well as plasticity—can start to be teased apart. This reflects the bidirectional causality that David Hamburg[2] and Jack Barchas[3] earlier in their careers championed at a time when it was not the model. The pendulum at one point was too psychological or psychodynamic, then it swung perhaps a little too much to the reductionistic side. Throughout this time, there were some saying "well, it's both," and people like Nancy Andreasen[4] being able to thoughtfully address the issues and categorize behaviors. Recently, the work of physician-scientists address mechanisms on the systems level (e.g., fronto-limbic dys-modulation)[5] and molecular level (e.g., val66met BDNF polymorphism).[6] Increasingly, such clinical and basic work is

doi: 10.1111/j.1749-6632.2010.05796.x

being integrated translationally. The work described by many of the presenters gives us a cross-section as well as a longitudinal sense of where we are.

In terms of posttraumatic stress disorder (PTSD), traumatic brain injury (TBI), depression, and anxiety, many of the same regions are implicated: amygdala, subgenual anterior cingulate, hippocampus, and entorhinal cortex.[7–10] There is a reason for that, a reason why there are so-called comorbidities, or common risk factors, and the more we understand about the circuitry and "connectivity,"[11] the more we will understand why certain symptoms and syndromes tend to co-occur, and why certain circuits underlying them are vulnerable. For instance, it is not a coincidence that in TBI there are brain regions that are particularly affected (e.g., orbitofrontal, anterior temporal),[12] that in PTSD there are brain regions (in the same areas) that are more vulnerable, and there are final common pathways of symptom expression[13] that allow us to increasingly diagnose based upon the functional/behavioral neuroanatomy. As we pinpoint which functions and networks are affected, we can zero in to achieve a greater understanding of the various etiologies that converge to produce the localized dysfunction. At the same time, we can work backward from the genetics/genomics, to identify candidate genes and single nucleotide polymorphisms that affect cellular and synaptic function in the implicated circuits. Novel therapeutics can then be developed that target the aberrant mechanisms biochemically/pharmacologically, or in terms of brain circuit modulation/stimulation.

With these approaches, we can think about our neuropsychiatric taxonomy in a more dimensional and mechanistic way, compared to the current DSM descriptive approach. This brings our field toward the rest of medicine, toward subtyping of illnesses, toward a notion of understanding our patients in terms of their risk and resilience profiles, in terms of the biomarker development that combines imaging with genetics/genomics, and increasingly with proteomics and metabolomics. We will be able to derive biological profiles, while not forgetting the clinical phenomenology, not forgetting the psychological reality from existentialism to executive functions, to the subjective aspects of fear and the objective autonomic components of arousal. The more we can measure such elements and their combinations in a way that allows us to predict who is at risk, the

closer we get to the "holy grail," which is to prevent or have early intervention, to have primary or secondary prevention, and to get to the point where we are not chasing at potential problems after the fact, but rather approach them more proactively.

We have heard about the medical and psychological approaches to TBI and PTSD, and about how it's not just psychotherapy or pharmacotherapy, but in some cases the evidence-based combination of the two. We did not hear much about brain stimulation. Some clinical researchers, exemplified by Niko Schiff at Weill Cornell are doing important work using brain stimulation to modulate some of these circuits. For instance, he and his colleagues have shown that stimulation of particular subnuclei of the reticular thalamus can improve mental functioning in people with the minimally conscious state[14] (that can result from head injury). They have even demonstrated initial evidence, unrelated to stimulation, of plasticity even late following TBI and white matter injury.[15] This opens up possibilities, beyond neuromodulation, of neural repair, as the underlying mechanisms are increasingly understood (whether involving neural stem cells, neurotrophic factors, gene therapy, or other elements mediating synaptogenesis, LTP/LTD, and myelination).[16–19]

We are increasingly able to think beyond categories or beyond turf battles among disciplines, and give a person D-cycloserine (a partial agonist of the NMDA receptor for glutamate) to enhance the effects of virtual reality or cognitive behavioral therapy;[20] to be able to think about neurophysiological extinction, or even reconsolidation,[21] of fear memories at the level of amygdala-hippocampal subregional activity and interactions; to be able to utilize computers and smartphones to extend therapeutic interactions; to be able to prescribe more specific medications, including neuroprotective agents,[17] and to be able to think exquisitely about the timing and critical periods for some of these neurodevelopmental and neurotoxic mechanisms, so that we may intervene more selectively and effectively.

All of these developments are swirling together in a very convergent and constructive fashion, such that our field will be no different than oncology or cardiology in terms of personalized medicine—but hopefully personalized in both senses: in the sense of biologic markers and intermediate phenotypes that allow us to better predict and direct an individual's treatment and monitor outcome[22] (with trajectory-altering therapeutics); and also personalized in the sense that in psychiatry and neuropsychiatry and related fields, we have the compassion, knowledge, and respect for the subjective experience of our patients, and can even see how the psychosocial experiential factors can be part of the causal mix,[23,24] the physiology of which was discussed.

And then going beyond the personal and medical issues affecting individual patients, we heard a number of discussions today relating to attempts to address the most destructive tendencies using public health tools. I remember not infrequently hearing one of my mentors say, "Well, we are an imperfect species." That wisdom was somewhat comforting, though it was quite a concerning statement about our species. I think we have heard that today. Leaders like David Hamburg are addressing problems, such as genocide, head on.[25] He is taking what we have learned, what the field has learned and what human beings have learned through history, and in a systematic way trying to get to solutions above and beyond descriptive aspects of the problem, or just the notion that the problems are always going to be thus. The stakes are higher now because we have potential nuclear terrorism, in which individuals or groups would have no hesitation causing untold misery and destruction. This produces a state of probabilistic uncertainty, since many positive developments can be counteracted by negative developments in a tiny minority of the population. The cusp of the solutions are there, so it's almost like a race: Is the species going to destroy itself before it figures itself out sufficiently to save itself?

What is the biology that evolved in us with our brain—lobes lopped on top of lobes—in situations where we needed fear circuitry and stress circuitry? We have these phylogenetically preserved systems that are highly interconnected with newer six-layer, heteromodal associative neocortex that supports abstraction and executive functions, and higher order control mechanisms, and ability to switch sets.[26] We are learning more and more about how these processes are interconnected. They are hooked up in a specific way that is unique in higher primates, and even more so in humans, and that can account for the phenomenology of what humans experience in health and in disease or dysfunction. It can also provide a mechanistic basis for our understanding of how to approach the disorders we've been hearing about today. The subcortical (brainstem projection, diencephalic, basal forebrain, and striato-palladal) and limbic (including hypothalamic) regions are associated with stereotyped, unconscious, and automatic processing. On the other end, the more dorsal, rostral, and the more lateral we go in the nervous system, one gets into processing that is more amenable to conscious modulation and volitional intention. The paralimbic regions in between mediate the interaction between the internal milieu/changing needs of the organism, and the changing contingencies of the environment (appetitive and approach, as well as aversive and avoidant and threat related, in a social/emotional context),[26,27] and we heard about the orbital frontal cortex and its importance in that regard.

I think it is almost ironic that these very regions in-between, which mediate these interactions, are almost like our Achilles heel as a species. One can almost advance the notion that the very brain areas, which get us into trouble in the first place (through overactivity and/or failure of local neuronal circuit and top–down, large-scale distributed circuit inhibition) and can contribute to violence and war, are themselves vulnerable to its effects; and also that such brain areas may be imperfectly developed or connected—at least on a population, bell-shaped curve basis—in a certain proportion of the population, with neurodevelopmental and adverse environmental contributions (including sociocultural, historical, educational, and resource factors). We need to understand more about this, especially with the increasing population in the world and all of the attendant stresses and limitations.

What are the brain regions that mediate the sense of a need for protection, retribution, preemptive action, threat,[28] belief, identity, hatred, absolutism, and honor—all of these—and how do they come together? For when they come together in a dysfunctional way, either biologically and/or environmentally mediated, and if only in a subpopulation of people, they end up causing damage to the brains of a lot of people in the very same brain areas that were dysfunctioning in the people who caused the trouble in the first place. While this is a speculation, it can serve as a heuristic device for considering the relevant interdisciplinary issues.

One may even go a step further and consider that this signature of regional brain dysfunction in the victims can predispose them to the emotional dysmodulation and hyperreactivity, aberrant stress–response, and to the lack of impulse control, that may perpetuate problematic interactions and behavior. There is some evidence for this pattern of subsequent (cortisol and excitotoxity mediated) effect in cytoarchitecture, spine density, and function in amygdale (increased), hippocampi and ventromedial prefrontal cortex (decreased) in animal models and human studies of abuse and neglect.[29] Thus, may violence beget violence.

Conversely, we are also learning more about the neural substrates of empathy, compassion,[30] and affiliative behavior. Such work may lead to advances and interventions that enhance these higher order capacities. Mechanisms that mediate the interactions among perception, emotion, cognition, and behavior are also being uncovered experimentally. Neurobiological sex differences are also being identified (this is relevant as violence is often initiated and perpetrated by men). As all of these strands of investigation converge, there is an opportunity to decrease human suffering.

I think that what's so hopeful about a conference like this and what's proximal is the ability to bring to bear the most basic understanding of the biological mechanisms, with the understanding of the pathophysiology of these disorders, with the inroads into treatment, and then the population level social and cultural[31–33] neuroscience. That gets us beyond mirror neurons, beyond theory of mind, and allows us to understand and cultivate the best of our evolutionary capacities—those that allowed us to cooperate in groups and therefore survive better, and those that (at the next level) can overcome even those tendencies that create in-group versus out-group distinctions that end up causing a lot of trouble.

At the risk of a sort of medicalization of these societal ills, it's worth realizing, as a number of our presenters pointed out, that we as clinicians, scientists, and educators have both a responsibility and perhaps an increasingly hopeful possibility for addressing some of these most difficult and important problems.

References

1. McEwen, E.L. 2010. Early life stress followed by subsequent adult chronic stress potentiates anxiety and blunts hippocampal structural remodeling. *Hippocampus*, September 16 [Epub ahead of print] http://www.ncbi.nlm.nih.gov/pubmed/20848608 (accessed September 29, 2010).

2. Board, F. *et al.* 1956. Psychological stress and endocrine functions. *Psychosom. Med.* **18:** 324–333.

3. Madden IV, J. *et al.* 1977. Stress-induced parallel changes in central opioid levels and pain responsiveness in the rat. *Nature* **265:** 358–360.

4. Andreasen, N.C. 2007. DSM and the death of phenomenology in America: an example of unintended consequences. *Schizophr. Bull.* **33:** 108–112.

5. Silbersweig, D. *et al.* 2007. Failure of frontolimbic inhibitory function in the context of negative emotion in borderline personality disorder. *Am. J. Psychiatry* **164:** 1832–1841.

6. Chen, Z.-Y. *et al.* 2006. Genetic variant BDNF (Val66Met) polymorphism alters anxiety-related behavior. *Science* **314:** 140–143.

7. Protopopescu, X. *et al.* 2005. Differential time courses and specificity of amygdala activity in posttraumatic stress disorder subjects and normal control subjects. *Biol. Psychiatry* **57:** 464–473.

8. Shin, L.M. *et al.* 2009. Resting metabolic activity in the cingulate cortex and vulnerability to posttraumatic stress disorder. *Arch. Gen. Psychiatry* **66:** 1099–1107.

9. Bremner, J.D. 2007. Functional neuroimaging in posttraumatic stress disorder. *Expert Rev. Neurother.* **7:** 393–405.

10. Hesdorffer, D.C. *et al.* 2009. Long-term psychiatric outcomes following traumatic brain injury: a review of the literature. *J. Head Trauma Rehabil.* **24:** 452–459.

11. Daniels, J.K. *et al.* 2010. Switching between executive and default mode networks in posttraumatic stress disorder: alternations in functional connectivity. *J. Psychiatry Neurosci.* **35:** 258–266.

12. McAllister, T.W. 1992. Neuropsychiatric sequelae of head injuries. *Psychiatr. Clin. North Am.* **15:** 395–413.

13. Silbersweig, D. & E. Stern. 1997. Symptom localization in neuropsychiatry. A functional neuroimaging approach. *Ann. N.Y. Acad. Sci.* **835:** 410–420.

14. Schiff, N.D. *et al.* 2007. Behavioural improvements with thalamic stimulation after severe traumatic brain injury. *Nature* **448:** 600–603.

15. Voss, H.U. *et al.* 2006. Possible axonal regrowth in late recovery from the minimally conscious state. *J. Clin. Invest.* **116:** 2005–2011.

16. Marr, R.A. *et al.* 2010. Insights into neurogenesis and aging: potential therapy for degenerative disease? *Future Neurol.* **5:** 527–541.

17. Lauterbach, E.C. *et al.* 2010. Psychopharmacological neuroprotection in neurodegenerative disease: assessing the preclinical data. *J. Neuropsychiatry Clin. Neurosci.* **22:** 8–18.

18. Ji, Y. *et al.* 2010. Acute and gradual increases in BDNF concentration elicit distinct signaling and functions in neurons. *Nat. Neurosci.* **13:** 302–309.

19. Filosa, A. *et al.* 2009. Neuron-glia communication via EphA4/Ephrin-A3 modulates LTP through glial glutamate transport. *Nat. Neurosci.* **12:** 1285–1292.

20. Ganasen, K.A. *et al.* 2010. Augmentation of cognitive behavioral therapy with pharmacotherapy. *Psychiatr. Clin. North Am.* **33:** 687–699.

21. Kim, J. *et al.* 2010. Reactivation of fear memory renders consolidated amygdala synapses labile. *J. Neurosci.* **30:** 9631–9640.

22. Mayberg, H.S. 2003. Modulating dysfunctional limbic-cortical circuits in depression: towards development of brain-based algorithms for diagnosis and optimised treatment. *Br. Med. Bull.* **65:** 193–207.

23. Miller, G.E. *et al.* 2009. Low early-life social class leaves a biological residue manifested by decreased glucocorticoid and increased proinflammatory signaling. *Proc. Natl. Acad. Sci. USA* **106:** 14716–14721.

24. Tyrka, A.R. *et al.* 2009. Interaction of childhood maltreatment with the corticotropin-releasing hormone receptor gene: effects on hypothalamic-pituitary-adrenal axis reactivity. *Biol. Psychiatry* **66:** 681–685.

25. Hamburg, D.A. 2008. *Preventing Genocide: Practical Steps Toward Early Detection and Effective Action.* 1st ed. Paradigm Publishers. Boulder, CO.

26. Mesulam, M.-M. 2000. *Principles of Behavioral and Cognitive Neurology.* 2nd ed. Oxford University Press. New York, N.Y.

27. Rolls, E.T. & F. Grabenhorst. 2008. The orbitofrontal cortex and beyond: from affect to decision-making. *Prog. Neurobiol.* **86:** 216–244.

28. Olsson, A. *et al.* 2005. The role of social groups in the persistence of learned fear. *Science* **309:** 785–787.

29. McEwan, B.S. 2010. Stress, sex, and neural adaptation to a changing environment: mechanisms of neuronal remodeling. *Ann. N.Y. Acad. Sci.* **1204**(Suppl.): E38–E59.

30. Lutz, A. *et al.* 2008. Regulation of the neural circuitry of emotion by compassion meditation: effects of meditative expertise. *PLoS One* **3:** e1897.

31. Forbes, C.E. & J. Grafman. 2010. The role of the human prefrontal cortex in social cognition and moral judgement. *Annu. Rev. Neurosci.* **33:** 299–324.

32. Kitayama, S. & J. Park. 2010. Cultural neuroscience of the self: understanding the social grounding of the brain. *Soc. Cogn. Affect. Neurosci.* **5:** 111–129.

33. Hackman, D.A. *et al.* 2010. Socioeconomic status and the brain: mechanistic insights from human and animal research. *Nat. Rev. Neurosci.* **11:** 651–659.